Data Mining in Medical and Biological Research

Edited by

Eugenia G. Giannopoulou

Published by In-Teh

In-Teh is Croatian branch of I-Tech Education and Publishing KG, Vienna, Austria.

www.in-teh.org
Additional copies can be obtained from:
publication@ars-journal.com

First published December 2008
Printed in Croatia

A catalogue record for this book is available from the University Library Rijeka under no. 120118041
Data Mining in Medical and Biological Research, Edited by Eugenia G. Giannopoulou
p. cm.
ISBN 978-953-7619-30-5
1. Data Mining in Medical and Biological Research, Eugenia G. Giannopoulou

For EU product safety concerns:
IN TECH d.o.o., Prolaz Marije Krucifikse Kozulić 3, 51000 Rijeka, Croatia,
info@intechopen.com or visit our website at intechopen.com.

Preface

Data mining is the research area involving powerful processes and tools that allow an effective analysis and exploration of usually large amounts of data. In particular, data mining techniques have found application in numerous different scientific fields with the aim of discovering previously unknown patterns and correlations, as well as predicting trends and behaviors.

In the meantime, during the current century of biomedical sciences, biology and medicine have undergone tremendous advances in their technologies and therefore have generated huge amounts of biomedical information. This book intends to bring together the most recent advances and applications of data mining research in the promising areas of medicine and biology from around the world. Seventeen chapters, twelve related to medical research and five focused on the biological domain, describe interesting applications, motivating progress and worthwhile results.

Chapter 1 presents a novel concept of improving the classification accuracy for common learning algorithms by uncovering the potential relevance of features through multivariate interdependent attribute preprocessing methods.

Chapter 2 introduces a hybrid approach, combining discrete wavelet transform and neural networks, for the classification of a complex dataset such as an electroencephalography time series and claims that a high degree of classification accuracy can be achieved.

Chapter 3 explores the possibility that DNA viruses play an important role in development of breast tumors, using artificial neural networks and agglomerative hierarchical clustering techniques.

Chapter 4 investigates the research hypothesis of developing certain domain ontology from discovered rules. To practically examine this assumption, the proposed approach integrates different data mining techniques to assist in developing a set of representative consensual concepts of the underlying domain.

Chapter 5 describes the process of medical knowledge acquisition and outlines the requirements for producing knowledge that can be trusted and applied in a clinical setting. This work demonstrates that the individual needs of medical professionals can be addressed and that data mining can be a valuable tool in the diagnostic and decision making toolkit.

Chapter 6 provides an overview of the various technologies in a radiology department that allow data mining, and describes case-examples utilizing data mining technologies.

Chapter 7 demonstrates the results of a nationwide study that applied data and text mining techniques to medical near-miss case data related to medicines and medical equipments. This study also analyzed the causal relationship of occurrences of the near-miss cases and the opinions on the counter measures against them.

Chapter 8 presents a complex clinical problem that has been addressed using particle swarm optimization, a suitable approach for data mining subject to a rule base which defines the quality of rules and constancy with previous observations.

Chapter 9 focuses on the description of a model for monitoring and planning of human resources in a nationwide public health-care system. The aim of the presented monitoring system is to assess performance and provide information for the management of a primary health-care network.

Chapter 10 summarizes the core technologies and the current research activities regarding the interoperability of information and knowledge extracted from data mining operations.

Chapter 11 describes a series of sensory vital-sign measurement technologies to facilitate data collection in the daily environment, and the application of data mining algorithms for the interpretation of comprehensive large-scale data.

Chapter 12 describes and suggests a mobile phone based intelligent electrocardiogram signal telemonitoring system that incorporates data mining and knowledge management techniques.

Chapter 13 suggests that using statistical measures of independence can indicate non-significant DNA motifs, whereas measures of significance based on shape distributions can be extremely informative.

Chapter 14 offers an explanatory review on the post genomic field and demonstrates representative and outstanding examples that highlight the importance of data mining methods in proteomics research.

Chapter 15 presents a variety of methods for a standard graph analysis, particularly oriented to the study of cellular networks, and indicates that the network approach provides a suitable framework for exploring the organization of biomolecules.

Chapter 16 demonstrates a framework for biomedical information extraction from text, which integrates a data mining module for extraction rule discovery.

Chapter 17 describes the attempt to exploit social data mining in order to improve results in bio-inspired intelligent systems, using a plethora of data mining techniques.

We are grateful to the authors of the chapters for their enthusiasm for contribution. We hope that the readers will benefit from this book and consider it as an excellent way to keep pace with the vast and diverse advances of new research efforts.

Editor

Eugenia G. Giannopoulou

Dept. of Computer Science and Technology

University of Peloponnese

Email:egian@uop.gr

Greece

Contents

Data Mining in Medical Research

1

Discovery of the Latent Supportive Relevance in Medical Data Mining

Sam Chao[1], Fai Wong[1], Qiulin Ding[2], Yiping Li[1] and Mingchui Dong[1]
[1]*University of Macau, Macau*
[2]*Nanjing University of Aeronautics and Astronautics, Nanjing, China*

1. Introduction

The purpose of a classification learning algorithm is to accurately and efficiently map an input instance to an output class label, according to a set of labeled instances. Decision tree is such a method that most widely used and practical for inductive inference in the data mining and machine learning discipline (Han & Kamber, 2000). However, many decision tree learning algorithms degrade their learning performance due to irrelevant, unreliable or uncertain data are introduced; or some focus on univariate only, without taking the interdependent relationship among others into consideration; while some are limited in handling the attributes[1] with discrete values. All these cases may be caused by improper pre-processing methods, where feature selection (FS) and continuous feature discretization (CFD) are treated as the dominant issues. Even if a learning algorithm is able to deal with various cases, it is still better to carry out the pre-processing prior the learning algorithm, so as to minimize the information lost and increase the classification accuracy accordingly. FS and CFD have been the active and fruitful fields of research for decades in statistics, pattern recognition, machine learning and data mining (Yu & Liu, 2004). While FS may drastically reduce the computational cost, decrease the complexity and uncertainty (Liu & Motoda, 2000); and CFD may decrease the dimensionality of a specific attribute and thus increase the efficiency and accuracy of the learning algorithm.
As we believe that, among an attributes space, each attribute may have certain relevance with another attribute, therefore to take the attributes relevant correlation into consideration in data pre-processing is a vital factor for the ideal pre-processing methods. Nevertheless, many FS and CFD methods focus on univariate only by processing individual attribute independently, not considering the interaction between attributes; this may sometimes loose the significant useful hidden information for final classification. Especially in medical domain, a single symptom seems useless regarding diagnostic, may be potentially important when combined with other symptoms. An attribute that is completely useless by itself can provide a significant performance improvement when taken with others. Two attributes that are useless by themselves can be useful together (Guyon & Elisseeff, 2003; Caruana & Sa, 2003). For instance, when learning the medical data for disease diagnostic, if

---

[1] In this paper, attribute has the same meaning as feature, they are used exchangeable within the paper.

a dataset contains attributes like patient *age, gender, height, weight, blood pressure, pulse, ECG result* and *chest pain*, etc., during FS pre-processing, it is probably that attribute *age* or *height* alone will be treated as the least important attribute and discarded accordingly. However, in fact attribute *age* and *height* together with *weight* may express potential significant information: whether a patient is *overweight*? On the other hand, although attribute *blood pressure* may be treated as important regarding classifying a cardiovascular disease, while together with a useless attribute *age*, they may present more specific meaning: whether a patient is *hypertension*? Obviously, the compound features *overweight* and/or *hypertension* have more discriminative power regarding to disease diagnostic than the individual attributes stated above. It is also proven that a person is *overweight* or *hypertension* may have more probabilities to obtain a cardiovascular disease (Jia & Xu, 2001).

Moreover, when processing CFD, the discretized intervals should make sense to human expert (Bay, 2000; Bay, 2001). We know that a person's *blood pressure* is increasing as one's *age* increasing. Therefore it is improper to generate a cutting point such as 140mmHg and 90mmHg for systolic pressure and diastolic pressure, respectively. Since the standard for diagnosing hypertension is a little bit different from young people (orthoarteriotony is 120-130mmHg/80mmHg) to the old people (orthoarteriotony is 140mmHg/90mmHg) (Gu, 2006). If the blood pressure of a person aged 20 is 139mmHg/89mmHg, one might be considered as a potential hypertensive. In contrast, if a person aged 65 has the same blood pressure measurement, one is definitely considered as normotensive. Obviously, to discretize the continuous-valued attribute *blood pressure*, it must take at least the attribute *age* into consideration. While discretizing other continuous-valued attribute may not take *age* into consideration. This demonstrates again that a useless attribute *age* is likely to be a potentially useful attribute once combined with attribute *blood pressure*. The only solution to address the mentioned problem is to use multivariate interdependent discretization in place of univariate discretization.

In the next section, we show the importance of attributes interdependence by describing in detail the multivatiate interdependent discretization method - MIDCA. Then in section 3, we demonstrate the significance of attributes relevance by specifying the latent utility of irrelevant feature selection - LUIFS in detail. The evaluations of our proposed algorithms to some real-life datasets are performed in section 4. In final section, we summarize our paper and present the future directions of our research.

2. Multivariate discretization

Many discretization algorithms developed in data mining field focus on univariate only, which discretize each attribute with continuous values independently, without considering the interdependent relationship among other attributes, at most taking the interdependent relationship with class attribute into account, more detail can be found in(Dougherty et al., 1995; Fayyad & Irani, 1993; Liu & Setiono, 1997; Liu et al., 2002). This is unsatisfactory in handling the critical characteristics possessed by medical area. There are few literatures discussed about the multivariate interdependent discreitzation methods. The method developed in (Monti & Gooper, 1998) concentrates on learning Bayesian network structure; hence the discretization is relied on the Bayesian network structure being evaluated only, which is unable to be applied in other structures, such as decision tree learning structure.

Multivariate interdependent discretization concerns the correlation between the attribute being discretized and the other potential interdependent attributes. Our MIDCA - Multivariate Interdependent Discretization for Continuous Attribute is based on the normalized relief (Kira & Rendell, 1992a; Kira & Rendell, 1992b) and information theory(Fayyed & Irani, 1993; Mitchell, 1997; Zhu, 2000), to look for the best correlated attribute for the continuous-valued attribute being discretized as the interdependent attribute to carry out the multivariate discretization. In order to obtain the good quality for a multivariate discretization, discovery of a best interdependent attribute against the continuous-valued attribute is considered as the primary essential task.

2.1 MIDCA method

MIDCA is interested mainly in discovering the best interdependent attribute relative to the continuous-valued attribute being discretized. As we believe that a good multivariate discretization scheme should highly rely on the corresponding perfect correlated attributes. If assume that a dataset $S = \{s_1, s_2, \ldots, s_N\}$ contains N instances, each instance $s \in S$ is defined over a set of M attributes (features) $A = \{a_1, a_2, \ldots, a_M\}$ and a class attribute $c \in C$. For each continuous-valued attribute $a_i \in A$, there exists at least one $a_j \in A$, such that a_j is the most correlated with a_i, or vice versa, since the correlation is measured symmetrically. For the purpose of finding out such a best interdependent attribute a_j for each continuous-valued attribute a_i, both gain information in equation (2) that derived from entropy information in equation (1) and relief measures in equation (3) depicted below are taken into account to capture the interaction among the attributes space.

$$Entropy(S) = -\sum_{i \in C} p(S_i) log(p(S_i)) \tag{1}$$

where $p(S_i)$ is the proportion of instances S belonging to class i; based on this measure, the most informative attribute A relative to a collection of instances S can be defined as:

$$Gain(S, A) = Entropy(S) - \sum_{v \in Values(A)} \frac{|S_v|}{|S|} Entropy(S_v) \tag{2}$$

where $Values(A)$ is the set of all distinct values of attribute A; S_v is the subset of S for which attribute A has value v, that is $S_v = \{s \in S \mid A(s) = v\}$. While the reformulated relief measure can be defined as to estimate the quality of an attribute over all training instances:

$$Relief_A = \frac{Gini'(A) \times \sum_{x \in X} p(x)^2}{(1 - \sum_{c \in C} p(c)^2) \sum_{c \in C} p(c)^2} \tag{3}$$

where C is the class attribute and *Gini'* is a variance of another attribute quality measure algorithm Gini-index (Breiman, 1996).

Then we use the symmetric relief and entropy information algorithms to calculate the interdependent weight for each attribute pair $\{a_i, a_j\}$ where $i \neq j$. However, the measures output from two symmetric measures are in different standards, the only way to balance them is to normalize the output values by using proportions in place of real values. Finally averaging the two normalized proportions as in equation (4) and chooses the best interdependent weight amongst all potential interdependent attributes as our target.

$$InterdependentWeight(a_i, a_j) = \left[\frac{SymGain(a_i, a_j)}{\sqrt{\sum_{M \neq i}^{A} SymGain(a_i, a_M)^2}} + \frac{SymRelief(a_i, a_j)}{\sqrt{\sum_{M \neq i}^{A} SymRelief(a_i, a_M)^2}} \right] / 2 \tag{4}$$

where

$$SymGain(A,B) = \left[Gain(A,B) + Gain(B,A)\right]/2$$

and

$$SymRelief(A,B) =$$

$$\left[\frac{Gini'(A) \times \sum_{x \in X} p(x)^2}{(1 - \sum_{b \in B} p(b)^2)\sum_{b \in B} p(b)^2} + \frac{Gini'(B) \times \sum_{y \in Y} p(y)^2}{(1 - \sum_{a \in A} p(a)^2)\sum_{a \in A} p(a)^2}\right]/2$$

The advantage of incorporating the measures of entropy information and relief in MIDCA algorithm is to minimize the uncertainty between the interdependent attribute and the continuous-valued attribute being discretized and at the same time to maximize their correlation by discovering the perfect interdependencies between them. However, if an interdependent attribute is a continuous-valued attribute too, it is first discretized with entropy-based discretization method (Dougherty et al., 1995; Fayyad & Irani, 1993). This is important and may reduce the bias of in favor of the attribute with more values. Furthermore, our method creates an interdependent attribute for each continuous-valued attribute in a dataset rather than using one for all continuous-valued attributes, this is also the main factor for improving the final classification accuracy.

MIDCA ensures at least binary discreatizaiton, which is different from other methods that sometimes the boundary of a continuous-valued attribute is [-∞, +∞]. We realized that if a continuous-valued attribute generates null cutting point means that the attribute is useless, hence increase the classification uncertainty. This may finally cause the higher error rate in the learning process. We believe that most continuous-valued attributes in medical domain have their special meanings, even though it alone seems unimportant, while it becomes useful when combining with other attributes. The before-mentioned examples are some typical ones. Furthermore, most figures express the degrees and seriousness of the specific illness, such as *blood pressure* may indicate the level of hypertension; higher *heart rate* may represent the existence of cardiovascular disease; while *plasma glucose* is an index for diabetes and so on, hence their discretization cannot be ignored.

The only drawback of MIDCA is its slightly heavy complexity. In the worst case, all N attributes in a dataset are numeric, but the interdependent weighting is calculated symmetrically, so there are $N/2$ attributes involved into calculations. For the first attribute taking into calculation, (N-1) times of executions are necessary; while for the second attribute taking into calculation, (N-3) times of executions should be carried out, and so on. Since such calculation is decreased gradually, so the total execution times are at most $(N-1)*N/2$, i.e., $O(N^2/2)$. However, such case is only a minority. Most real life datasets have low percentage of numeric attributes, then the execution time of the algorithm becomes less influential compared with classification accuracy.

2.2 MIDCA algorithm

Different from other discretization algorithms, MIDCA is carried out with respect to the best interdependent attribute that discovered from equation (4) in addition to the class attribute. Moreover, we assume that the interdependent attribute INT has T discrete values; as such each of its distinct value identifies a subset in the original data set S, the probability should be generated relative to the subset in place of the original data set. Therefore, the combinational probability distribution over the attribute space $\{C\} \cup A$ can be redefined based on equation (2) as well as the information gain algorithm as following:

$$MIDCAInfoGain(A, P; INT_T, S) = \\ Entropy(S \mid INT_T) - \sum_{v \in Values(A) \mid INT_T} \frac{|S_v|}{|S|} Entropy(S_v) \quad (5)$$

where P is a collection of candidate cutting points for attribute A under the projection of value T for the interdependent attribute INT, the algorithm defines the class information entropy of the partition induced by P. In order to emphasize the importance of the interaction respect to the interdependent attribute INT, $Entropy(S)$ is replaced by the conditional entropy $Entropy(S \mid INTT)$. Consequently, $v \in Values(A) \mid INT_T$ becomes the set of all distinct values of attribute A of the cluster induced by T of interdependent attribute INT; and S_v is the subset of S for which attribute A has value v and under the projection of T for INT, i.e., $S_v = \{s \in S \mid A(s) = v \wedge INT(s) = T\}$.

Now we compendiously present our MIDCA algorithm as below and the evaluation for such algorithm is illustrated in section 4:

1. Sort the continuous-valued attributes for the data set in ascending order;
2. Discovery the best interdependent attributes pair by algorithm INTDDiscovery;
3. Calculate the MIDCAInfoGain measure and select the best cutting point;
4. Evaluate whether stopping the calculation according to MDLP;
5. Repeat step 3 if the test failed. Else, order the best cutting points to generate the discretized data set.

INTDDiscovery algorithm

    If the interdependent attribute is a continuous-valued attribute
        Discretize using entropy-based method and select the best cutting point;
        Test to stop using MDLP;
    Calculate the symmetric entropy information measure for the pair of attributes;
    Calculate the symmetric relief measure for the pair of attribute;
    Normalize the symmetric entropy information and relief measure;
    Average the two normalized measures;
    Select the one with the highest average measure;

End algorithm;

3. Feature selection

More features no longer mean more discriminative power; contrarily, they may increase the complexity and uncertainty of an algorithm, thus burden with heavy computational cost. Therefore various feature selection algorithms have been introduced in (Liu & Motoda, 2000) as well as their evaluations and comparisons in (Hall & Holmes, 2003; Molina et al., 2002; Dash & Liu, 1997). Feature selection can be defined as a process of finding an optimal subset of features from the original set of features, according to some defined feature selection criterion (Cios et al., 1998).

Suppose a dataset D contains a set of M original attributes $OriginalA = \{a_1, a_2, \ldots, a_M\}$ and a class attribute $c \in C$, i.e., $D = OriginalA \cup C$. The task of feature selection is to find such a subset of N attributes among M that $OptimalA = \{a_1, a_2, \ldots, a_N\}$, where $N \leq M$ and $OptimalD =$

OptimalA $\cup$ *C*, hence the *ClassificationErrorRate*(*OptimalD*)≤*ClassificationErrorRate*(*D*). Features can be defined as relevant, irrelevant or redundant. A relevant feature is neither irrelevant nor redundant to the target concept; an irrelevant feature does not affect the target concept in any way, and a redundant feature does not add anything new to the target concept (John et al., 1994).
Many feature selection algorithms generate the optimal subset of relevant features by ranking the individual attribute or subset of attributes. Each time the best single attribute or attributes subset will be selected, the iteration will be stopped when some pre-defined filtering criteria has been matched. For instance, a forward selection method recursively adds a feature x_i to the current optimal feature subset *OptimalA*, among those have not been selected yet in *OriginalA*, until a stopping criterion is conformed to. In each step, the feature x_i that makes evaluation measure *W* be greater is added to the optimal set *OptimalA*. Starting with *OptimalA* = {}, the forward step consists of:

$$\begin{aligned} OptimalA &:= OptimalA \cup \{OriginalA \setminus OptimalA \mid \\ &W(OptimalA \cup \{x_i\}) \text{ is maximum}\} \end{aligned} \tag{6}$$

Nevertheless, this method does not have in consideration certain basic interactions among features, i.e., if x_1 and x_2 are such interacted attributes, that $W(\{x_1, x_2\}) >> W(\{x_1\}), W(\{x_2\})$, neither x_1 nor x_2 could be selected, in spite of being very useful (Molina et al., 2002). Since most feature selection methods assume that the attributes are independent rather than interactive, hence their hidden correlations have been ignored during feature generation like the one above. As before-mentioned, in medical domain, sometimes a useless symptom by itself may become indispensable when combined with other symptom. To overcome such problem, our LUIFS (latent utility of irrelevant feature selection) method takes interdependence among attributes into account instead of considering them alone.

3.1 LUIFS

LUIFS mainly focuses on discovering the potential usefulness of supportive irrelevant features. It takes the inter-correlation between irrelevant attributes and other attributes into consideration to measure the latent importance of those irrelevant attributes. As we believe that in medical field an irrelevant attribute is the one that providing neither explicit information nor supportive or implicit information. In (Pazzani, 1996), Pazzani proposed a similar method to improve the Bayesian classifier by searching for dependencies among attributes. However, his method has several aspects that are different from ours: (1) it is restricted under the domains on which the naïve Bayesian classifier is significantly less accurate than a decision tree learner; while our method aims to be a preprocessing tool for most learning algorithms, no restrictions on the learner. (2) It used wrapper model to construct and evaluate a classifier at each step; while a simpler filter model is used in our method, which minimized computational complexity and cost. (3) His method created a new compound attribute replacing the original two attributes in the classifier after joining attributes. This may result in a less accurate classifier, because joined attributes have more values and hence there are fewer examples for each value, as a consequence, joined attributes are less reliable than the individual attributes. Contrarily, our method adds the potential useful irrelevant attributes to assist increasing the importance of the valuable attributes, instead of dynamically joining the attributes. Our experimental evidence in the corresponding section will show that there are additional benefits by including the latent useful irrelevant attributes.

LUIFS generates an optimal feature subset in two phases: (1) Attribute sorting: a general feature ranking process by sorting the attributes according to the relevance regarding the target class, and filters the ones whose weight is below a pre-defined threshold σ; (2) Latent utility attribute searching: for each filtered irrelevant and unselected attribute, determine its supportive importance by performing a multivariate interdependence measure that combined with another attribute. There are two cases that an irrelevant attribute in the second phase becomes a potentially supportive relevant attribute and will be selected into the optimal feature subset: (1) if a combined attribute is a relevant attribute and already be selected, then the combinatorial measure should be greater than the measure of such combined attribute; (2) if a combined attribute is an irrelevant attribute too and filtered out in the first phase, then the combinatorial measure should be greater than the pre-defined threshold σ, such that both attributes become relevant and will be selected. Two hypotheses have been conducted from our method LUIFS as below:

Hypothesis1. If a combined attribute helps in increasing the importance of a yet important attribute; including such combined attribute into the optimal feature subset may most probably improve the final class discrimination.

Hypothesis2. If a combined attribute helps an ignored attribute in reaching the importance threshold; including both attributes into the optimal feature subset may most probably improve the class discrimination

3.2 Attribute sorting

In this phase, we first sort all *N* features according to the importance respect to the target class. Information gain theory in equation (2) is used as the measurement, which may find out the most informative (important) attribute *A* relative to a collection of examples *S*. Attributes are sorted in descending order, from the most important one (with the highest information gain) to the least useful one. In LUIFS, we introduced a threshold ϖ to distinguish the weightiness of an attribute. The value of a threshold either too high or too low may cause the attributes insufficient or surplus. Therefore it is defined as a mean value excluding the ones with maximum and minimum weights, in order to eliminate as much bias as possible. Equation (7) illustrates the threshold.

$$\begin{aligned}\varpi = mean(\sum_{i=1}^{N} InfoGain(S, A_i) - \max(InfoGain) \\ - \min(InfoGain))\end{aligned} \tag{7}$$

Then, an attribute *A* will be selected into the optimal feature subset if $Gain(S, A) > \varpi$. In addition, if an attribute *A* is a numeric type, it is discretized first by using the method of (Fayyad & Irani, 1993). This phase requires only linear time in the number of given features *N*, i.e. $O(N)$.

3.3 Latent utility attribute searching

This phase is the key spirit in LUIFS, since our objective is to uncover the usefulness of the latent or supportive relevant attributes, particularly those specifically owned in medical domain. It is targeted at the irrelevant attributes that filtered out from the Attribute sorting phase, to look for their latent utilities in supporting other relevant attributes. To determine whether an irrelevant attribute is potentially important or not, we measure the interdependence weight between it and another attribute regarding the class attribute. We use Relief theory (Kira & Rendell, 1992a; Kira & Rendell, 1992b), which is a feature weighting algorithm for estimating the quality of attributes such that it is able to discover the interdependencies between attributes. It randomly picks a sample, for each sample it finds *near hit* and *near miss* sample based on distance measure. Relief works for noisy and correlated features, and requires only linear time in the number of features and the number of samples (Dash & Liu, 1997). Our method adopts the combinatorial relief in equation (8), which measures the interdependence between a pair of attributes and the class attribute rather than a single attribute. It approximates the following probability difference:

$$\begin{aligned} W[a_i + a_j] = {} & P(\text{different value of } a_i + a_j | \\ & \text{nearest instances from different class } C) \\ & \text{- } P(\text{different value of } a_i + a_j | \\ & \text{nearest instances from same class } C) \end{aligned} \qquad (8)$$

where a_i is an irrelevant attribute, whose information gain measure in equation (2) is less than the mean threshold ϖ in equation (7) and is filtered out in Attribute sorting phase; a_j is a combined attribute either relevant or irrelevant. $W[a_i+a_j]$ is the combinatorial weighting between attributes a_i and a_j regarding the class attribute C, and P is a probability function. Equation (8) measures the level of hidden supportive importance for an irrelevant attribute to another attribute, hence the higher the weighting, the more information it will provide, such that the better the diagnostic results. According to our hypotheses, an irrelevant attribute a_i may become latent relevant if there exists another attribute a_j, where $a_i \neq a_j$, so that the combinatorial measure $W[a_i+a_j] > W[a_j]$ if a_j is an explicit relevant attribute and already be selected into the optimal feature subset; or $W[a_i+a_j] > \varpi$ (a pre-defined threshold) if a_j is an irrelevant attribute also.

Unlike the Attribute sorting phase, the complexity of this searching phase is no longer simple linear in time. In the worst case, if there is only one important attribute was selected after Attribute sorting phase, that is, there are $(N\text{-}1)$ irrelevant attributes were ignored and unselected. For each irrelevant attribute $a_i \in$ *UnselectedAttributes*, calculate its interdependent weight with another attribute. Again in the worst case, if a_i could not encounter an attribute that makes it becoming useful, then the searching algorithm should be repeated for $(N\text{-}1)$ times. Whereas the algorithm is symmetric, i.e. $W[a_i+a_j] = W[a_j+a_i]$, so the total times of searching should be in half respect to the number of *UnselectedAttributes*, which equals to $(N\text{-}1)/2$. Therefore, the complexity of such Latent utility attribute searching for irrelevant attributes is $(N\text{-}1)*(N\text{-}1)/2$ for the worst case, i.e. $O((N\text{-}1)^2/2)$. Nevertheless the feature selection is typically done in an off-line manner (Jain & Zongker, 1997), in the meantime, the capacity of the hardware components increase while the price of them decrease. Hence, the execution time of an algorithm becomes less important compared with its final class discriminating performance.

3.4 LUIFS algorithm

In this section, the pseudo code of LUIFS algorithm is illustrated as following. First, several variables are defined, and then the program body are sketched subsequently.

Mean – the threshold value for picking the relevant attributes
selectedlist – list of attributes that are treated as important and used in final classification
unselectedlist – list of attributes that are treated as useless and are ignored
N – the total number of attributes in a dataset
A_i – the ith attribute in a dataset
M – the total number of attributes in *unselectedlist*
Map – an array of boolean values indicating whether an attribute is processed multivariate interdependent attributes mapping or not

MIFS algorithm
```
    selectedlist := {};
    unselectedlist := {};
    -- phase one processing
    for i := 1 to N do
   if InformGain(Ai) >= Mean then
           selectedlist := selectedlist + {Ai};
       else
           unselectedlist := unselectedlist + {Ai};
       end if;
    end for;
    -- phase two processing
    for i := 1 to M do
       for j := 1 to N do
         if {Aj} is in selectedlist and {Ai} <> {Aj} then
           if Measure[Ai+Aj] > Measure[Aj] then
              selectedlist := selectedlist + {Ai};
              unselectedlist:=unselectedlist-{Ai};
              Map[Ai] := true;
           end if;
         elseif {Aj} is in unselectedlist and
         {Ai} <> {Aj} then
           if Measure[Ai+Aj]>Mean and
           Map[Aj] = false then
              selectedlist := selectedlist + {Ai};
              selectedlist := selectedlist + {Aj};
              unselectedlist:=unselectedlist-{Ai};
              unselectedlist:=unselectedlist-{Aj};
              Map[Ai] := true;
              Map[Aj] := true;
           end if;
         end if;
       end for;
    end for;
end algorithm;
```

4. Experiments

In this section, we have verified the superiority of our before-mentioned theories by evaluating the effectiveness of proposed pre-processing methods: MIDCA and LUIFS. The solid evidences demonstrate our belief: by uncovering potential attributes relevance during pre-processing step (either FS or CFD) and taking them into the data mining task, the learning performance can have significant improvement. The experiments are carried out individually with learning algorithms into two subsections, and are performed on several real life datasets from UCI repository (Blake & Merz, 1998). Both experiments adopt ID3 (Quinlan, 1986) from (Blake & Merz, 1998) and C4.5 (Quinlan, 1993; Quinlan, 1996) as the learning algorithms for the comparisons to be performed. Table 1 depicts the detailed characteristics of various datasets, while the datasets beneath the double line separator are only involved in the experiment of LUIFS.

4.1 Experiment of MIDCA

The last four datasets in Table 1 are not considered in this experiment, since they do not have numeric attributes, so there are eight datasets to take performance in the experiment of MIDCA. In order to make comparisons between different discretization methods, we downloaded the discretization program - *Discretize* (a discretization program that downloaded from UCI repository, here it is used as a preprocessing tool for ID3 learning algorithm only). On the other hand, since C4.5 is embedded with the discretization function in the learning algorithm, *Discretize* is not applicable to this algorithm. Table 2 shows the results in classification error rate obtained by using ID3 learning algorithm with *Discretize* and MIDCA pre-processing methods respectively; while Table 3 shows the results in classification error rate obtained by using C4.5 learning algorithm without/with MIDCA pre-processing method respectively.

Dataset	Feature Type		Instance size	Class
	Numeric	Nominal		
Cleve	6	7	303	2
Hepatitis	6	13	155	2
Hypothyroid	7	18	3163	2
Heart	13	0	270	2
Sick-euthyroid	7	18	3163	2
Auto	15	11	205	7
Breast	10	0	699	2
Diabetes	8	0	768	2
Mushroom	0	22	8124	2
Parity5+5	0	10	1124	2
Corral	0	6	64	2
Led7	0	7	3200	10

Table 1. Bench-mark datasets from UCI repository

Dataset	Discretize (%)	MIDCA (%)
Cleve	26.733±4.426	17.822±3.827
Hepatitis	19.231±5.519	9.615±4.128
Hypothyroid	1.232±0.340	0.000±0.000
Heart	15.556±3.842	17.778±4.053
Sick-euthyroid	3.697±0.581	0.000±0.000
Auto	26.087±5.325	25.373±5.356
Breast	3.863±1.265	4.292±1.331
Diabetes	25.781±2.739	32.031±2.922
Average	15.27	13.36

Table 2. Results in classification error rate of ID3 algorithm with various discretization methods

The experiments reveal that our method MIDCA decreases the classification error rate for ID3 learning algorithm on all but three datasets among eight; similarly MIDCA decreases the classification error rate for C4.5 learning algorithm on all but two out of eight datasets. For the rest of the datasets, MIDCA provides a significant improvement in classification accuracy, especially on two data sets: *Hypothyroid* and *Sick-euthyroid*, which approached to zero error rates for both learning algorithms. As observed from Table 2 and Table 3, MIDCA slightly decreases the performance on two and three datasets out of eight for C4.5 and ID3 algorithms respectively, and all these datasets contain only continuous attributes. This is

Dataset	C4.5 (%)	MIDCA (%)
Cleve	24.8	17.8
Hepatitis	17.3	9.6
Hypothyroid	0.9	0.0
Heart	17.8	21.1
Sick-euthyroid	3.1	0.0
Auto	29.0	23.9
Breast	5.6	3.9
Diabetes	30.9	31.6
Average	16.18	13.49

Table 3. Results in classification error rate of C4.5 algorithm without/with MIDCA method

due to the MIDCA algorithm needs to perform a univariate discretization once prior the multivariate discretization if an interdependent attribute is a continuous-valued attribute also. Such step increases the uncertainty of the attribute being discretized, hence increases the error rate accordingly. Although it is inevitable that a continuous-valued attribute to be selected as a best interdependent attribute regarding the attribute being discretized, our theories DO work in most cases. From the average error rate results described in Table 2 and

Table 3, obviously our method MIDCA indeed decreases the classification error rate from 15.27% down to 13.36% for ID3 algorithm; and from 16.18% down to 13.49% for C4.5 algorithm. The improvements relative to both algorithms reach to approximately 12.5% and 16.6% respectively. The comparisons under various situations are clearly illustrated in Figure 1 and Figure 2 respectively.

4.2 Experiment of LUIFS

In this experiment, all twelve datasets in Table 1 are used. In order to make clear comparison, experiments on two learning algorithms without feature selection (NoFS) and with information gain attribute ranking method (ARFS) are performed, as well as LUIFS. Table 4 and Table 5 summarize the results in error rates of ID3 and C4.5 algorithms without/with feature selection respectively. The last column LRA in Table 4 indicates the number of irrelevant attributes becoming useful and is selected in LUIFS method, which further demonstrates the importance of supportive attributes.

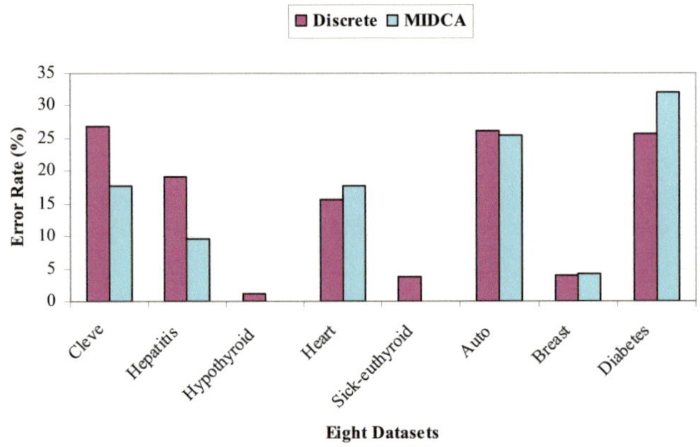

Fig. 1. Comparisons in classification error rate of ID3 algorithm with different discretization methods

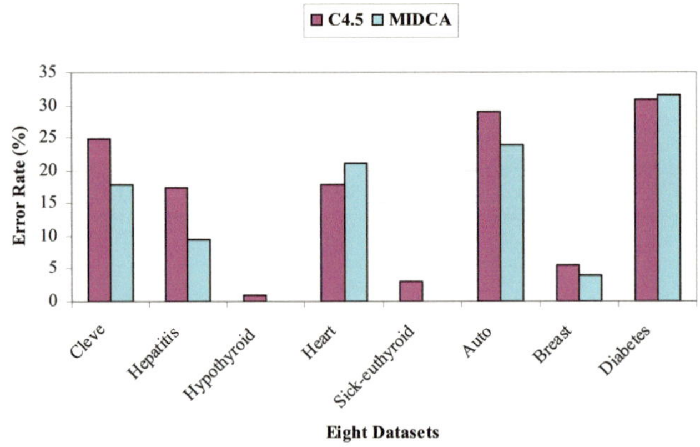

Fig. 2. Comparisons in classification error rate of C4.5 algorithm without/with MIDCA method

As observed from the results in Table 4 and Table 5, LUIFS slightly increases the classification error rate in compared with ARFS for both learning algorithms on only one dataset - *Heart*, amongst all twelve datasets; but its results are still better than the learning algorithms with NoFS. This is because the dataset *Heart* contains numeric attributes only, which needs prior discretized to the latent utility attribute searching being carried out. Such step increases the uncertainty to the attribute being correlated, hence increases the error rate accordingly.

Nevertheless, LUIFS may still help in obtaining quite good classification accuracy, even for the simplest learning algorithm. The average results from Table 4 and Table 5 reveal that LUIFS does improve on the final classification accuracy significantly. Especially with ID3 algorithm, which the accuracy growth rate relative to NoFS and ARFS are 10.79% and 11.09% respectively; while with C4.5 method, the corresponding growth rates are not as good as with ID3, they are only 8.51% and 7.86% respectively. Even so, the classification accuracy with LUIFS in Table 5 is still the highest. The vast improvements made by LUIFS in ID3 learning algorithm is due to ID3 is a pure decision tree algorithm, without any built-in pre-processing functions, such as FS or CFD, hence there is still certain rooms for improving; while C4.5 is embedded with its own feature selection and pruning functions already, it filters the useless features from its own point of view, no matter additional feature selection algorithm attached or not, hence limiting the great improvements. The comparisons under various situations are apparently portrayed in Figure 3 and Figure 4 respectively.

Dataset	NoFS	ARFS	LUIFS	LRA
Cleve	35.64	23.762	22.772	2
Hepatitis	21.154	15.385	13.462	7
Hypothyroid	0.948	0.190	0.190	8
Heart	23.333	13.333	18.889	2
Sick-euthyroid	3.791	0	0	7
Auto	26.087	18.841	18.841	3
Breast	5.579	6.438	5.579	2
Diabetes	Error[2]	35.156	32.131	3
Mushroom	0	0	0	1
Parity5+5	49.291	50	49.291	4
Corral	0	12.5	0	2
Led7	33.467	42.533	32.8	1
Average	18.12	18.18	16.16	3.5

Table 4. Results in classification error rate of ID3 algorithm without/with various feature selections

[2] Error refers to the program error during execution, hence no result at all. Therefore, the corresponding average error rate with NoFS is only approximated without taking such result into calculation.

5. Conclusion and future research

5.1. Conclusions

In this paper, we have proposed a novel concept of improving the classification accuracy for common learning algorithms by uncovering the potential attributes relevance through multivariate interdependent attribute pre-processing methods. However, many common pre-processing methods ignored the latent inter-correlation between attributes, this sometimes may loose the potential hidden valuable information, thus limit the performance of the learning algorithms. Especially in medical domain, diagnostic accuracy is treated as the most important issue, in order to approach to the highest accuracy, qualities of the pre-processing methods are quite essential, thereby finding out the most useful attributes relevance is a key factor for a successful method.

Dataset	NoFS	ARFS	LUIFS
Cleve	20	22.2	19.3
Hepatitis	15.6	7.9	7.9
Hypothyroid	1.1	0.4	0.4
Heart	17.8	14.4	15.6
Sick-euthyroid	2.5	2.5	2.4
Auto	27.1	21.9	21.8
Breast	5.7	5.6	5.4
Diabetes	30.9	30.1	30.1
Mushroom	0	0	0
Parity5+5	50	50	50
Corral	9.4	12.5	9.4
Led7	32.6	43.7	32.3
Average	17.72	17.6	16.21

Table 5. Results in classification error rate of C4.5 algorithm without/with various feature selections

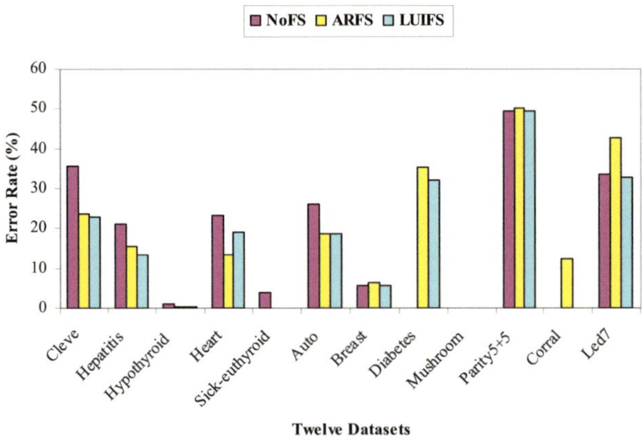

Fig. 3. Comparisons in classification error rate of ID3 algorithm without/with various feature selections

Two pre-processing methods MIDCA and LUIFS have been presented in detail, to verify the superiority of our theories. The empirical evaluation results from various experiments further demonstrated their effectiveness by applying two different classification algorithms on the datasets with and without MIA-Processing. The significant performance improvement by using MIDCA method indicates that it can accurately and meaningfully discretize a continuous-valued attribute by discovering its perfect matched interdependent attribute. In addition, the usage of LUIFS method on the other hand can minimize the classification error rate as well, even for the learning algorithm with built-in feature selection and discretization capabilities.

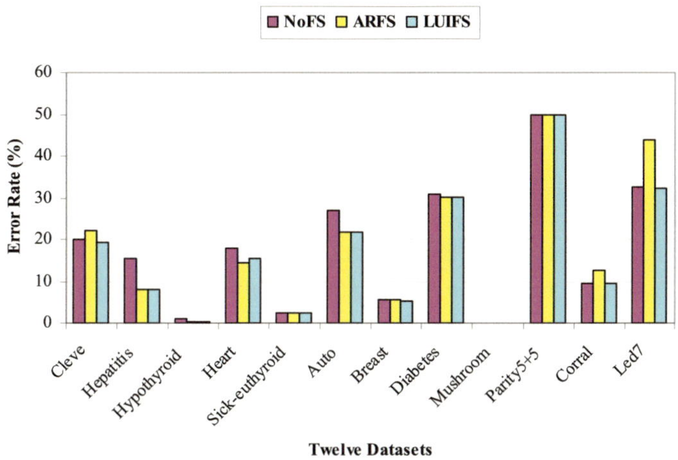

Fig. 4. Comparisons in classification error rate of C4.5 algorithm without/with various feature selections

Finally, the purpose of our methods to incorporate relief theory with information measure is to minimize the uncertainty and at the same time maximize the classification accuracy. Although the methods are designed for using in medical domain, they still can be applied to other domains, since the models do not rely on any background knowledge to be constructed.

5.2 Future research

The future work of our research can be substantially extended to include more factors into comparisons; they may be summarized into the following aspects:

1. Involve more learning algorithms in data mining, such as Naïve-Bayes (Langley et al., 1992), 1R (Holte, 1993), ANNs (Hand et al., 2001; Kasabov, 1998) or Gas (Melanie, 1999), etc. This may validate the practicability of our proposed MIA-Processing methods.
2. Implement the existing pre-processing methods, such as ReliefF (Kononenko, 1994), Focus (Almualim & Dietterich, 1992) or MLDM (Sheinvald et al., 1990), etc. This may allow us to discover the weakness of our current methods, and then improve accordingly.
3. Include different types of real-life or artificial datasets into the experiments, to enrich the usability of our MIA-Processing methods.

Furthermore, our next principal direction for the future research is focused on the optimization of both MIA-Processing methods. A feasible solution should be investigated to eliminate the uncertainties and to reduce the complexities as much as possible, in order to adapt to the future development trend in data mining. Besides, the existing weaknesses of our methods should be found out and reimplemented. They should not decrease the accuracy in learning on a dataset contains all numeric attributes; and should handle high dimensional or large datasets efficiently.

6. References

J. Han, and M. Kamber, *Data Mining - Concepts and Techniques,* Morgan Kaufmann Publishers, 2000.

L. Yu, and H. Liu, "Efficient Feature Selection via Analysis of Relevance and Redundancy", *Journal of Machine Learning Research, Vol. 5,* 2004, pp. 1205-1224.

H. Liu, and H. Motoda, *Feature Selection for Knowledge Discovery and Data Mining,* Kluwer Academic Publisher, 2000.

I. Guyon, and A. Elisseeff, "An Introduction to Variable and Feature Selection", *Journal of Machine Learning Research, Vol. 3,* 2003, pp. 1157-1182.

R. Caruana, and V.R. Sa, "Benefitting from the Variables that Variable Selection Discards", *Journal of Machine Learning Research, Vol. 3,* 2003, pp. 1245-1264.

L. Jia, , and Y. Xu, *Guan Xing Bing De Zhen Duan Yu Zhi Liao,* Jun Shi Yi Xue Ke Xue Chu Ban She, 2001.

S.D. Bay, "Multivariate Discretization of Continuous Variables for Set Mining", In Proceedings of the Sixth ACM SIGKDD International Conference on Knowledge Discovery and Data Mining, 2000, pp. 315–319.

S.D. Bay, "Multivariate Discretization for Set Mining", *Knowledge and Information Systems, Vol. 3(4),* 2001, pp. 491-512.

W.Q. Gu, "Xin Xue Guan Ji Bing Jian Bie Zhen Duan Xue", Xue Yuan Chu Ban She, 2006

J. Dougherty, R. Kohavi, and M. Sahami, "Supervised and Unsupervised Discretization of Continuous Features", *In Proceedings of the Twelfth International Conference on Machine Learning,* Morgan Kaufmann Publishers, San Francisco, CA., 1995.

U.M. Fayyad, and K.B. Irani, "Multi-interval Discretization of Continuous-valued Attributes for Classification Learning", *In Proceedings of the Thirteenth International Joint Conference on Artificial Intelligence,* 1993, pp. 1022–1027.

H. Liu, and R. Setiono, "Feature Selection via Discretization", *Technical report,* Dept. of Information Systems and Computer Science, Singapore, 1997.

H. Liu, F. Hussain, C. Tan, and M. Dash, "Discretization: An Enabling Technique", *Data Mining and Knowledge Discovery,* 2002, pp. 393–423.

S. Monti, and G.F. Cooper, "A Multivariate Discretization Method for Learning Bayesian Networks from Mixed Data", *In Proceedings of 14th Conference of Uncertainty in AI,* 1998, pp. 404-413.

K. Kira, and L. Rendell, "A Practical Approach to Feature Selection", *In Proceedings of International Conference on Machine Learning,* Morgan Kaufmann, Aberdeen, 1992a, pp. 249-256.

K. Kira, and L. Rendell, "The Feature Selection Problem: Traditional Methods and New Algorithm", *In Proceedings of AAAI'92*. San Jose, CA, 1992b.

T.M. Mitchell, *Machine Learning*, McGraw-Hill Companies, Inc., 1997.

X.L. Zhu, *Fundamentals of Applied Information Theory*, Tsinghua University Press, 2000.

L. Breiman, "Technical Note: Some Properties of Splitting Criteria", *Machine Learning Vol. 24,* 1996, pp. 41–47.

M.A. Hall, and G. Holmes, "Benchmarking Attributes Selection Techniques for Discrete Class Data Mining", *IEEE Transactions on Knowledge and Data Engineering Vol. 15(3),* 2003, pp. 1-16.

L.C. Molina, L. Belanche, and A. Nebot, "Feature Selection Algorithms: A Survey and Experimental Evaluation", *In Proceedings of the IEEE International Conference on Data Mining*, 2002.

M. Dash, and H. Liu, "Feature Selection for Classification", *Intelligent Data Analysis, Vol. 1(3),* 1997, pp. 131-156.

K.J. Cios, W. Pedrycz, and R. Swiniarski, *Data Mining Methods for Knowledge Discovery*, Kluwer Academic Publisher, 1998.

G.H. John, R. Kohavi, and K. Pfleger, "Irrelevant Features and the Subset Selection Problem", *In Proceedings of the Eleventh International Conference on Machine learning,* 1994, pp. 121-129.

M.J. Pazzani, "Searching for Dependencies in Bayesian Classifiers", *In Proceedings of the Fifth International Workshop on AI and Statistics*, Springer-Verlag, 1996, pp. 424-429.

A. Jain, and D. Zongker, "Feature Selection: Evaluation, Application and Small Sample Performance", *IEEE Transactions on Pattern Analysis and Machine Intelligence Vol. 19(2),* 1997, pp. 153–158.

C.L. Blake, and C.J. Merz, "UCI Repository of Machine Learning Databases", Irvine, CA: University of California, Department of Information and Computer Science, 1998. [http://www.ics.uci.edu/~mlearn/MLRepository.html]

J.R. Quinlan, "Induction of Decision Trees", *Machine Learning Vol. 1(1)*, 1986, pp. 81-106.

J.R. Quinlan, *C4.5: Programs for Machine Learning*, Morgan Kaufmann, San Mateo, CA, 1993.

Quinlan, J. R. Improved use of continuous attributes in C4.5. Journal of Artificial Intelligence Research 4, 1996, 77-90.

P. Langley, W. Iba, and K. Thompsom, "An Analysis of Bayesian Classifiers", *In Proceedings of the tenth national conference on artificial intelligence,* AAAI Press and MIT Press, 1992, pp. 223-228.

R.C. Holte, "Very Simple Classification Rules Perform Well on Most Commonly Used Datasets", *Machine Learning Vol. 11*, 1993.

D. Hand, H. Mannila, and P. Smyth, *Principles of Data Mining*, The MIT Press, 2001.

N.K. Kasabov, *Foundations of Neural Networks, Fuzzy Systems, and Knowledge Engineering*, The MIT Press, Cambridge, Massachusetts London, England, 1998.

M. Melanie, *An Introduction to Genetic Algorithms*, MIT Press, Cambridge, Massachusetts, London, England, 1999.

I. Kononenko, "Estimating Attributes: Analysis and Extension of RELIEF", *In Proceedings of the European Conference on Machine Learning*, Springer-Verlag, Catania, Italy, Berlin, 1994, pp. 171-182.

H. Almualim, and T.G. Dietterich, "Learning with Many Irrelevant Features", *In Proccedinggs of the Ninth National Conference on Artifical Intelligence,* AAAI Press/The MIT Press, Anaheim, California, 1992, pp. 547-552.

J. Sheinvald, B. Dom, and W. Niblack, "A Modeling Approach to Feature Selection", *In Proceedings of the Tenth International Conference on Pattern Recognition,* 1990, pp. 535-539.

2

Intelligent Decision Support System for Classification of Eeg Signals using Wavelet Coefficients

Pari Jahankhani and Vassilis Kodogiannis
School of Computer Science, University of Westminster, London HA1 3TP, UK

1. Introduction

The human brain is obviously a complex system, and exhibits rich spatiotemporal dynamics. Among the non-invasive techniques for probing human brain dynamics, electroencephalography (EEG) provides a direct measure of cortical activity with millisecond temporal resolution. Early on, EEG analysis was restricted to visual inspection of EEG records. Since there is no definite criterion evaluated by the experts, visual analysis of EEG signals is insufficient. For example, in the case of dominant alpha activity delta and theta, activities are not noticed. Routine clinical diagnosis needs to analysis of EEG signals. Therefore, some automation and computer techniques have been used for this aim (Guler et al., 2001). Since the early days of automatic EEG processing, representations based on a Fourier transform have been most commonly applied. This approach is based on earlier observations that the EEG spectrum contains some characteristic waveforms that fall primarily within four frequency bands—delta (1–4 Hz), theta (4–8 Hz), alpha (8–13 Hz), and beta (13–30 Hz). Such methods have proved beneficial for various EEG characterizations, but fast Fourier transform (FFT), suffer from large noise sensitivity. Parametric power spectrum estimation methods such as AR, reduces the spectral loss problems and gives better frequency resolution. AR method has also an advantage over FFT that, it needs shorter duration data records than FFT (Zoubir et al., 1998). A powerful method was proposed in the late 1980s to perform time-scale analysis of signals: the wavelet transforms (WT). This method provides a unified framework for different techniques that have been developed for various applications. Since the WT is appropriate for analysis of non-stationary signals and this represents a major advantage over spectral analysis, it is well suited to locating transient events, which may occur during epileptic seizures. Wavelet's feature extraction and representation properties can be used to analyse various transient events in biological signals. (Adeli et al., 2003) gave an overview of the discrete wavelet transform (DWT) developed for recognising and quantifying spikes, sharp waves and spike-waves. Wavelet transform has been used to analyze and characterise epileptiform discharges in the form of 3-Hz spike and wave complex in patients with absence seizure. Through wavelet decomposition of the EEG records, transient features are accurately captured and localised in both time and frequency context. The capability of this mathematical microscope to analyse different scales of neural rhythms is shown to be a powerful tool for investigating small-scale oscillations of the brain signals. A better understanding of the dynamics of the human brain through EEG analysis can be obtained through further analysis of such EEG records.

Numerous other techniques from the theory of signal analysis have been used to obtain representations and extract the features of interest for classification purposes. Neural networks and statistical pattern recognition methods have been applied to EEG analysis. Neural network (NN) detection systems have been proposed by a number of researchers. (Pradhan et al. 1996) used the raw EEG as an input to a neural network while (Weng and Khorasani ,1996) used the features proposed by Gotman with an adaptive structure neural network, but his results show a poor false detection rate. (Petrosian et al., 2000) showed that the ability of specifically designed and trained recurrent neural networks (RNN) combined with wavelet pre-processing, to predict the onset of epileptic seizures both on scalp and intracranial recordings only one-channel of electroencephalogram. In order to provide faster and efficient algorithm, (Folkers et al., 2003) proposed a versatile signal processing and analysis framework for bioelectrical data and in particular for neural recordings and 128-channel EEG. Within this framework the signal is decomposed into sub-bands using fast wavelet transform algorithms, executed in real-time on a current digital signal processor hardware platform. Neuro-fuzzy systems harness the power of the two paradigms: fuzzy logic and NNs by utilising the mathematical properties of NNs in tuning rule-based fuzzy systems that approximate the way human process information. A specific approach in neuro-fuzzy development is the adaptive neuro-fuzzy inference system (ANFIS), which has shown significant results in modelling nonlinear functions. In ANFIS, the membership function parameters are extracted from a data set that describes the system behaviour. The ANFIS learns features in the data set and adjusts the system parameters according to a given error criterion. Successful implementations of ANFIS in EEG analysis have been reported (Guler et al., 2004).

As compared to the conventional method of frequency analysis using Fourier transform or short time Fourier transform, wavelets enable analysis with a coarse to fine multi-resolution perspective of the signal. In this work, DWT has been applied for the time–frequency analysis of EEG signals and NNs for the classification using wavelet coefficients. EEG signals were decomposed into frequency sub-bands using discrete wavelet transform (DWT). A neural network system was implemented to classify the EEG signal to one of the categories: epileptic or normal. The aim of this study was to develop a simple algorithm for the detection of epileptic seizure, which could also be applied to real-time.

In this study, an alternative approach based on the multiple-classifier concept will be presented for epileptic seizure detection. A neural network classifier, Learning Vector Quantisation (LVQ2.1), is employed to classify unknown EEGs belonging to one set of signal.

Here we investigated the potential of statistical techniques, such as Rough Set and Principal Component Analysis (PCA) that capture the second-order statistical structure of the data. Fig. 1 shows overall computation scheme.

2. Data selection and recording

We have used the publicly available data described in (Andrzejak *et al.*). The complete data set consists of two sets (denoted A and E) each containing 100 single-channel EEG segments. These segments were selected and cut out from continuous multi-channel EEG recordings after visual inspection for artefacts, e.g., due to muscle activity or eye movements. Sets A consisted of segments taken from surface EEG recordings that were carried out on five healthy volunteers using a standardised electrode placement scheme (Fig. 2).

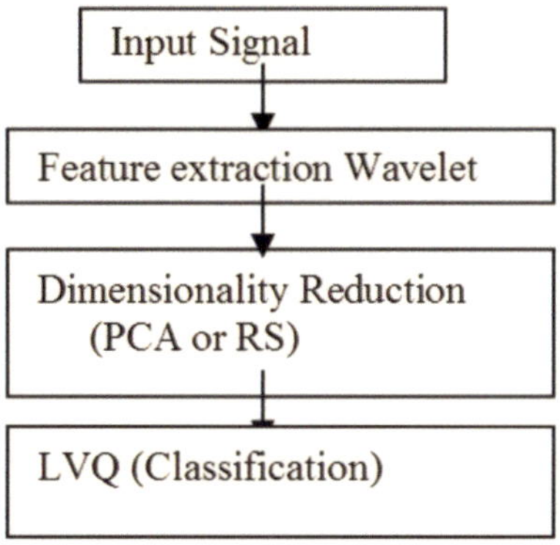

Fig. 1. Computation scheme for classifying signals

Brain Area	Left Hemisphere	Midline	Right Hemisphere
Pre-Frontal	Fp1		Fp2
Frontal	F3		F4
Inferior Frontal	F7		F8
Mid-Frontal		Fz	
Mid-Temporal	T3		T4
Posterior Temporal	T5		T6
Central	C3		C4
Vertex (Mid-Central)		Cz	
Parietal	P3		P4
Mid-Parietal		Pz	
Occipital	O1		O2
Ear (Auricular)	A1		A2
Ground		G	

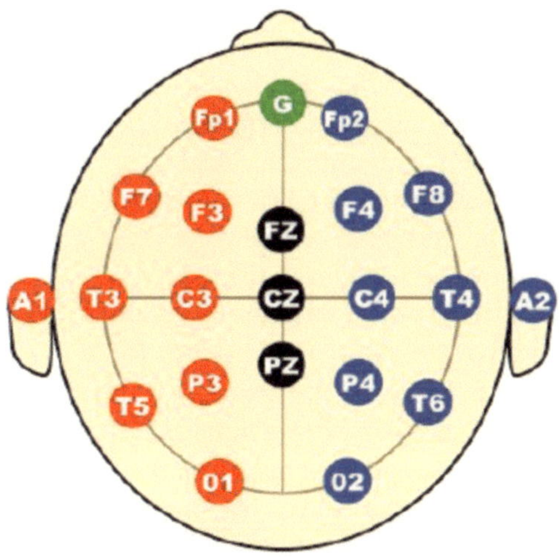

Fig. 2. The 10–20 international system of electrode placement c images of normal and abnormal cases.

Volunteers were relaxed in an awake-state with eyes open (A). Sets E originated from EEG archive of pre-surgical diagnosis. EEGs from five patients were selected, all of who had achieved complete seizure control after resection of one of the hippocampal formations, which was therefore correctly diagnosed to be the epileptogenic zone. Segments, set E only contained seizure activity.

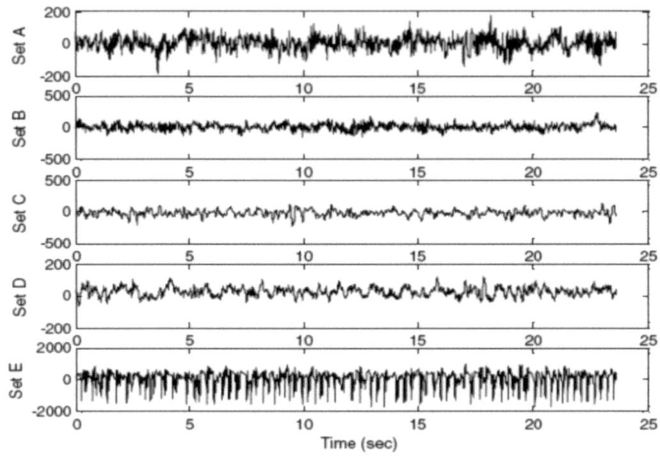

Fig. 3. Examples of five different sets of EEG signals taken from different subjects.

Here segments were selected from all recording sites exhibiting ictal activity. All EEG signals were recorded with the same 128-channel amplifier system, using an average common reference. The data were digitised at 173.61 samples per second using 12-bit resolution. Band-pass filter settings were 0.53–40 Hz (12dB/oct). In this study, we used two dataset (A and E) of the complete dataset (Jahankhani et al 2005) . Typical EEGs are depicted in Fig. 3.

3. Analysis using Discrete Wavelet Transform (DWT)

Wavelet transform is a spectral estimation technique in which any general function can be expressed as an infinite series of wavelets. The basic idea underlying wavelet analysis consists of expressing a signal as a linear combination of a particular set of functions (wavelet transform, WT), obtained by shifting and dilating one single function called a mother wavelet. The decomposition of the signal leads to a set of coefficients called wavelet coefficients. Therefore the signal can be reconstructed as a linear combination of the wavelet functions weighted by the wavelet coefficients.

DWT is a time-frequency analysis technique that is most suited for non-stationary signal. It was chosen as the feature extraction method for these signals, since the important feature may be in the time domain, in the frequency domain, or in both domains. DWT also has other properties, such as providing a substantial amount of data reduction. DWT analyses the signal at different frequency bands with different resolution by decomposing the signal into coarse approximation and detail information. DWT using two sets of functions, called scaling functions and wavelet functions, which are associated with low-pass and high-pass filter. The original signal x[n] is first passed through a half-band high-pass filter g[n] and a low-pass filter h[n].after the filtering, half of the samples can be eliminated according to

Nyquist's rule, since the signal now has a highest frequency of $\pi/2$ radians instead of π. The signal can therefore be sub sampled by 2, simply by discarding every other sample. In general when dealing with stationary signals, whose statistical properties are invariant over time, the ideal tool is the Fourier transform. The Fourier transform is an infinite linear combination of dilated cosine and sine waves. When we encounter non-stationary signals, we ca represent these signals by linear combinations of atomic decompositions known as wavelet.

In order to obtain an exact reconstruction of the signal, adequate number of coefficients must be computed. The key feature of wavelets is the time-frequency localisation. It means that most of the energy of the wavelet is restricted to a finite time interval. Frequency localisation means that the Fourier transform is band limited. When compared to STFT, the advantage of time-frequency localisation is that wavelet analysis varies the time-frequency aspect ratio, producing good frequency localization at low frequencies (long time windows), and good time localisation at high frequencies (short time windows). This produces a segmentation, or tiling of the time-frequency plane that is appropriate for most physical signals, especially those of a transient nature. The wavelet technique applied to the EEG signal will reveal features related to the transient nature of the signal, which are not obvious by the Fourier, transform. In general, it must be said that no time-frequency regions but rather time-scale regions are defined [Subasi, 2005). The operators h and g are called perfect reconstruction or quadrature mirror filters (QMFs) if they satisfy the orthogonality conditions:

$$G(z)G(z^{-1}) + G(-z)G(-z^{-1}) = 1 \tag{1}$$

Where G(z) denotes the z-transform of the filter g. Its complementary high-pass filter can be defined as

$$H(z) = zG(-z^{-1}) \tag{2}$$

A sequence of filters with increasing length (indexed by i) can be obtained

$$\begin{aligned} G_{i+1}(z) &= G(z^{2^i})G_i(z), \\ H_{i+1}(z) &= H(z^{2^i})G_i(z) \end{aligned} \tag{3}$$

With the initial condition $G_0(z) = 1$. It is expressed as a two-scale relation in time domain

$$\begin{aligned} g_{i+1}(k) &= [g]_{\uparrow 2^i} g_i(k), \\ h_{i+1}(k) &= [h]_{\uparrow 2^i} g_i(k) \end{aligned} \tag{4}$$

where the subscript $[.]_{\uparrow m}$ indicates the up sampling by a factor of m and k is the equally sampled discrete time.

The normalised wavelet and scale basis functions $\varphi_{i,l}(k), \psi_{i,l}(k)$ can be defined as

$$\varphi_{i,l}(k) = 2^{\frac{i}{2}} h_i(k - 2^i l)$$
$$\psi_{i,l}(k) = 2^{\frac{i}{2}} g_i(k - 2^i l) \tag{5}$$

where the factor $2^{i/2}$ is inner product normalization, i and l are the scale parameter and the translation parameter, respectively. The DWT decomposition can be described as:

$$a_i(l) = x(k)\varphi_{i,l}(k)$$
$$d_i(l) = x(k)\psi_{i,l}(k) \tag{6}$$

where $a_i(l)$ and $d_i(l)$ are the approximation coefficients and the detail coefficients at resolution, i, respectively (Daubechies,1990 and 1992), (Solttani, 2002).

One area in which the DWT has been particularly successful is the epileptic seizure detection because it captures transient features and localises them in both time and frequency content accurately. DWT analyses the signal at different frequency bands, with different resolutions by decomposing the signal into a coarse approximation and detail information. DWT employs two sets of functions called scaling functions and wavelet functions, which are related to low-pass and high-pass filters, respectively. The decomposition of the signal into the different frequency bands is merely obtained by consecutive high-pass and low-pass filtering of the time domain signal. The procedure of multi-resolution decomposition of a signal x[n] is schematically shown in Fig 4. Each stage of this scheme consists of two digital filters and two down-samplers by 2. The first filter, h[.] is the discrete mother wavelet, high-pass in nature, and the second, g[.] is its mirror version, low-pass in nature. The down-sampled outputs of first high-pass and low-pass filters provide the detail, D1 and the approximation, A1, respectively. The first approximation, A1 is further decomposed and this process is continued as shown in Fig 4

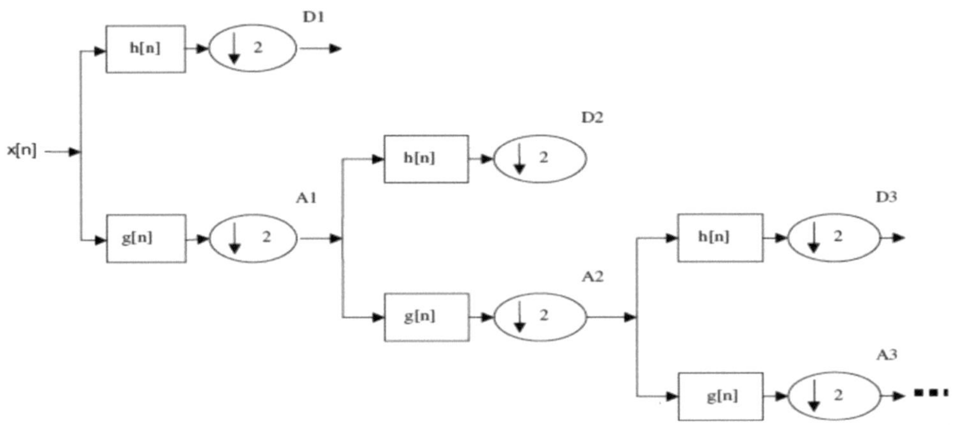

Fig. 4. Sub-band decomposition of DWT implementation; h[n] is the high-pass filter, g[n] the low-pass filter.

Selection of suitable wavelet and the number of decomposition levels is very important in analysis of signals using the DWT. The number of decomposition levels is chosen based on the dominant frequency components of the signal. The levels are chosen such that those parts of the signal that correlates well with the frequencies necessary for classification of the signal are retained in the wavelet coefficients.
It should also be emphasized that the WT is appropriate for analyses f non-stationary signals, and this represents a major advantage over spectral analysis.
One area in which the DWT has been particularly successful is the epileptic seizure detection because it captures transient features and localises them in both time and frequency content accurately. DWT analyses the signal at different frequency bands, with different resolutions by decomposing the signal into a coarse approximation and detail information. DWT employs two sets of functions called scaling functions and wavelet functions, which are related to low-pass and high-pass filters, respectively. The decomposition of the signal into the different frequency bands is merely obtained by consecutive high-pass and low-pass filtering of the time domain signal. The procedure of multi-resolution decomposition of a signal x[n] is schematically shown in Fig. 3. Each stage of this scheme consists of two digital filters and two down-samplers by 2. The first filter, h[.] is the discrete mother wavelet, high-pass in nature, and the second, g[.] is its mirror version, low-pass in nature. The down-sampled outputs of first high-pass and low-pass filters provide the detail, D1 and the approximation, A1, respectively.
Selection of suitable wavelet and the number of decomposition levels is very important in analysis of signals using the DWT. The number of decomposition levels is chosen based on the dominant frequency components of the signal. The levels are chosen such that those parts of the signal that correlates well with the frequencies necessary for classification of the signal are retained in the wavelet coefficients. In the present study, since the EEG signals do not have any useful frequency components above 30 Hz, the number of decomposition levels was chosen to be 4. Thus, the EEG signals were decomposed into details D1–D4 and one final approximation, A4. Usually, tests are performed with different types of wavelets and the one, which gives maximum efficiency, is selected for the particular application. The smoothing feature of the Daubechies wavelet of order 2 (db2) made it more appropriate to detect changes of EEG signals. Hence, the wavelet coefficients were computed using the db4 in the present study. The proposed method was applied on both data sets of EEG data (Sets A and E). Fig. 5 shows approximation (A4) and details (D1–D4) of an epileptic EEG signal (Jahankhani et al (2005a),.

3.1 Feature extraction

The extracted wavelet coefficients provide a compact representation that shows the energy distribution of the EEG signal in time and frequency. Table 1 presents frequencies corresponding to different levels of decomposition for Daubechies order-2 wavelet with a sampling frequency of 173.6 Hz. In order to further decrease the dimensionality of the extracted feature vectors, statistics over the set of the wavelet coefficients was used (Kandaswamy et al, 2004). The following statistical features were used to represent the time frequency distribution of the EEG signals:

- Maximum of the wavelet coefficients in each sub-band.
- Minimum of the wavelet coefficients, in each sub-band.
- Mean of the wavelet coefficients in each sub-band
- Standard deviation of the wavelet coefficients in each sub-band

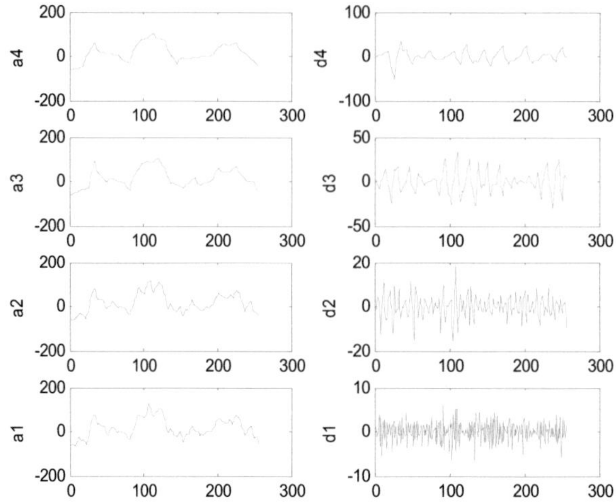

Fig. 5. Approximate and detailed coefficients of EEG signal taken from unhealthy subject (epileptic patient).

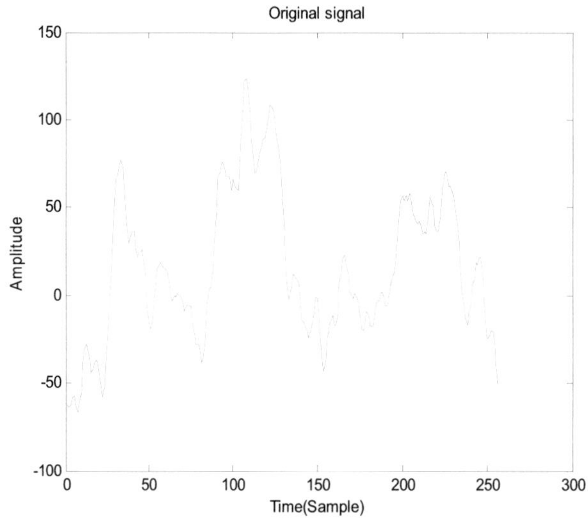

Extracted features for two-recorded class A and E shown in Table 2. The data was acquired using a standard 100 electrode net covering the entire surface of the calvarium Fig. 1).

Decomposed signal	Frequency range (Hz)
D1	43.4–86.8
D2	21.7–43.4
D3	10.8–21.7
D4	5.4–10.8
D5	2.7–5.4
A5	0–2.7

Table 1. Frequencies corresponding to different levels of decomposition

The total recording time was 23.6 seconds, corresponding to a total sampling of 4,096 points. To reduce the volume of data, the sample (time points) was partitioned into 16 windows of 256 times points each. From these sub-samples, we performed the DWT and derived measures of dispersion statistics from these windows (each corresponding to approximately 1.5 seconds). The DWT was performed at 4 levels, and resulted in five sub-bands: d1-d4 and a4 (detail and approximation coefficients respectively). For each of these sub-bands, we extracted four measures of dispersion, yielding a total of 20 attributes per sample window. Since our classifiers use supervised learning, we must also provide the outputs, which was simply a class label (for the experiments presented in this paper (Jahankhani et al (2005b), and (Jahankhani et al (2005c), there were 2, corresponding to classes A and E).

Data	Extracte d features	Sub-band D1	Sub-band D2	Sub-band D3	Sub-band D4	Approxi-mation
Set A	Max.	28.1094	101.757	131.0846	124.377	114.138
	Min.	-28.4010	-60.813	-149.072	-158.797	-109.521
	Mean	-0.0022	0.0058	-0.0035	0.0388	3.7950
	Std dev.	5.1818	13.6442	23.3685	24.7933	35.1465
Set E	Max	123.3921	278.924	429.6621	375.0564	582.3167
	Min	-90.7055	-238.51	-417.120	-468.064	-361.2154
	Mean	0.0131	-0.0281	-0.0359	-0.0071	-5.5526
	Std dev.	11.8488	35.9941	73.7659	78.1432	180.4493

Table 2. The extracted features of two windows from A & E classes

4. Intelligent classifiers

Recently, the concept of combining multiple classifiers has been actively exploited for developing highly reliable "diagnostic" systems [12]. One of the key issues of this approach is how to combine the results of the various systems to give the best estimate of the optimal result. A straightforward approach is to decompose the problem into manageable ones for several different sub-systems and combine them via a gating network. The presumption is that each classifier/sub-system is "an expert" in some local area of the feature space. The sub-systems are local in the sense that the weights in one "expert" are decoupled from the weights in other sub-networks. In this study, 16 subsystems have been developed, and each of them was associated with the each of the windows across each electrode (16/electrode). Each subsystem was modelled with an appropriate intelligent learning scheme. In our case, two alternative schemes have been proposed: the classic MLP network and the RBF network using the orthogonal least squares learning algorithm. Such schemes provide a degree of certainty for each classification based on the statistics for each plane. The outputs of each of these networks must then be combined to produce a total output for the system

4.1 Learning Vector Quantization (LVQ) network

LVQ algorithm is one of the popular quantization algorithms. LVQ is a method for training competitive layers in a supervised manner. Vector Quantization (VQ) is a form of data compression that represents data vectors by set of codebook vectors. This is the basic idea of

VQ theory, the motivation of which is dimensionality reduction or data compression. Each data vector is then its nearest codebook vector then represents vector. VQ methods are closely related to certain paradigms of self-organising Neural Networks. LVQ can be understood as a special case of an artificial NN, more precisely, it applies a winner-take-all Hebbian learning-based approach.
In effect, the error of the VQ approximation is the total squared distance

$$D = \sum_{x} \| x - w_{I(x)} \|^2 \tag{7}$$

Between the input vectors $\{x\}$ and their codebook vectors$\{w_{Ix}\}$, and we clearly wish to minimize this.
Among the many prototype-based learning algorithm proposed recently, LVQ algorithms developed by Kohonen are a family of training algorithms for the nearest-neighbour classifications, which include LVQ1, LVQ2 and its improved versions LVQ2.1, LVQ3 algorithms (Kohonen.T et al, 1988), (Kohonen.T et al, 2001) and (Kohonen.T et al, 2001) The family of LVQ algorithms is widely used for pattern classification, and found a very important role in statistical pattern classification (Kohonen.T et al, 1988), (Kohonen.T et al, 2001) and signal processing achieved satisfactory results than other neural network classifiers in spite of their simple and time efficient training process.
A competitive layer automatically learns to classify input vectors. However, the classes that the competitive layer finds are dependent only on the distance between input vectors. If two input vectors are very similar, the competitive layer probably will put them in the same class. There is no mechanism in a strictly competitive layer design to say whether or not any two input vectors are in the same class or different classes.
A neural network for learning VQ consists of two layers: an input layer and an output layer. It represents a set of reference vectors, the coordinates of which are the weights of the connections leading from the input neuron to an output neuron.
Advantages of LVQ are as follows:

- The model is trained significantly faster than other neural network techniques like Back Propagation.
- Reducing large datasets to a smaller number of codebook vectors for classification
- There is no limit in the number of dimensions in the codebook vectors like nearest neighbour techniques.
- Normalisation of input data is not required.
- Can handle data with missing values.

LVQ has some disadvantages

- Generate useful distance measures for all attributes
- The accuracy is highly depends on the initialisation of the model as well as the learning parameters such as learning rate and training iteration
- Also accuracy is depending on the class distribution in the training dataset.
- It is difficult to determine a good number of codebook vectors for a given problem.

4.1.1 LVQ algorithms

Assume for a one-dimensional case, there are two classes C_1 and C_2 with mean vectors (reference vectors) m_k and an input vector x belong to the same class to which the nearest reference vector belongs.

The learning method of LVQ is often called competition learning, because it works as follows:
For each training pattern the reference vector that is closest to it is determined.
For each data point, the neuron that is closest to its determined called the winner neuron
The weight of the connections to this neuron and winner neuron is then adapted, ie made closer if it correctly classifieds the data point (winner, takes all).
The movement of the reference vector is controlled by a parameter called the learning rate.
The VQ methods are closely related to certain paradigms of self-organising Neural Networks.
LVQ Kohonen ,T,1988), found a very important role in statistical pattern classification (Kohonen ,T,2001).
A detailed description of LVQ training algorithm can be found in (Crammer et al 2002).
LVQ can be included in a broad family of learning algorithms based on Stochastic Gradient Descent In the 1980's, Kohonen proposed a number of improvements in his algorithm generating the LVQ1, LVQ2, LVQ2.1, and LVQ3 (Crammer et al 2002 and Kohonen ,T(2001),
Categorisation of signal patterns is one of the most usual Neural Network (NN) applications.

4.1.2 LVQ2.1

LVQ2.1 is an improved version of LVQ2, which aims at eliminating the detrimental effect described in previous section.
The nearest neighbours, m_1 and m_2, are updated simultaneously; one of them must belong to the correct class and other to wrong class, respectively. Moreover, x must fall into a "window", which is defined around the mid plane of $m_1$and m_2 .

$$m_i \leftarrow m_i + \alpha(t)(x - m_i) \tag{8}$$

$$m_j \leftarrow m_j - \alpha(t)(x - m_j) \tag{9}$$

The "window" is defined using a relative window width w as follows:

$$\min(\frac{d_i}{d_j}, \frac{d_j}{d_i}) > s \tag{10}$$

$$s = \frac{1 - w}{1 + w} \tag{11}$$

Where $d_i = || x - m_i ||, d_j = || x - m_j ||$

4.1.3 LVQ3

The LVQ2.1 has a drawback that reference vectors diverge during learning. In LVQ3 algorithm, corrections are introduced to the LVQ2.1 algorithm to ensure that the reference vectors continue approximating the class distributions.

$$m_i \leftarrow m_i + \alpha(t)(x - m_i) \tag{12}$$

$$m_j \leftarrow m_j - \alpha(t)(x - m_j) \tag{13}$$

Where m_i and m_j are the two nearest neighbours, where by x and m_i belong to the same class, while x and m_j belong to different classes, respectively, also x must be fall into the "window"

$$m_k \leftarrow m_k - \varepsilon\alpha(t)(x - m_k), \varepsilon > 0 \tag{14}$$

For $\kappa\varepsilon\{i, j\}$, if x, m_i and m_j belong to the same class.

In this study we used LVQ2.1 algorithm to locate the nearest two exemplars to the training case.

Step1: Initialise the codebook (centre) vector.

Step2: Find

$$\min\left(\frac{d_i}{d_j}, \frac{d_j}{d_i}\right) > s \tag{15}$$

$$s = \frac{1 - w}{1 + w} \tag{16}$$

where d_i and d_j are the Euclidean distances from 2 classes and window(w) in range 0.2 to 0.3 around the mid-plane of neighbouring codebook vectors m_i and m_j and m_i belong to class C_i and m_j to class C_j respectively.

Step3: Update the centres (codebook vectors) at each step, namely, the "winner" and the "runner-up"

$$m_i(t+1) \leftarrow m_i(t) + \alpha(t)(x(t) - m_i(t)) \tag{17}$$

$$m_j(t+1) \leftarrow m_j(t) - \alpha(t)(x(t) - m_j(t)) \tag{18}$$

where x is the input vector.

5. Rough sets

Rough set theory is a relatively new data-mining technique used in the discovery of patterns within data first formally introduced by (Pawlak, 1982 ,Pawlak, 1991). It's deals with the classificatory analysis of data tables. The data can be acquired from measurements and in principle it must be discrete. The main goal of the rough set theory is the " automated transformation of data into knowledge".

It has a wide range of uses, such as medical data analysis, stock market prediction and financial data analysis, information retrieval systems, voice recognition, and image processing. Rough sets are especially helpful in dealing with vagueness and uncertainty in decision situations.

The overall modelling process typically consists of a sequence of several sub steps that all require various degrees of tuning and fine-adjustments. An important feature of rough sets is that the theory is followed by practical implementations of toolkits that support interactive model development.

The first step in the process of mining any dataset using rough sets is to transform the data into a decision table. In a decision table (DT), each row consists of an observation (also called an object) and each column is an attribute, One attribute is chosen or created for the decision attribute (or dependent attribute). The rest of the attributes are the condition attributes (independent attributes).

Formally, a DT is a pair A = (*U*, A∪{d}) where d ϖ A is the *decision attribute, U* is a finite non-empty set of objects called the *universe* and A is a finite non-empty set of attributes such that $a:U \rightarrow V_a$ is called the value set of a. Once the DT has been produced, the next stage entails cleansing the data.

There are several issues involved in small datasets - such as missing values, various types of data (categorical, nominal and interval) and multiple decision classes. Each of these potential problems must be addressed in order to maximise the information gain from a DT. Missing values is very often a problem in biomedical datasets and can arise in two different ways. It may be that an omission of a value for one or more subject was intentional - there was no reason to collect that measurement for this particular subject (i.e. 'not applicable' as opposed to 'not recorded'). In the second case, data was not available for a particular subject and therefore was omitted from the table. We have 2 options available to us: remove the incomplete records from the DT or try to estimate what the missing value(s) should be. The first method is obviously the simplest, but we may not be able to afford removing records if the DT is small to begin with. So we must derive some method for filling in missing data without biasing the DT. In many cases, an expert with the appropriate domain knowledge may provide assistance in determining what the missing value should be - or else is able to provide feedback on the estimation generated by the data collector. In this study, we employ a conditioned mean/mode fill method for data imputation. In each case, the mean or mode is used (in the event of a tie in the mode version, a random selection is used) to fill in the missing values, based on the particular attribute in question, conditioned on the particular decision class the attribute belongs to. There are many variations on this theme, and the interested reader is directed to (Pawlak, 1982 ,Pawlak, 1991) for an extended discussion on this critical issue. Once missing values are handled, the next step is to discretise the dataset. Rarely is the data contained within a DT all of ordinal type - they generally are composed of a mixture of ordinal and interval data. Discretisation refers to partitioning attributes into intervals - tantamount to searching for "cuts" in a decision tree. All values that lie within a given range are mapped onto the same value, transforming interval into categorical data. As an example of a discretisation technique, one can apply equal frequency binning, where a number of bins *n* is selected and after examining the histogram of each attribute, n-1 cuts are generated so that there is approximately the same number of items in each bin. See the discussion in (Pawlak, 1991) for details on this and other methods of discretisation that have been successfully applied in rough sets. Now that the DT has been pre-processed, the rough sets algorithm can be applied to the DT for the purposes of supervised classification.

Rough sets generates a collection of 'if..then..' decision rules that are used to classify the objects in the DT. These rules are generated from the application of reducts to the decision table, looking for instances where the conditionals match those contained in the set of reducts and reading off the values from the DT. If the data is consistent, then all objects with the same conditional values as those found in a particular reduct will always map to the same decision value. In many cases though, the DT is not consistent, and instead we must contend with some amount of indeterminism. In this case, a decision has to be made regarding which decision class should be used when there are more than 1 matching conditioned attribute values. Simple voting may work in many cases, where votes are cast in proportion to the support of the particular class of objects. If the rules are too detailed (i.e. they incorporate reducts that are maximal in length), they will tend to overfit the training set and classify weakly on test cases. What are generally sought in this regard are rules that possess low cardinality, as this makes the rules more generally applicable.

6. Principal Component Analysis (PCA)

Dimensionality reduction techniques aim to determine the underlying true dimensionality of a discrete sampling X of an n-dimensional space. That is if X embedded in a subspace of dimensionality m, where m<n, then we can find a mapping F: X→Y such that $Y \subset B$ is a m dimensional manifold. The commonly used method to find such mapping is Principal Component Analysis (PCA).

Reducing the dimensionality of the problem simplifies the task of the classifier, and alleviates the generalization problems due to the curse of dimensionality. Depending on the nature of a given classification problem: the raw data, the chosen features, and classifier. Dimensionality reduction is almost essential when time-frequency representation is used as feature basis. There are numerous books and articles reviewed traditional and current state-of-the art dimension reduction methods published in the statistics and signal processing and machine learning literature (Jollife,2002), (Holtell, 1933), (Lay,2000).

The basic idea is to reduce the dimensionality of dataset $D=\{x_i\ ,\ i=1..n\}$ from k features (attributes) in D to some m<k, in an optimal way. PCA is a well-known technique in statistics and data compression. PCA is also known as Karhunen_Loeve transformation

The main use of PCA is to reduce the dimensionality of a data set while retaining the most information. PCA's effectiveness in pattern recognition is due to its ability to eliminate linear dependencies and uncorrelated noise in the data.

The importance of PCA is due to several factors.

By capturing directions of maximum variance in the data, the principal component offers a way to compress the data with minimum information loss.

The principal components are uncorrelated, which can aid with interpretation or subsequent statistical analysis.

One limitation of PCA is that it does not model non-linear relationships among variables efficiently.

Computation of the principal components can be presented with the following algorithm:

Calculate the covariance matrix from the input data.

$$Cov(X_j, X_k) = \frac{\sum_{i=1}^{n}(X_{ij} - \overline{X}_j)(X_{ik} - \overline{X}_k)}{(n-1)} \tag{19}$$

Where

$$\bar{X} = \frac{\sum_{i=1}^{n} X_{ij}}{n} \quad \text{and } j, k = 1, 2, \ldots\ldots, p \tag{20}$$

The covariance matrix then has the following form:

$$C = \begin{bmatrix} C_{11}C_{12}C_{13}\ldots\ldots C_{1p} \\ C_{21}C_{22}C_{23}\ldots\ldots C_{2p} \\ \ldots\ldots\ldots\ldots\ldots\ldots \\ \ldots\ldots\ldots\ldots\ldots\ldots \\ \ldots\ldots\ldots\ldots\ldots\ldots \\ C_{p1}C_{p2}C_{p3}\ldots\ldots C_{pp} \end{bmatrix}$$

Where C is the covariance matrix, C_{jk} is the covariance of variable X_j and X_k when $j \neq k$ and the diagonal element C_{jk} is the variance of variable X_j when j=k.
There are several properties of covariance matrix Cx:
Cx is a squre symmetric $m \times m$ matrix.
The diagonal terms of Cx are the variance of particular measurement types.
The off-diagonal terms of Cx are the covariance between measurement types.
PCA is finding the eigenvalues and eigenvectors of the sample correlation matrix. Eigenvectors (PCs) and their associated eigenvalues can be calculated from the correlation matrix.
The basic equation in eigen value is

$$Ax=\lambda x \tag{21}$$

This can only hold if

$$\text{Det } |A-\lambda I| = 0 \tag{22}$$

Where λ is an eigenvalue of the matrix A and x the corresponding eigenvector.
Equation 21 can be expressed in matrix form with a matrix V whose columns contain the eigenvectors and diagonal matrix D with the eigenvalues in the diagonal:

$$AV=VD$$

Compute the eigenvalues and eigenvectors and then sort them in a descending order with respect to eigenvalues. Each eigenvalue represents the amount of variance that has been captured by one component.
The first principal component PC_1 is then a linear combination of the original variables X1, $X_2, \ldots\ldots\ldots\ldots X_p$

$$PC_1 = a_{11}X_1 + a_{12}X_2 + a_{13}X + \ldots\ldots a_{1p}X_p = \sum_{j=1}^{p} a_{ij}X_j \tag{23}$$

That varies as much as possible for the individuals, subject to the condition that

$$a_{11}^{2}+a_{12}^{2}+a_{13}^{2}+........a_{1p}^{2}=1 \quad (24)$$

where $a_{11}, a_{12}, ..., a_{1p}$ are coefficients assigned to the original p variables for PC_1. Therefore, the eigenvalue of PC_1 is as large as possible given this constrain on the constant a. Constrain must be imposed in order to avoid the increasing of the eigenvalue of PC_1 by simply increasing one or more of the values.
Similarly, the second principal component,

$$PC_2 = a_{21}X_1 + a_{22}X_2 + a_{23}X + ...a_{2p}X_p \quad (25)$$

Is such that eigenvalues of PC_2, is as large as possible subject to the constraint that:

$$a_{21}^{2}+a_{22}^{2}+a_{23}^{2}+........a_{2p}^{2}=1 \quad (26)$$

and also on the condition that PC2 is uncorrelated with PC1. Other principal components can be expressed in a similar way. There can be up to p principal components if there are p variables.
If our p variables share considerable variance, several of the p components should have large eigenvalues and others have small eigenvalues. To decide how many components to retain, one of the rule is to retain only components with eigenvalues of one or more, and drop any component that account for less variance than does a single variable. Another method for deciding on the number of components to retain is the screen plot. This is a plot with eigenvalues on the ordinate and component number on the abscissa. The plot provides a visual aid for deciding at what point including additional components no longer increases the amount of variance accounted for by a nontrivial amount. Fig. 6 shows the screen plot produced by SPSS.

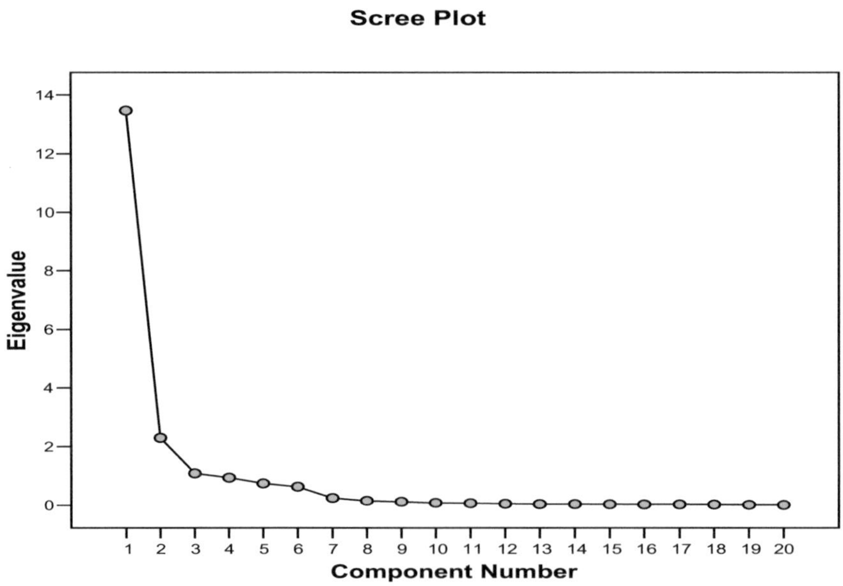

Fig. 6. Screen plot of the correlation matrix, using SPSS.

The lower-dimensional (reduced) matrix can be obtained by multiply the original feature space with the obtained transition matrix (number of component).
The PCA dimensionality reduction method is fast to compute, simple to implement, and since the optimisation do not involve local minima. One of the limitations of PCA is that their effectiveness is limited by the fact that PCA is globally linear method.
Computation of the principal components can be presented with the following algorithm:
Calculate the covariance matrix from the input data.
Compute the eigenvalues and eigenvectors and then sort them in a decending order with respect to the eigenvalues.
From the actual transition matrix by taking the predefined number of components (eigenvectors)
The lower-dimensional matrix can be obtained by multiply the original feature space with the obtained transition matrix.
Table 3 shows how the variation is partitioned between the 8 factors.

7. Results

The proposed diagnostic system consists of a pre-processing /feature selection and one classifier subsystem. Duabechies Wavelets order-2 with 4 levels has been used for pre-processing in order to achieve the same dimensionality reduction of wavelet coefficients. In this work, the 100 time series of 4096 samples for each class partitioned by a rectangular window composed of 256 discrete data and then training and test sets were formed by 3200 vectors (1600 vectors from each class) of 20 dimensions (dimension of the extracted feature vectors). The proposed multi-classifier scheme consists of 16 sub-systems/classifiers. For each one of these sub-systems, LVQ network structure has been utilized. The average concept of combining the individual output of the 16 classifiers has been adopted in this study. The architecture of LVQ is based on straightforward approach with 20 input and two outputs, with 2000 epochs training. The 20 inputs correspond to the four features times the number of wavelet decomposition (D1-D4 & A4).

Component	Initial Eigenvalues			Extraction Sums of Squared Loadings		
	Total	% of Variance	Cumulative %	Total	% of Variance	Cumulative %
1	13.404	67.019	67.019	13.404	67.019	67.019
2	2.302	11.509	78.528	2.302	11.509	78.528
3	1.125	5.624	84.152	1.125	5.624	84.152
4	.905	4.525	88.677	.905	4.525	88.677
5	.818	4.092	92.769	.818	4.092	92.769
6	.620	3.098	95.867	.620	3.098	95.867
7	.213	1.066	96.933	.213	1.066	96.933
8	.148	.741	97.674	.148	.741	97.674

Table 3. This table displays the total variance for the first 8 principle components contained within the original dataset.

	Component Matrix (a)							
	1	2	3	4	5	6	7	8
D1	.926	-.008	-.040	-.028	.244	-.025	-.151	-.115
D1	-.945	.002	.070	-.008	-.172	.032	.109	.112
D1	.164	.896	-.054	-.028	-.137	-.373	-.013	.010
D1	.948	.002	-.018	.044	.240	-.047	.116	.111
D2	.953	-.019	-.043	-.019	.225	-.003	-.097	-.019
D2	-.959	.002	.079	-.015	-.183	.030	.081	.015
D2	-.116	-.965	-.113	.104	.000	.141	.010	-.004
D2	.956	.007	-.032	.047	.209	-.036	.143	.115
D3	.970	.000	-.031	-.008	.141	.005	-.006	-.013
D3	-.973	.006	.063	-.016	-.088	.016	-.001	-.013
D3	-.083	.733	.084	.096	.136	.648	-.010	.013
D3	.972	.006	-.021	.033	.085	-.004	.194	.067
D4	.943	.001	.023	-.079	-.236	.060	.037	-.141
D4	-.937	.009	-.010	.016	.273	-.076	-.047	.103
D4	.021	-.114	.767	-.611	.151	-.008	.023	-.005
D4	.923	.016	.002	-.041	-.246	.054	.214	-.127
A	.885	-.021	.106	.005	-.369	.065	-.125	.076
A	-.920	.113	-.070	.071	.206	-.036	.151	-.152
A	.153	-.032	.685	.700	.025	-.113	-.008	-.040
A	.927	-.058	.075	.015	-.281	.063	-.044	.118

Table 4. Principal Component Analysis, displaying the first 8 components that were extracted (in the form of a component matrix). The symbols in the left most column refer to the level of the detail (D) or approximation (A) coefficients. The order is the following: Max, Min, Mean, and Standard Deviation.

LVQ Applied to	Class A	Class E
All A & E Attributes	1600	1558
Attribute MaxD4	1600	1596
8 attributes using PCA	1568	1558
Rough sets	1600	1600

Table 5. Summary of the correctly classified objects in the testing set for each of the classification algorithms employed in this study (note the maximum number was 1,600)

8. Conclusions

The results from this study indicate that the hybrid approach to the classification of a complex dataset such as an EEG time series can be achieved with a high degree of accuracy. This dataset contains both a spatial and a temporal component – the electrodes are placed on spatially distinct regions of the calvarium. There are several diseases that yield a characteristic signature that can be detected reproducibly using standard EEG equipment. For instance epilepsy yields a characteristic change in the power spectrum within the temporal lobe region. This would indicate that there would be a spatial signal that requires proper spatial localisation within the appropriate brain region. In addition, symptoms may change over time - and thus the temporal resolution of the recording must be such that it is samples at the correct frequency - without yielding Nyquist or other sampling errors. In the present work, we employed a discrete wavelet transform to the dataset in order to extract temporal information in the form of changes in the frequency domain over time - that is they are able to extract non-stationary signals embedded in the noisy background of the human brain. In this study, we examined the difference(s) between normal and epileptic EEG signals - over a reasonable duration of approximately 24 seconds. We extracted statistical information from the wavelet coefficients, which we used as inputs to a set of supervised learning algorithms - LVQ 2.1 based neural networks. The attributes (inputs) used were measures of dispersion - which captured the statistical variations found within the particular time series. The results from this preliminary study will be expanded to include a more complete range of pathologies. In this work, we focused on the extremes that are found within the EEG spectrum - normal and epileptic time series. These two series were chosen as they would more than likely lead to the maximal dispersion between the 2 signals and is amenable for training of the classifiers. In the next stage of this research, we have datasets that are intermediate in the signal changes they present. This will provide a more challenging set of data to work with - and will allow us to refine our learning algorithms and/or approaches to the problem of EEG analysis. In a future work, we will also investigate additional pre-processing steps such as clustering techniques.

9. Acknowledgements

The authors wish to thank Andrzejak et al., 2001 for making the data publicly available at (http://www.meb.uni-bonn.de/epile-ptologie/science/physik/eegdata.html

10. References

Adeli H, Zhou Z, Dadmehr N.(2003) Analysis of EEG records in an epileptic patient using wavelet transform. J Neurosci Methods;123(1):69–87.

Andrzejak RG, Lehnertz K, Mormann F, Rieke C, David P, Elger CE. Indications of nonlinear deterministic and finite-dimensional structures in time series of brain electrical activity: dependence

Daubechies I (1992), Ten Lectures on Wavelets, CBMS-NSF Regional , Conference Series in Applied Mathematics, Vol. 61, Capital City Press, Montpelier, Vermont

Daubechies I, (1990), The wavelet transform, time-frequency localization and signal analysis. IEEE T Inform Theory ; 36(5); pp 961-1005.

Folkers, A., Mosch, F., Malina, T., & Hofmann, U. G.(2003) Real-time bioelectrical data acquisition and processing from 128 channels utilizing the wavelet-transformation. Neurocomputing, 52–54, 247–254.

Guler I, Ubeyli ED.(2004) Application of adaptive neuro-fuzzy inference system for detection of electrocardiographic changes in patients with partial epilepsy using feature extraction. Expert Syst Appl;27(3):323–30.

Guler, I., Kiymik, M. K., Akin, M., & Alkan, A. (2001) AR spectral analysis of EEG signals by using maximum likelihood estimation. Computers in Biology and Medicine, 31, 441–450.

Jahankhani[1], K. Revett[2], V. Kodogiannis[1] , (2005 a), Automatic Detection Of EEG Abnormalities Using Wavelet Transforms, [1]Mechatronics Group, [2]Artificial Intelligent and Multimedia School of Computer ScienceUniversity of Westminster,

London HA1 3TP UNITED KINGDOM WSEAS Transactions on Signal Processing Issue 1, Volume 1, ISSN 1790-5022, pp 55-61

Jahankhani [1], Ken Revett[2], Lynne Spackman3, Vassilis Kodogiannis [1]and Stewart Boyd[3,] (2005 b) An Automated Anomaly EEG Detection Algorithm Using Discrete Wavelet Transforms Proceeding of the 2nd Indian International Conferrence on Aritficial Intelligence, ISBN 0-9727412-1-6 1.Mechatronics Group, School of Computer Science, University of Westminster, London HA1 3TP, UK 2. Artificial Intelligent and Multimedia, School of Computer Science, University of Westminster,London HA1 3TP, UK 3. Great Ormond Street Hospital for Children NHS Trust, Great Ormond Street, London WC1N 3JH, UK

Jahankhani [1], Kenneth Revett[2], Vassilis Kodogiannis [1], (2005 c) Detecting Clinically Relevant EEG Anomalies Using Discrete Wavelet Transforms [1]Mechatronics Group, [2]Artificial Intelligent and Multimedia School of Computer Science, University of Westminster, London HA1 3TP, UK Proceedings of the WSEAS International Conference 5TH WSEAS Int.Conf. on WAVELET ANALYSIS AND MULTIRATE SYSTEMS (WAMUS'05), Sofia, Bulgaria, October 27-29, ISBN: 960-8457-36-X

Jolliffe, T.(2002). Principal Component Analysis, (2nd ed.), New York: Springer-Verlag. Kandaswamy, A., Kumar, C. S., Ramanathan, R. P., Jayaraman, S., & Malmurugan, (2004) Neural classification of lung sounds using wavelet coefficients. Computers in Biology and Medicine, 34(6), 523–537.

Kohonen ,T,(2001), self-Organising Maps, Berlin Heidelberg: Springer-Verlag, third ed.

Kohonen. T,(1988), An Introduction to Neural Computing, Neural Networks pp. 3-16

Crammer,K., R. Gilad-Bachrach, and A.Tishby, (2002) Marging Analysis of the LVQ Algorithm, Proc. 15th Ann.Conf. Neural Information Processing systems.

Bottou,L., (2004), Stochastic Learning, Lecture Notes in Artificial Intelligence, Vol. 3176, pp 146-168

Lay, David, (2000), Linear Algebra and its Applications. Addison-Wesley, New York

Boulougoura,M., E. Wadge, V.S. Kodogiannis, H.S. Chowdrey,(2004), Intelligent systems for computer-assisted clinical endoscopic image analysis, 2nd IASTED Int. Conf . on BIOMEDICAL ENGINEERING, Innsbruck, Austria, pp. 405-408.

Pawlak, Z. (1991): Rough sets - Theoretical aspects of reasoning about data.

Pawlak, Z. (1982), Rough Sets, International Journal of Computer and Information Sciences, 11, pp. 341-356.

Petrosian, A., Prokhorov, D., Homan, R., Dashei, R., & Wunsch, D.(2000) Recurrent neural Network based prediction of epileptic seizures in intraand extracranial EEG. Neurocomputing, 30, 201–218.

Pradhan, N., Sadasivan, P. K., & Arunodaya, G. R.(1996) Detection of seizure activity in EEG by an artificial neural network: A preliminary study. Computers and Biomedical Research, 29, 303–313.

Soltani S.(2002), On the use of the wavelet decomposition for time series prediction. Neurocomputing ; 48:267-77

Subasi, A.(2005), Automatic recognition of alertness level from EEG by using neural network and wavelet coefficients. Expert Systems with Applications, 28, 701–711.

Weng, W., & Khorasani, K. (1996) An adaptive structure neural network with application to EEG automatic seizure detection. Neural Networks, 9, 1223–1240.

Zoubir, M., & Boashash, B., (1998), Seizure detection of newborn EEG using a model approach. IEEE Transactions on Biomedical Engineering, 45, 673–685.

3

Data Mining for DNA Viruses with Breast Cancer and its Limitation

Ju-Hsin Tsai
Central Taiwan University of Science and Technology, and Surgical Department, Shian-De General Hospital, No. 420. Yichang Rd., Taiping City, Taichung County 411, Taiwan

1. Introduction

Breast cancer is very common worldwide, with 800,000 new cases diagnosed each year [Parkin et al,1999]. Among Taiwanese women, breast cancer is the second most common form of cancer (Cancer Registry Annual Report in Taiwan, 1998-2002) and the fourth leading cause of cancer-related death (Public Health Annual Report in Taiwan, 2002). The risk factors for development of breast cancer in Taiwan, a low incidence area, are similar to those in a moderate-to-high risk area [Yang et al,1997]. Although there are recognized factors that increase the risk of breast cancer, its causes are still unknown and thus there is no way of preventing it. This paper explores the possibility that viruses play a role in development of breast tumors. DNA viruses have been recognized as oncogenic in humans: Examples include EBV, which is associated with Burkitt lymphoma and nasopharyngeal carcinoma, HPV, which is associated with cervical cancer, and hepatitis B virus, which is associated with hepatocellular cancer. Viral DNA sequences have been found in breast tumors [Tsai et al,2005, ue et al,2003. Fina et al,2001. Labecque et al,1995. Horiuchi et al,1994. Kleer et al,2002], but it is not certain that the presence of the virus is related to development of breast tumors because similar sequences have been found in normal mammary tissue Tsai et al,2005. Pogo et al,1997].

Breast cancer is a multistep disease, and infection with a DNA virus could play a role in one or more of the steps in this pathogenic process [Labecque et al,1995]. In addition, it has been hypothesized that familial breast cancer and sporadic breast cancer are caused by different mechanisms. More recently, the differences between familial and sporadic breast cancers have be shown to be compatible with Knudson's 'two - hit' hypothesis [Knudson,1971. Richardson,1997],which suggests that at least two mutations are required before a cell becomes malignant. The reason thatwomen with familial predisposition to breast cancer are likely to develop it at a younger age and are also morelikely to develop bilateral disease is because they have inherited one of the two genetic defects (such as mutation of p53) that are required for breast cancer. These women require only one 'hit' to get breast cancer, whereas women with non-familial breast cancer start with no major mutations and thus need two'hit' Thisobservation is consistent with the hypothesis that breast cancer is caused in part by a virus. One of the 'hit'required for development of breast cancer may be infection with a breast cancer virus. There are a few reports about the relationship between fibroadenoma and virus infection [Kleer et al,2002. Lau et al,2003], but they only investigated EBV andfibroadenoma. As far as we know, we are the first to report about relationships among multiple viruses and fibroadenoma [Tsai et al,2005]. Thus, the question arises whether or not breast tumors (either benign - fibroadenoma - or malignant - breast cancer) are influenced by infection with oncogenic viruses.

2. Materials and methods

In the current study, we explored possible relationships among DNA viruses with breast cancer, fibroadenoma, and normal mammary tissue with 106 data points (tissue samples), including 62 specimens of non- familial invasive ductal breast cancer from women and 32 mammary fibroadenomas and 12 normal mammary tissues from women cared for at Chung-Shan Medical University Hospital, with tissues collected as previously described [3]. DNA extraction, Polymerase Chain Reaction (PCR) assay, and Southern Hybridization as described previously [Tsai et al , 2005] were applied here. Genome regions, primers, and thermal cycler programs for iden- tification of each virus (e.g., HSV-1, EBV, CMV, HPV, and HHV-8) were listed in the previous report [Tsai et al , 2005].
Using PCR and Southern hybridization, 69 breast cancer and 44 non-breast cancer specimens were screened for the presence of, β-globin, the internal control. However, five breast cancer tissue samples had negative results for β-globin, and the two breast cancer specimens from patients with familial histories of breast cancer were excluded from the study. All 44 non-breast cancer specimens were positive for. β-globin. Among the 62 breast cancer samples, 8 (12.90%) were positive for HSV-1, 28 (45.16%) for EBV, 47 (75.81%) for CMV, 8 (12.90%) for HPV, and 28 (45.16%) for HHV-8. In the non-breast cancer control groups, 8/12 (66.67%) were CMV-positive normal samples, whereas the results for fibroadenoma samples (total, 32) were 20 (62.50%)HSV-1-positive, 16 (50.00%) EBV-positive, 20 (62.50%) CMV-positive, 2 (6.25%) HPV-positive, and 28 (87.50%) HHV-8-positive.
We submitted a data mining approach to the current research that included artificial neural networks (ANNs) and agglomerative hierarchical clustering techniques (AHCTs). With the proposed data mining approach (named ANN-AHCT hereafter), the different combinations of DNA viruses possible in breast cancer, fibroadenoma, and normal mammary tissue were classified by ANNs; then, AHCTs clustered the common characteristic during the same classification.

2.1 Artificial neural networks (ANNs) model

ANNs are composed of processing elements (nodes or neurons) and their connections. The nodes are inter- connected layer-wise among themselves. Each node in each successive layer receives the inner product of synaptic weights with the outputs of the nodes in the previous layer. The operation of single node is shown in Fig. 1. ANNs have been shown to be effective for addressing complex nonlinear problems. The two types of learning networks are supervised and unsupervised. For a supervised learning network, a set of training input vectors with a corresponding set of target vectors is trained to adjust weights in the ANN. For an unsupervised learning network, a set of input vectors is proposed; however, no target vectors are specified. In this study, a supervised learning network was thought to be more suitable for the classification problem. Several well-known supervised learning ANNs are the back-propagation (BP), learning vector quantization, and counter propagation network. The BP model is used most extensively and can provide better solutions for many applications [Lippmann,1987. Dayhoff,1990]. Therefore, the BP model was selected for the current study.

A BP neural network consists of three or more layers, including an input layer, one or more hidden layers, and an output layer. Fig. 2. illustrates a basic BP neural network with three layers. BP neural network learning works on a gradient-descent algorithm [Funahashi, 1989]. The BP neural network initially receives the input vector and directly passes it into the hidden layer(s). Each element of the hidden layer(s) is used to calculate an activation value by summing up the weighted input, and the sum of the weighted input will be transformed into an activity level by using a transfer function. Each element of the output layer is then used to calculate an activation value by summing up the weighted inputs attributed to the hidden layer. Next, a transfer function is used to calculate the network output. The actual network output is then compared with the target value. The BP neural network algorithm refers to the propagation of errors of nodes from the output layer to nodes in the hidden layer(s).These errors are used to update the network weights. The amount of weights to be added to or subtracted from the previous weight is governed by the delta rule. After the knowledge representation is determined, the BP neural network will be trained to attempt the classification behavior. The number of hidden layers and the number of nodes in each hidden layer are determined during the training phase. In this study, a fully connected feedforward neural network was used, and its network parameters and stopping criterion were set.

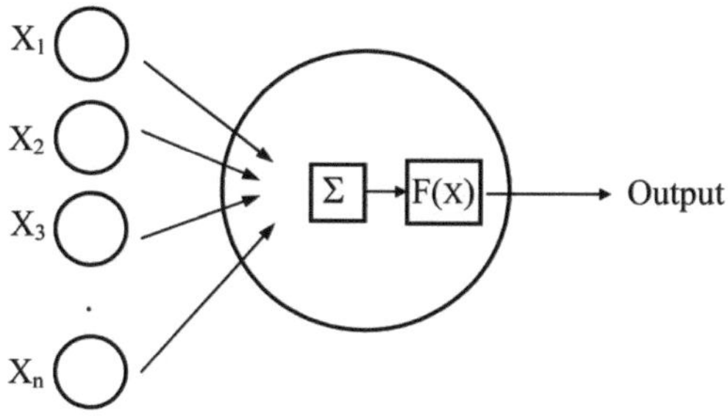

Fig. 1. Node operation

To be able to attempt the classification behavior, a learning rule needs to be used in the BP neural network. In the case of a multi-layer perception, this rule should also be able to adapt the weights of all connections in order to model a nonlinear function. The learning rule used most frequently for this purpose is the BP rule. It acts through the following two steps. First, the generalized difference D *(t) is calculated by

$$D_i^*(t) = (A_i^*(t) - A_i(t)) * A_i(t) \quad (1 - A_i(t)), \tag{1}$$

where A_i^* is the desired activation of output unit i, and $A_i^*(t)$ is the generated activation of this unit. In order to obtain the generalized difference the calculated difference $A_i^*(t)$ - $A_i(t)$ is multiplied by the simplified derivative of the activation function $A_i(t)$* (1 -$A_i(t)$). Second, the generalized differences of the units in the output layer are propagated back through the weighted connections to the units of the hidden layer(s). The generalized difference collected from a hidden unit is multiplied by the simplified derivative of the unit's activation function in order to obtain the generalized difference of the hidden unit

$$D_j^*(t) = \sum_{i=1}^{n} (W_{ij}(t) * D_i^*(t)) * A_j(t) * (1 - A_j(t)). \quad (2)$$

Using the generalized difference D*(t), the weights are adjusted by

$$W_{ij}(t+1) = W_{ij}(t) + C * D_i^*(t) * A_j(t). \quad (3)$$

The adaptation size of the weight Wij(t) of the connection used to send information from unit j to unit i is influenced by the existing weight Wij(t), the learning rate C, the generalized difference D_i^* (*t*), and the actual activation Aj(t) of unit j. To reduce the probability of weight change oscillation, a weight momentum term is added to adjust the weight. The weight momentum term is constructed by previous adjustment of the weight $D^*W_{ij}(t)$ and a constant value B, so

$$W_{ij}(t+1) = W_{ij}(t) + C * D_i^*(t) * A_j(t) + B * D * W_{ij}(t). \quad (4)$$

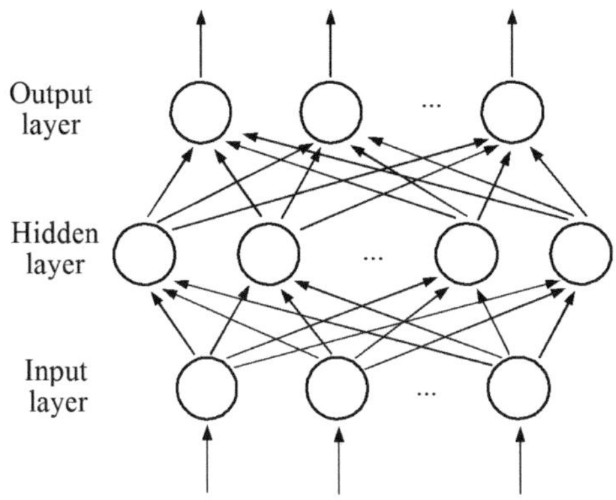

Fig. 2. A back-propagation (BP) neural network

If more hidden layers are implemented, the BP rule will use the generalized differences of the hidden units of the BP neural network to get the hidden units of the hidden layer closer to the input layer. To test the network, test set data are assigned to the networks, and then the output is evaluated. The network should be able to interpolate and, possibly, extrapolate.

In this study, through the above-mentioned principle for construction of a BP model, we collected training and testing patterns by randomly selecting data from the total number of 106 (specimens, or data points) to correlate the presence of DNA viruses with breast cancer, fibroadenoma, and normal mammary tissue to develop a BP model that could obtain underlying relationships. The BP model can be constructed without requiring any assumptions concerning the functional form of the relationship among the DNA viruses with breast cancer, fibroadenoma, or normal mammary tissue. The developed BP model can classify the behavior of all possible combinations of DNA viruses. Then, all possible DNA virus combinations in the developed classification model would be presented and the estimated probability of breast tumor (benign or malignant) would be computed.

2.2 Agglomerative hierarchical clustering techniques (AHCTs)

AHCTs are a statistical method that serially fuses n individuals into groups in order to obtain partitions. When AHCTs have placed two individuals into the same group, the two individuals cannot subsequently appear in different groups, that is, the AHCT procedure is irreversible. AHCTs' main objective is to organize data in order to form clusters that contain all individuals. In this project, AHCTs were applied to cluster DNA viruses that belong to the same classification based on the ANN's classification behavior. The decision- maker's duty is to seek the 'best' fitting number of clusters needed to decide how to organize data. The AHCT procedure is as follows [Salton,1989]:

P_n, $P_{n\,1}$, ... , P_1 represents a series of partitions of data. The first, Pn, includes n single member clusters, and the last, P1, includes a single group that contains all n individuals. The basic operation to form P_n, $P_{n\,1}$, ... , P_1 is similar.

STEP 0: Each cluster C_1, C_2, ... , C_n includes a single individual.

STEP 1: To find the nearest pair of distinct clusters, say C_i and C_j, then to merge C_i and C_j, and to delete C_j, decrease the number of clusters by one.

STEP 2: If the number of clusters equals one then stop, or else return to STEP 1.

Three inter-group measures of AHCTs differ primarily in the distances between or similarity of two clusters.

One is single linkage clustering (5), another is complete linkage clustering (Eq. 6), and the other is average linkage clustering (Eq. 7) [Bunke & Shearer,1998. Wallis et al,2001].

$$d_{AB} = \min_{\substack{i \in A \\ i \in B}} (d_{ij}), \tag{5}$$

$$d_{AB} = \max_{\substack{i \in A \\ i \in B}} (d_{ij}) \tag{6}$$

where d_{AB} is the distance between two clusters A and B, and d_{ij} is the distance between individuals i and j. (This could be a Euclidean distance or one of a variety of other distance measures.)

$$d_{AB} = \frac{1}{n_A n_B} \sum_{i \in A} \sum_{i \in B} d_{ij}, \tag{7}$$

where n_A and n_B are the number of individuals in clusters A and B.

The average linkage cluster is the same as single linkage or complete linkage. However, the cluster criterion of the average linkage cluster is the average distance from all individuals in one cluster to all individuals in another. Unlike single linkage clustering and complete linkage clustering, average linkage clustering does not depend on extreme values to partition all members of the cluster. The other merit for using the average linkage approach is to form clusters with small within-cluster variation. Average linkage clustering also tends to be biased toward production of clusters with approximately the same variance. So, the authors of the current work considered the average linkage cluster's advantages and the steps of computing Eq. (7) to further cluster the DNA viruses in the ANN-AHCT approach.

2.3 The proposed ANN-AHCT approach

In order to obtain the relationship among combinations of DNA viruses with breast cancer, fibroadenoma, and normal mammary tissue, an effective and feasible data mining method, the ANN-AHCT approach, was proposed. It includes two phases that are summarized in Fig. 3, which shows the structure of the ANN-AHCT approach flow chart.

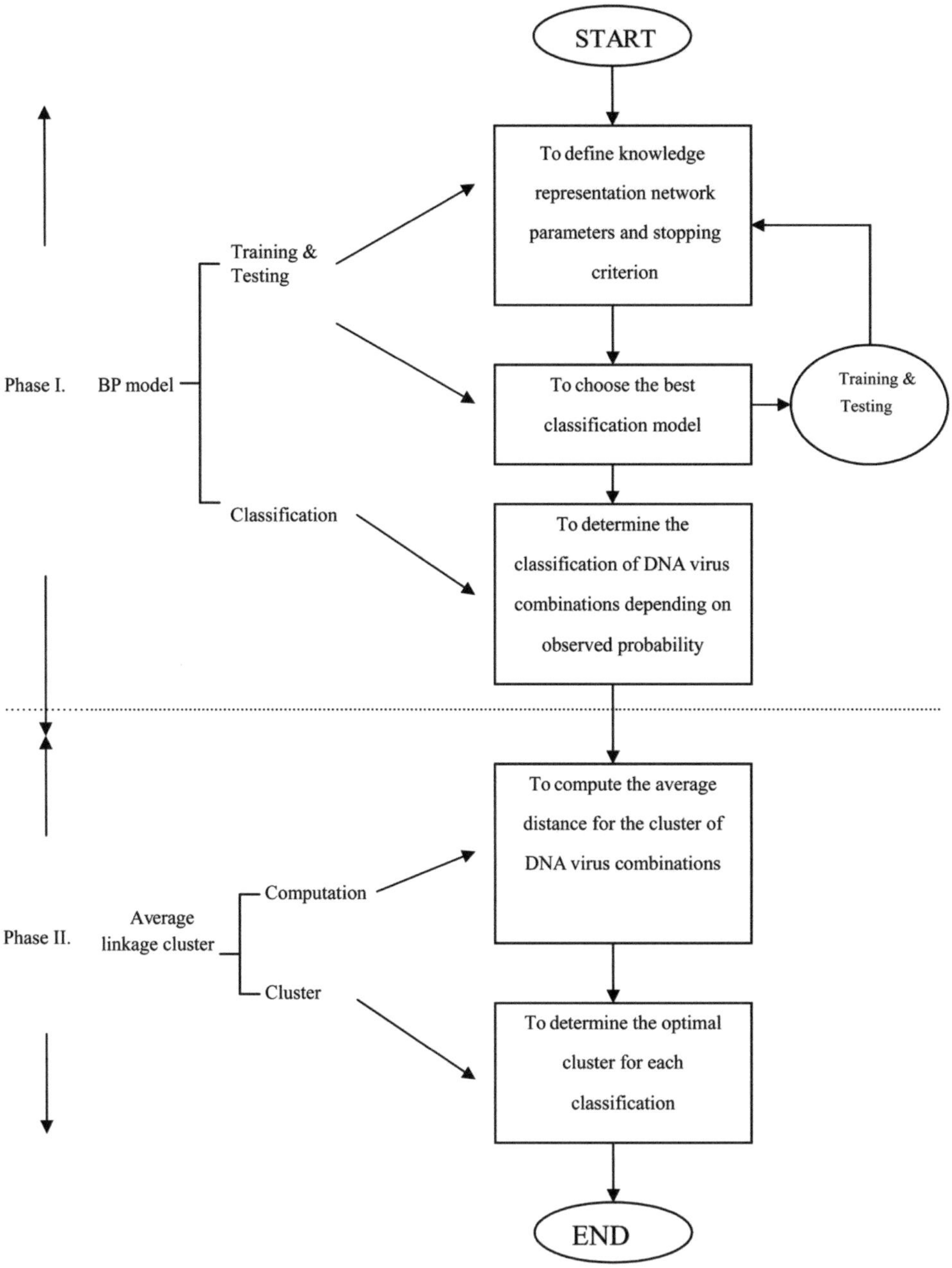

Fig. 3. The flow chart ANN-AHCT approach.

Phase I. Using the BP model to classify all combinations of DNA viruses.

To define the knowledge representation, network parameters and stopping criterion is most important to obtain the best classification BP model. The knowledge representation defines the relationship among the DNA viruses with breast cancer, fibroadenoma, and normal mammary tissue. The number of input nodes is equal to the number of DNA viruses (five, HSV-1, EBV, CMV, HPV, HHV-8); the input values are the value of (positive, negative) DNA viruses. In addition, the number of output nodes is three (breast cancer, fibroadenoma, and normal mammary tissue); the output values are the code. This means that if breast cancer is present, the code is 1, otherwise, the code is 0; similarly, if fibroadenoma is present, the code is 1, otherwise, the code is 0; if normal mammary tissue is present, the code is 1, otherwise, the code is 0. In addition, the network parameter-learning rate and moment will be set to assist the trained network to attempt convergence andstabilization in classification behavior.

The stopping criterion is set to lower the root mean square error (RMSE) in the training and testing processes. In this study, in order to obtain the appropriate BP model, the iteration was set to 10,000 and the learning rate was set to dynamically auto-adjust from 0.01 to 0.3 for rapid effective learning and stable behavior as observed by mildly varying values of RMSE. Table 1 lists these appropriate BP architectures and their momentums.

In order to obtain the best BP model from Table 1, selection of the best classification model is done through selecting the lowest RMSE of training and testing or the highest classification correction rate. The architecture (input nodes-hidden nodes-output nodes) 5-2-3 was selected to obtain a better performance. In order to obtain the relationship among each different combination of DNA viruses with breast cancer, fibroadenoma, and normal mammary tissue, the total number 32 (2 * 2 * 2 * 2 * 2, the combination of DNA viruses) was inputted into the architecture 5-2-3, and then the classification of breast tumor and occurrence probability could be obtained. Placement of all DNA virus combinations into Tables 2–5 depended on the possible occurrence probability of breast cancer, fibroadenoma, and normal mammary tissue.

In Table 2, 10 DNA virus combinations would result in the highest probability of fibroadenoma; in Table 3, 15 DNA virus combinations would result in the highest probability of breast cancer; and in Table 4, 4 DNA virus combinations would result in a higher probability of breast cancer than of normal mammary tissue, a value that was also higher than the probability of fibroadenoma. In Table 5, 3 DNA virus combinations resulted in a higher probability of breast cancer or fibroadenoma, that is, a breast tumor.

Phase II. Using average linkage clustering to obtain different clusters during each classification.

In order to obtain the common combination for each classification, further clustering of each classification was necessary. This study used average linkage clustering to obtain different clusters in each classification. In Tables 2 and 3, the results of average linkage clustering were computed and depicted the possible cluster results shown in Tables 6 and 7. To decide the best number of clusters in Table 6, a medical expert in breast tumors at the Chung-Shan Medical University Hospital suggested that three clusters would be best. The first cluster is labeled 10 and 12. The second cluster is labeled 26, 28, 30, and 32. The third cluster is labeled 18, 20, and 24. The label 27 was clustered in the three clusters with difficulty. In addition, to decide the best number of clusters in Table 7, the medical expert suggested that four clusters would be best. The first cluster is labeled 2,4, 6, and 8. The second cluster is labeled 9 and 11. The third cluster is labeled 13, 15, 29, and 31. The fourthcluster is labeled 17, 19, 21, and 23.

The label 14 was clustered in the four clusters with difficulty. In Table 3, where the combination included only four situations, it was not necessary to further cluster. Similarly, in Table5, the combination included only three situations, so it was not necessary to further cluster.

Using used Kendall's tau-b test to examine the correlation between number of virus infections and survivals in breast cancer patients. The results suggest that the number of infecting viruses is related to the overall and relapse-free survivals of breast cancer patients (correlation coefficient=-0.275; P=0.021). In order to further investigate the relationship between viral factors and overall and relapse-free survivals in our sample of breast cancer patients, univariate log-rank analysis was used. Both overall and relapse-free survival rates were significantly different (P=0.001 and P=0.000, respectively; Table 9) comparing V0, V1, V2, V3 and V4 subgroups (zero, one, two, three and four virus infections, respectively).

Architecture (nodes) input-hidden-output	Momentum	RMSE		Correction rate (%)
		Training	Testing	
5-1-3	0.52	0.02358	0.02334	89
5-2-3	0.45	0.02227	0.02241	93
5-3-3	0.63	0.02587	0.02432	85
5-4-3	0.43	0.02262	0.02258	93
5-5-3	0.60	0.02428	0.02518	85
5-6-3	0.55	0.02344	0.02488	89

Iteration 10,000.

Learning rate 0.01−0.

Table 1. Network options for current study

Label	HSV-1	EBV	CMV	HPV	HHV-8	Breast cancer	Normal mammary tissue	Fibroadenoma
10	-	+	-	-	+	0.10	0.00	0.90
12	- -	+	-	+	+	0.02	0.00	0.98
26	+	+	-	-	+	0.00	0.00	1.00
28	+	+	-	+	+	0.00	0.00	1.00
30	+	+	+		+	0.00	0.00	1.00
32	+	+	+	+	+	0.00	0.00	1.00
18	+	-	-	-	+	0.01	0.00	0.99
20	+	-	-	+	+	0.00	0.00	1.00
24	+	-	+	+	+	0.16	0.00	0.84
27	+	+	-	+	-	0.28	0.00	0.72

Table 2. DNA virus combinations for fibroadenoma

Label	HSV-1	EBV	CMV	HPV	HHV-8	Breast cancer	Normal mammary tissue	Fibroadenoma
2	-	-	-	-	+	0.96	0.00	0.04
4	-	-	-	+	+	0.90	0.00	0.10
6	-	-	+	-	+	1.00	0.00	0.00
8	-	-	+	+	+	0.99	0.00	0.01
9	-	+	-	-	-	0.99	0.00	0.01
11	-	+	-	+	-	0.99	0.00	0.01
13	-	+	+	-	-	0.99	0.00	0.01
15	-	+	+	+	-	0.99	0.00	0.01
29	+	+	+	-	-	0.97	0.00	0.03
31	+	+	+	+	-	0.92	0.00	0.08
17	+	-	-	-	-	0.98	0.00	0.02
19	+	-	-	+	-	0.98	0.00	0.02
21	+	-	+	-	-	0.99	0.00	0.01
23	+	-	+	+	-	0.99	0.00	0.01
14	-	+	+	-	+	0.79	0.00	0.21

Table 3. DNA virus combinations for breast cancer

Label	HSV-1	EBV	CMV	HPV	HHV-8	Breast cancer	Normal mammary tissue	Fibroadenoma
1	-	-	-	-	-	0.59	0.28	0.12
3	-	-	-	+	-	0.69	0.21	0.10
5	-	-	+	-	-	0.50	0.36	0.14
7	-	-	+	+	-	0.61	0.27	0.12

Table 4. DNA virus combinations and probability for breast cancer

Label	HSV-1	EBV	CMV	HPV	HHV-8	Breast cancer	Normal mammary tissue	Fibroadenoma
16	-	+	+	+	+	0.50	0.00	0.50
22	+	-	+	-	+	0.43	0.00	0.57
25	+	+	-	-	-	0.60	0.00	0.40

Table 5. DNA virus combinations and probability of breast cancer or fibroadenoma

Cluster (total)	{Label}
1	{24, 20, 18, 32, 30, 28, 26, 12, 10}
2	{24, 20, 18} {32, 30, 28, 26, 12, 10}
3	{24, 20, 18} {32, 30, 28, 26} {12, 10}

Table 6. Possible total number of clusters for fibroadenoma

Cluster (total)	{Label}
1	{23, 21, 19, 17, 31, 29, 15, 13, 11, 9, 8, 6, 4, 2}
2	{23, 21, 19, 17, 31, 29, 15, 13, 11, 9} {8, 6, 4, 2}
3	{23, 21, 19, 17} {31, 29, 15, 13, 11, 9} {8, 6, 4, 2}
4	{23, 21, 19, 17} {31, 29, 15, 13} {11, 9} {8, 6, 4, 2}

Table 7. Possible total number of clusters for breast cancer

Moreover, as shown in Table 9, significant differences were also demonstrated in comparisons of the respective survival rates for the virus infection subgroups: V(0,1), V2, V3 and V4; V(0, 1), V2, V(3, 4), V(0, 1), V(2, 3), V4, and, V(0, 1) and V(2, 3, 4) (P<0.005 or <0.001) (n, n+1.., indicates virus number). Except for the V0 vs. V1 vs. V2 vs. V3 vs. V4 variable, only when V(0,1) was grouped for comparison with other multiply virus-infected subgroups, however, were the overall and relapse-free survivals significantly different. These results suggest that the number of virus infections is related to the overall and relapse-free survivals in our sample of breast cancer patients, moreover, the overall and relapse-free survivals of multiply (more than two) virus-infected breast cancer patients group is significantly different from the no virus- or one virus-infected group.

3. Discussion

Previous studies have provided direct evidence that viruses exist in human breast tumors and suggest that viruses are one risk factor for breast tumors [Tsai et al,2005. Pogo et al,1997. Brower, 2004]. However, some of these studies are disputed [Gopalkrishna et al,1996. McCall et al,2001]. From the sample data, this study detected DNA of the five viruses HSV-1, HPV, CMV, EBV, and HHV-8 in some tissue samples from patients with breast cancer or fibroadenoma or women with normal mammary tissue. Only CMV was detected in some normal mammary tissue samples. In contrast, breast cancer and fibro- adenoma had a much higher frequency for the presence of DNA belonging to two or more viruses (76.90% and 100.00%, respectively) than the presence of DNA from one virus (23.10% and 0.00%, respectively). This suggests that multiple viral infection is closely associated with benign or malignant breast tumors. Lawson et al. speculated that EBV may enhance the action of the human homologue of the mouse mammary tumor virus (HHMMTV) because it is known that some viruses remain dormant unless activity is promoted by the activity of another virus [Mckeating et al,1990. Biegalke, Geballe,1991]. Therefore, different viruses have different oncogenic potencies in mammary gland tissue.

In Table 2 showing data from this study, both the HSV-1 and HHV-8 positive group (clusters 2 and 3) with or without EBV infection nearly always had the pathological diagnosis of fibroadenoma (nearly 99.00%). The first cluster of Table 2 has the same result, but with the conditions HSV-1(-), EBV(+), CMV(-), HHV-8(+). In Table 8, the individual effect of HSV-1 and HHV-8 is seen between fibroadenoma and breast cancer. The HSV-1(+) group shows OR (Odds Ratio) = 0.09, 95%CI (Confidence Interval) = 0.03–0.25, P (P-value) < 0.001. The HHV-8(+) group shows OR = 0.12, 95%CI = 0.04–0.38, P < 0.001. The individual effect of HSV-1 and HHV-8 between fibroadenoma and breast cancer shows that both HSV-1 and HHV-8 positive groups appear to show a strongly protective effect against the progression from fibroadenoma to breast cancer. When the combination

HSV-1(-), HHV-8(+) is compared with HSV-1(+), HHV-8(+) for fibroadenoma and breast cancer cases, OR = 20.83, 95%CI = 4.88–88.87, $P < 0.001$. There is a similar difference between cluster 1 of Table 2 and cluster 1 of Table 3: Apart from the combination HSV-1(-), HHV-8(+),the other condition found to be present was EBV(+), CMV(-), which was associated with a roughly 99.00% probability of fibroadenoma. In our previous report [Tsai et al , 2005], when we took the comparative results of the mammary fibroadenoma group with normal tissues into account (data not shown), EBV was closely related to fibroadenoma ($P < 0.01$). Kleer et al. suggested that EBV was associated with fibroadenoma in an immunosuppressed population, with infection localized specifically to epithelial cells. Gandhi et al. suggested that the replication of CMV in the absence of an effective immune response is central to pathogenesis of disease. Therefore, complications such as tumor formation are primarily seen in individuals whose immune systems are immature or are suppressed by drug treatment or coinfection with other pathogens. In this study,EBV appears to be related closely to fibroadenomas in non-immunosuppressed women. In this classification,the prerequisite was CMV(+) or CMV(-). When HSV-1(-), HHV-8(+) accompanied EBV(-) (cluster 1 of Table 3), there was a greater than 96.00% probability of breast cancer.

DNA viruses have been recognized as oncogenic in humans, and viral DNA sequences have been found in breast tumors [Tsai et al,2005. Kleer et al,2002]. Different viruses have different carcinogenicity, as has been shown in models of mouse mammary cancer induced by 7.12-dimethylbenz(a)anthrance (DMBA). Qing et al. gave the classical dosage (1mg DMBA give once a week for six weeks) intragastrically to female SENCAR mice, with resulting high toxicity; the major tumor type was lymphoma. Lowering the dose to 60 mcg/day produced less toxicity; in terms of tumor type, there was a 75% incidence of lymphoma and a 30% incidence of mammary carcinoma. However, 20mcg DMBA given five times per week for six weeks resulted in a 65–70% incidence of mammary carcinoma. It is known that some viruses remain dormant unless activity is promoted by the presence of another virus [Mckeating et al,1990. Biegalke et al,1991]. In contrast, some virus activity may be diminished by the presence of another virus. This may be the basis for the different result between HSV-1(-), HHV-8(+) with EBV(+) or EBV(-), CMV(-).

In Table 3, cluster 2 shows HSV-1(-), EBV(+), CMV(-), HHV-8(-). In Table 8, comparing HSV-1(-), HHV-8(-) to HSV-1(+), HHV-8(+) yields OR = 48.33, 95%CI = 9.75–239.65, $P < 0.001$, showing that the combined effect of HSV-1 and HHV-8 is more likely to be breast cancer than fibroadenoma. In this cluster, other prerequisites were EBV(+), CMV(-). Labecque et al. and Bonnet et al. , who detected the presence of EBV by PCR, found the virus more frequently in malignant tumors than in non-malignant tumors. Disputes surrounding some of these studies [Gopalkrishna et al,1996. Chu et al,1998] may be due to the focus on the relationship of a single virus with breast cancer. In Table 3, cluster 3 shows EBV(+), CMV(+), HHV-8(-) events. Late expo-sure to a common virus, such as human CMV [Richardson,1997], or delayed exposure to EBV [Yasui et al,2001] has been suggested as a risk factor of breast cancer. In Table 6, the individual effect of HHV-8(+) suggests a strongly protective effect on progression from fibroadenoma to breast cancer (OR = 0.12, 95%CI = 0.04–0.38, $P < 0.001$). These pre- requisites resulted in a nearly 97.00% probability of breast cancer. Cluster 4 of Table 3 shows that HSV-1(+), EBV(-), HHV-8(-) was a prerequisite. In Table 8, which compares HSV-1(+), HHV-8(-) to HSV-1(+), HHV-8(+), there is OR = 25.00, 95%CI = 5.92–105.58, $P < 0.001$ for the combined effect of HSV-1 and HHV-8 with the greater likelihood of breast cancer than fibroadenoma. Beside these factors, EBV as a negative condition showed a nearly 98.00% possibility of breast cancer. Bonnet et al., who detected EBV by PCR, found EBV was detected more frequently in breast tumors that were hormone-receptor negative (P = 0.01). However, it may still be necessary in the study of breast tumors to investigate hormonal influences.Moore et al. indicated that a virus was oncogenic in the estrogen milieu of female mice of a strain with genetic susceptibility to mammary tumors.

There is experimental evidence that insulin, glucocorticoids, estrogen, and progestins synergize with MMTV in genetically susceptible female mice to cause mammary cancer [McGrath et al,1978]. However, insulin and glucocor-ticoids are physiologically required in certain amounts and consistently over time. Therefore, there is particular importance in estrogen and progesterone and their correlation to breast cancer [McGrath et al,1978]. Mastopathia cystica (fibrocystic disease, mammary dysplasia) was induced by DMBA in neonatally androgenized female Spraque-Dawley rats [Yoshida, 1994]. In these androgenized rats, no corpora lutea were found in the ovaries. The rat mastopathia cystica condition varied widely, with two kinds of macroscopically detectable tumor-forming lesions (solid and cystic). The development of rat mastopathia cystica was dependent on estrogen [Yoshida, 1994]. Although mammary car-cinoma occurred more frequently in neonatally non-androgenized rats than did fibroadenoma [Yoshida, 1994. Yoshida et al,1980], it seems even mammary tissues induced by the same carcinogen require a specific hormonal state to result in a benign or malignant condition.

In Table 4, the prerequisite was negative status for HSV-1, EBV, and HHV-8. For the three combinations either CMV or HPV, neither CMV nor HPV, or both CMV and HPV in the absence of any of the first three viruses, carcinogenic potency was not linked absolutely to a malignant or benign tumor. Different studies of HPV in breast cancer present conflicting results [Gopalkrishna et al,1996. Morimoto et al,1999]. Yu et al. [Morimoto et al,1999], who detected HPV-33 by PCR, suggested that it may be involved in human breast cancer. However, the positive rate of HPV-33 in China was 43.75% (14/32), while in Japan it was only 8.33% (1/12). Richardson et al. hypothesized that some breast cancers might be caused by late exposure to a common virus such as CMV. According Richardson's hypothesis, in breast cancer exposure to the virus could be a "hit," while other "hits" [Knudson,1971] could be genetic susceptibility (such as an inherited mutation of p53) or uninterrupted exposure to a combination of estrogen and progesterone. Therefore, absent an enhancing factor (HSV-1, EBV, HHV-8), the incidence of breast cancer in this group was only 60.00%.

In Table 5, there is no prerequisite: Random virus infection in the mammary tissue produces an incidence of either breast cancer or fibroadenoma that is almost the same (50.00%). However, despite lack of specificity in resulting pathology, viruses are clearly a tumorigenesis factor in the mammary gland. Endogenous estrogens are central to the etiology of breast cancer [Adami et al,1998] because in the absence of estrogens breast cancer does not occur. A recent prospective study of Japanese women indicated that levels of serum estrogens were positively correlated with risk of breast cancer. In humans, there are strong associations between dietary pattern and level of circulating estrogen, with energy-rich diets correlated with high circulating estrogen levels [Kabuto et al,1998].Well-conducted case–control and ecological studies in populations with a low risk of breast cancer such asthose in China, Japan, and Indonesia, have shown that the risk of breast cancer is up to seven times higher in women who consume the highest level of fats and energy within those populations [Goldin et al,1986. Hirayama,1978]. Chen and Liaw [2002], who conducted an ecological study of dietary fat intake and mortality rates from breast cancer and colorectal cancer in Taiwan, found a positive correlation between fat and both breast cancer and colorectal cancer. Lawson et al. [2001] hypothesized that viruses such

as HPV and EBV act as cofactors with diet, estrogen, and other hormones in initiation and promotion of some types of breast cancer in genetically susceptible women.
Triple negative breast cancers have more aggressive clinical course than other forms of breast cancer and the incidence was 10-15% [Sorlie et al,200 and 2003. Iwase and Yamamoto,2008]. In the current study, the viral prereguisites for breast carcinogenesis almost showed the single virus-infected events and the incidence was two folds(27.3%) of previous studies (data not shown). In the author unpublished data showed that the overall and relapse - free survivals of multiple (more than two) virus - infected breast cancer patients group is significantly better than the no virus - or one virus infected group. It suggest that current method only detect the aggressive factors of the viral prereguisites for breast carcinogenesis.

HSV-1				
Negative (-)	12	54	1	
Positive (+)	20	8	0.09 (0.03–0.25)	P < 0.001
HHV-8				
Negative (-)	4	34	1	
Positive (+)	28	28	0.12 (0.04–0.38)	P < 0.001
HSV-1(+) HHV-8(+)	20	3	1	
HSV-1(-) HHV-8(+)	8	25	20.83 (4.88–88.87)	P < 0.001
HSV1(+) HHV-8(+)	20	3	1	
HSV1(+) HHV-8(-)	8	30	25.00 (5.92–105.58)	P < 0.001
HSV1(-) HHV-8(-)	4	29	48.33 (9.75–239.65)	P < 0.001

Table 8. Odds ratios and P-values from sample data (breast cancer and fibroadenoma)

Variable	Overall survival	Relapse-free survival
	P value	P value
V0 vs. V1 vs. V2 vs. V3 vs. V4	0.001*	<0.001*
V0 vs. V(1, 2) vs. V(3, 4)	0.359	0.189
V0 vs. V(1, 2, 3) vs. V4	0.645	0.598
V0 vs. V(1, 2, 3, 4)	0.515	0.979
V(0,1) vs. V2 vs. V3 vs. V4	0.013*	<0.001*
V(0, 1) vs. V2 vs. V(3, 4)	0.005*	<0.001*
V(0, 1) vs. V(2, 3) vs. V4	0.005*	<0.001*
V(0, 1) vs. V(2, 3, 4)	0.001*	<0.001*
V(0, 1, 2) vs. V3 vs. V4	0.543	0.187
V(0, 1, 2) vs. V(3, 4)	0.288	0.078
V(0, 1, 2, 3) vs. V4	0.539	0.312

Table 9. Results of log-rank analysis for overall and relapse-free survival

4. Conclusion

In previous research on the relationships among DNA viruses and breast cancer, fibroadenoma, and normal mammary tissue, only statistical analysis was used. However, when using statistical methods to classify DNA viruses and predict their probability in breast cancer, fibroadenoma, and normal mammary tissue,the assumption of statistics is necessary. Thus, statistics may become inappropriate to deal with problems of prediction, classification, and cluster in this study setting. In order to overcome this difficulty, our approach used an ANN and AHCTs to achieve the research objective.

Our findings suggest that in Taiwan, at least, the viral prerequisites of HSV-1(-); EBV(-), HHV-8(+);HSV-1(-), EBV(+), CMV(-), HHV-8(-); EBV(+), CMV(+,) HHV-8(-); and HSV-1(+); EBV(-), HHV-8(-) have a role in breast carcinogenesis. HSV-1(+) and HHV-8(+) have a strongly protective effect on progression from fibroadenoma to breast cancer. ANN and AHCTs seems to be a contributory method for detecting aggressive viral factors but not the better one. However, it is likely that infection by multiple viruses is important in development of either benign or malignant breast tumors. Further investigation is required to clarify which oncogenic viruses have protective effects and to clarify correlation of viral factors and hormone status with development of benign and malignant breast tumors.

5. References

D. M. Parkin, P. Pisani, J. Ferlay, Global cancer statistics, Ca. Cancer. J. Clin. 49 (1999) 33–64.

P. S. Yang, T. L. Yang, C. L. Liu, C. W. Wu, C. Y. Shen, A case-control study of breast cancer in Taiwan - a low incidence area, Br. J. Cancer 75 (1997) 752–756.

J. H. Tsai, C. H. Tsai, M. H. Chang, S. J. Lin, F. L. Xu, C. H. Yang, Association of viral factors with non-familial breast cancer in Taiwan by comparison with non-cancerous, fibroadenoma, and thyroid tumor tissues, J. Med. Virol. 75 (2005) 276–281.

S. A. Xue, I. A. Lampert, J. S. Haldane, J. E. Bridger, B. E. Griffin, Epstein-Barr virus gene expression in human breast cancer: protagonist or passenger? Br. J. Cancer 89 (2003) 113–119.

F. Fina, S. Romain, L. H. Ouafik, J. Palmari, A. F. Ben, S. Benharkat, P. Bonnier, F. Spyratos, J. A. Foekens, C. Rose, M. Buisson, H. Gerard, M. O. Reymond, J. M. Seigneurin, P. M. Martin, Frequency and genome load of Epstein-Barr virus in 509 breast cancer from different geographical area, Br. J. Cancer 84 (2001) 783–790.

L. G. Labecque, D. M. Barnes, I. S. Fentiman, B. E. Griffin, Epstein-Barr virus in epithelial cell tumors: A breast cancer study, Cancer Res. 55 (1995) 39–45.

K. Horiuchi, K. Mishima, M. Ohasawa, K. Aozasa, Carcinoma of stomach and breast with lymphoid stroma: Localization of Epstein-Barr virus, J. Clin. Pathol. 47 (1994) 538–540.

C. G. Kleer, M. D. Tseng, D. E. Gutsch, R. A. Rochford, Z. Wu, L. K. Joynt, M. A. Helvie, T. Chang, K. L. Van Golen, S. D. Merajver, Detection of Epstein-Barr virus in rapid growing fibroadenomas of the breast in immunosuppressed hosts, Mod. Pathol. 15 (2002) 759–764.

B. G. Pogo, J. F. Holland, Possibilities of a viral etiology for human breast cancer. A review, Biol. Trace Elem. Res. 56 (1997) 131–142.

A. G. Knudson, Mutation and cancer: statistical study of retinoblastoma, Proc. Natl. Acad. Sci. USA 68 (1971) 820–823.

A. Richardson, Is breast cancer caused by late exposure to a common virus? Med. Hypotheses 48 (1997) 491–497.

S. K. Lau, Y.-Y. Chen, G. J. Berry, S. A. Yousem, Epstein-Barr virus infection is not associated with fibroadenomas of the breast in immunosuppressed patients after organ translation, Mod. Pathol. 16 (12) (2003) 1242–1247.

R. P. Lippmann, An introduction to computing with neural nets, IEEE ASSP Mag. (1987) 4–12. April.

J. E. Dayhoff, Neural Network Architecture, Van Nostrand Reinhold, New York, 1990.

K. Funahashi, On the approximate realization of continuous mappings by neural networks, Neural Networks 2 (1989) 183–192.

G. Salton, Automatic Text Processing: The Transformation, Analysis, and Retrieval of Information by Computer, Addison-Wesley, Reading, MA, 1989.

H. Bunke, K. Shearer, A graph distance metric based on the maximal common subgraph, Pattern Recognit. Lett. 19 (1998) 255–259.

M. L. Fernandez, G. Valiente, A graph distance metric combing maximum common subgraph and minimum common supergraph, Pattern Recognit. Lett. 22 (2001) 753–758.

W. D. Wallis, P. Shoubridge, M. Kraetz, D. Ray, Graph distances using graph union, Pattern Recognit. Lett. 22 (2001) 701–704.

V. Brower, Accidental passenger or perpetrators? Current virus-cancer research, J. Natl. Cancer Inst. 96 (2004) 257–258.

V. Gopalkrishna, U. R. Singh, P. Sodhani, J. K. Sharma, S. T. Hedau, A. K Mandal, B. C. Das, Absence of human papillomavius DNA in breast cancer are revealed by polymerase chain reaction, Breast Cancer Res. Treat. 39 (1996) 197–202.

J. S. Chu, C. C. Chen, K. J. Chang, In situ detection of Epstein-Barr virus in breast cancer, Cancer Lett. 124 (1998) 53–57.

S. A. McCall, J. H. Lichy, K. E. Bijwaard, N. S. Aguilera, W. S. Chu, J. K. Taubenberger, Epstein-Barr virus detection in ductal carcinoma of breast, J. Natl. Cancer Inst. 93 (2001) 48–150.

J. S. Lawson, D. Tran, W. D. Rawlinson, From Bittner to Barr: a viral, diet and hormone breast cancer aetiology hypothesis, Breast Cancer Res. 3 (2001) 81–85.

J. A. Mckeating, P. D. Griffith, R. A. Weiss, HIV susceptibility conferred to human fibroblasts by Cytomegalovirus-induced FC receptor, Nature 343 (1990) 659–661.

B. J. Biegalke, A. P. Geballe, Sequence requirements for activation of the HIV-1 LTR by human cytomegalovirus, Virology 183 (1991) 381–385.

M. K. Gandhi, R. Khanne, Human Cytomegalovirus: clinical aspects, immune regulation, and emerging treatment, Lancet Infect. Dis. 4 (2004) 725–738.

W. G. Qing, C. J. Conti, M. LaBati, D. Johnston, T. J. Slaga, M. C. MacLeod, Induction of mammary cancer and lymphoma bymultiple, low oral doses of 7.12-dimethylbenz(a)anthrance in SENCAR mice, Carcinogenesis 18 (1997) 553–559.

M. Bonnet, J. M. Guinebretiere, E. Kremmer, V. Grunewald, E. Benhamon, G. Contesso, I. Joab, Detection of Epstein-Barr virus in invasive breast cancer, J. Natl. Cancer Inst. 91 (1999) 1376–1381.

Y. Yasui, J. D. Potter, J. L. Stanford, M.A. Rossing, M. D. Winget, M. Bronner, J. Daling, Hypothesis: breast cancer risk and "delay" primary Epstein-Barr virus infection, Cancer Epidemiol. Biomark. Prevent. 10 (2001) 9–16.

D. H. Moore, J. Charney, B. Kramarsky, E. Y. Lasbraques, N. H. Sarkar, M.J. Brennan, J. H. Burrows, S. M. Sirsat, J. C. Paymaster, A. B. Vaidya, Search for a human breast cancer virus, Nature 229 (1971) 611–615.

C. M. McGrath, R.F. Jones, Hormonal induction of mammary tumor viruses and its implication for carcinogen, Cancer Res. 38 (1978) 4112–4125.

H. Yoshida, Experimental study of pathogenesis of mastopathia cystica, Jpn. J. Breast Cancer 9 (1994) 185–193 (Japanese withEnglish summary).

H. Yoshida, R. Fukunish, Y. Kato, K. Matsumoto, Progesterone-stimulated growth of mammary carcinomas induced by 7,12-dimethylbenz(a)anthracene in neonatally androgenized rats, JNCI 65 (1980) 823–828.

Y. Yu, T. Morimoto, M. Sasa, K. Okazaki, Y. Harada, T. Fujiwara, Y. Irie, E. Takahashi, A. Tanigami, K. Izumi, HPV33DNA in premalignant and malignant breast lesions in Chinese and Japanese population, Anticancer Res. 19 (1999) 5057–5062.

H.-O. Adami, L.B. Signorello, D. Trichopoulos, Toward an understanding of breast cancer etiology, Cancer Biol. Semin. 8 (1998) 255–262.

M. Kabuto, S. Akiba, R.G. Stevens, K. Neriishi, C.E. Land, A prospective study of estradiol and breast cancer in Japanese women, Cancer Epidemiol. Biomark. Prev. 9 (2000) 575–579.

B. R. Goldin, H. Aldercreutz, S.L. Gorbach, M. N. Woods, J. T. Dwyer, T. Conlon, E. Bohn, S. N. Gershoff, The relationship between estrogen levels and diets of Caucasian American and Oriental immigration women, Am. J. Clin. Nutr. 44 (1986) 945–953.

J. M. Yuan, O. S. Wang, R.K. Ross, B. E. Henderson, M. C. Yu, Diet and breast cancer in Shanghai and Tianjin, China, Br. J. Cancer 71 (1995) 1353–1358.

T. Hirayama, Epidemiology of breast cancer with special reference to the role of diet, Prev. Med. 7 (1978) 173–195.

K. Wakai, D. S. Dillon, Y. Ohno, J. Prihartono, S. Budiningsih, M. Ramli, I. Darwis, D. Tjindarbumi, G. Tjahjadi, E. Soestrisno, E.S. Roostini, G. Sakamoto, S. Herman, S. Cornain, Fat intake and breast cancer risk in an area where fat intake is low: a case control study in Indonesia, Int. J. Epidemiol. 29 (2000) 20–28.

K.-J. Chen, Y.-P. Liaw, An ecological study of dietary fat intake and mortality rates from breast cancer and colorectal cancer in Taiwanese women, Nutr. Sci. J. 27 (2002) 202–210 (Chinese with English summary).

J. H. Tsai, C. S. Hsu, C. H. Tsai, J. M. Su, Y. T. Liu, M. H. Cheng, J. C. C. Wei, F.L hen, C. C. Yang: Relationship between viral factors , axillary lymph node status and survival in breast cancer. J Cancer Res Clin Oncol (2007)133:13-21

T. Sorlie, C . M Perou, R. Tibshirani, T. Aas, S. Geisler, H. Johnsen, T. Hastie, M.B. Eisen, M. van de Rijn, S. S. Jeffrey, T. Thorsen, H. Quist, J. C. Matese, P. O. Brown, D. Botstein, P. E. Lonning, and A-L Borresen-Dale: Gene expression patterns of breast carcinomas distinguish tumor subclasses with clinical implications.: Proc Natl Acad Sci USA 98(2001)10869-10874.

T. Sorlie, R. Tibshirani, J. Parker, T. Hastie, J. S. Marron, ANobel, S. Deng, H.Johnsen, R. Pesich, S. Geisler, J. Demeter, C. M. Perou, P. E. Lonning, P. O. Brown, A-L. Borresen-Dale, and D. Botstrin. Repeated observation of breast tumor subtypes in independent gene expression data sets : Proc Natl Acad Sci 100(2003)8418-8423

H. I wase and Y. Yamamoto: Biological characteristico of triple negative breast cancer. Jpn J Breast Cancer 23(2008)75-80

4

Building Ontology from Knowledge Base Systems

Faten Kharbat[1] and Haya El-Ghalayini[2]
[1]*Zarqa Private University*,
[2]*Petra University*
Jordan

1. Introduction

In the last decade, ontologies have been considered as the backbone technology in most knowledge-based applications. As ontologies have become more common, their applicability has ranged from artificial intelligence areas such as knowledge representation and natural language processing to different fields such as information integration and retrieval systems, requirements analysis, and lately in semantic web applications.
In the literature, several methodologies and methods have been introduced for building ontologies. Some of these methods allow the development of ontologies from existing ontologies or data sources. However, the proposed method for building ontologies integrates different data mining techniques to assist in developing a given domain ontology. Thus, the extracted and representative rules generated from the original dataset can be utilised in developing ontology elements.
The main research hypothesis in this chapter is that ontology can be developed from discovered hidden and interesting rules. In order to practically investigate this assumption, this chapter presents a complete developing discovery structure using one of the well known breast cancer test sets.
The chapter is organised into five sections. A general overview is found in section two with a brief description of the main components of this research. The development engine framework is introduced in the section three. Section four demonstrates proposed method using Wisconsin Breast Cancer dataset as a case study. Finally, this practical investigation ends by presenting the learned lessons and conclusions.

2. Background

2.1 What is ontology?

In the last decade, ontologies have been considered as the backbone technology in most knowledge-based applications. As ontologies have become more common, their applicability has ranged from artificial intelligence areas such as knowledge representation and natural language processing to different fields such as information integration and retrieval systems, requirements analysis, and lately in semantic web applications.
What is an ontology? This question may be answered from two viewpoints: philosophical and computing. From the philosophical viewpoint, *Ontology* (with an upper case 'O') is an

ancient branch of enquiry, initiated by the Ancient Greeks and continued through the Middle Ages till the Modern Age. Ontology is the study of what exists in the world: *beings, their nature, and essential properties.* In Ontology, philosophers try to answer questions such as what are things or beings, and how things can be classified.

The second viewpoint of *ontology* (with a lower case 'o') has been emerging into the discipline of computer science during the last 10-20 years. Ontology was initially proposed by the artificial intelligence community to model declarative knowledge for knowledge-based systems and shared with other systems. Recently, the utilisation of ontologies attracted attention in the development of information systems (Guarino, 1998). Also, the evolution of the semantic web has encouraged the development of ontologies. This is because an ontology represents the shared understanding and the well-defined meaning of a domain of interest, thereby enabling computers and people to collaborate better (Gómez-Pérez et al., 2004).

The most popular definition of ontology was proposed by Gruber (1993), who defined it as "*...a formal, explicit specification of a shared conceptualisation*". In this definition, Gruber placed emphasis on formalising the specification of concepts and relations, which in turn allows for knowledge representation and sharing among different agents. Studer et al. (1998) analysed this definition, and identified four main concepts: *formal, explicit, shared, and conceptualisation.* The term *formal* means that an ontology should be machine readable; *explicit* implies that all concepts and constraints used are explicitly defined; *shared* indicates that an ontology should capture consensual knowledge accepted by the communities involved; and *conceptualisation* refers to an abstract model of phenomena in the real world arrived at by identifying the relevant concepts of those phenomena. Another relevant definition of an ontology was introduced by Guarino (1998): "*a set of logical axioms designed to account for the intended meaning of a vocabulary*". In this definition, Guarino highlighted the role of logic theory as a means of representing an ontology.

As a conclusion, ontologies formalise the semantics of the domain explicitly by describing their elements; and thus, they consist of concepts that describe the internal features of the concepts, and the properties that describe the relationships between these concepts. Ontologies are based on a shared and consensual domain knowledge agreed by a community. Because of these properties, ontologies can support a wide variety of tasks in diverse research areas. Here are some examples:

1. The integration of heterogeneous data sources can benefit from the use of a domain ontology to overcome semantic heterogeneities (Lacroix and Critchlow, 2003).
2. An ontology enables explicit and consensual knowledge to be shared and reused between human and software agents (Uschold and Jasper, 1999).
3. An ontology can be used to build knowledge bases - a knowledge base being an ontology with a set of instances (Noy and McGuinness, 2001). Also, ontologies can be used in deriving aspects of information systems at development or run time (Guarino, 1998). For example, ontology-based retrieval systems can assist users to browse and understand domain concepts, and therefore, formulate better specialised queries (Baker et. al, 1999).

2.1.1 Types of ontology

Different kinds of ontologies exist that have been specified for different application domains thereby representing different types of knowledge. This section classifies ontologies along the following three dimensions: level of formality, level of generality, and primitive types.

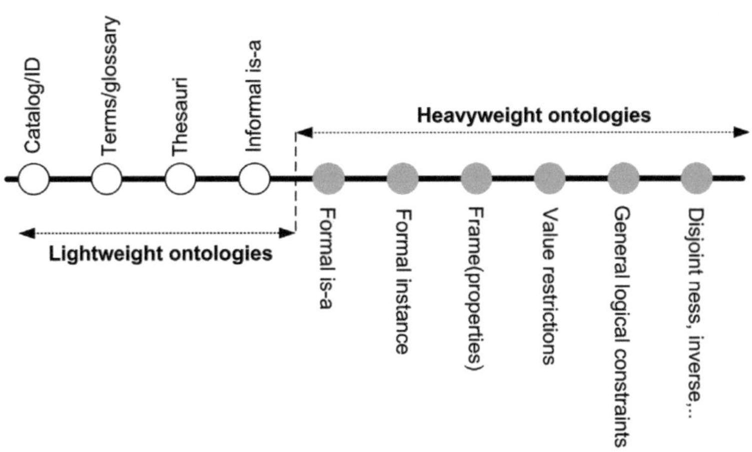

Fig. 1. An Ontology Expressiveness Spectrum adapted from McGuinness (2003)

In the first dimension, Uschold & Grüninger (1996) proposed distinguishing ontologies according to the degree of formality in the specification of the concepts. The basic types in this dimension are: *informal* ontologies comprising a set of concepts written in a natural language and organised in a hierarchy; *semi-formal* ontologies consisting of a hierarchy of concepts such as taxonomies defined by simple axiomatisation; and *formal ontologies* defining the semantics of the vocabulary in a formal language using complete axioms. McGuinness (2003) took his classification further by adding a number of levels of formality and expressiveness. The ontology spectrum in Fig. 1 depicts both the level of semantic expressiveness and the distinction between heavyweight and lightweight ontologies. Corcho et al. (2003) introduced *lightweight* ontologies as a set of concepts, properties and concept taxonomies, whereas *heavyweight* ontologies include, in addition, axioms and constraints.

In the second dimension (i.e., level of generality), Van Heijst et al. (1997) and Guarino (1998) classified ontologies according to their levels of conceptualisation. These are: *general* ontologies (or top-level ontologies) which define very general concepts that are independent of a particular domain such as space, time, thing, event, or property; *domain* ontologies which define concepts for a specific domain; *task* ontologies which describe concepts for specific task activities; *application* ontologies which describe concepts relating to both domain and the task activities; and *representation* ontologies which describe representation entities that are used in knowledge representation formalisms.

Finally, the third dimension for the classification of ontologies was proposed by Jurisica et al. (2004), which may be considered as the basis for capturing primitive concepts for large scale applications. This allows for a further classification of ontologies to cover the *static, dynamic, intentional,* and *social* aspects of the real world. A *static* ontology describes static aspects of the world which includes what things exist, their attributes and their relationships. Its main aim is to unify the domain concepts to enable information sharing and system cooperation. A *dynamic* ontology is concerned with the changing aspects of the world in terms of its states, state transitions, and processes. An *intentional* ontology covers the world of things that agents believe in, prove or disprove, and argue about, in terms of concepts such as issue, and goal. Finally, a *social* ontology involves social settings in terms of the key concepts of actor, position, and commitment.

After having introduced ontologies and their different classifications along with the potential support for them in different application areas, the next section introduces the different methodologies and methods for developing ontologies.

2.1.2 Methods and methodologies for developing ontologies

Ontologies have received much attention from researchers in different application areas in the computer science community. Therefore, different approaches have been reported for developing ontologies. This section presents methods and methodologies for developing ontologies from two perspectives: (1) Building ontology from scratch, and (2) Building ontologies from existing ontologies or from different data sources

In what follows a set of approaches related to the first perspective are introduced. In 1995 Grüninger & Fox (1995) proposed a methodology based on TOVE (TOronto Virtual Enterprise) project and Uschold & King (1995) proposed a method built upon the experience assembled from developing the Enterprise ontology. The two approaches were used to build ontologies about enterprise modelling processes (Pinto & Martins, 2004). The first activity in Grüninger and Fox methodology identifies the main scenarios that describe the purpose of the ontology with respect to the intended applications. Then, a set of competency questions are used to identify the scope of the ontology, thereby extracting the main concepts, properties, axioms of the underlying scope. After that, the elements of the ontology are expressed in first order logic. The Uschold and King's method proposes the following activities: (1) Identify the purpose of the ontology, (2) build the ontology by capturing knowledge and identifying key concepts and properties in the domain, coding knowledge, and reusing other ontologies inside the current one, (3) Evaluate the ontology, and (4) document the ontology. In 1996, the methodology METHONTOLOGY (Gomez-Perez et al., 1996) for building ontologies from scratch or from reusing other ontologies was proposed and influenced by software engineering methodologies. It identifies the ontology development process where the life cycle is based on evolving prototypes. In 2001, Noy and McGuinness proposed an iterative approach to ontology development. The approach starts with a rough first pass at the ontology. This is followed by revising and refining the evolving ontology and filling in the details.

Since building ontologies from scratch is not a simple task and is a time-consuming process, next we introduce the research work related to the second perspective, which studies the approaches for developing ontologies either from reusing existing ontologies or from reusing different data sources. For example, the developed ontology at Kactus (Bernaras et al, 1996) is built on the basis of an application knowledge base. In other words, the approach starts by building a knowledge base for an application. After that, when another knowledge base in a similar domain is needed, the first knowledge base can be generalized into an ontology. The output of repeating this process can lead to the development of an ontology that represents the consensual knowledge needed in all applications (Corcho et al, 2003). Also, Swartout and colleagues (1997) proposed an approach for deriving domain specific ontologies Sensus ontology (which contains more than 70,000 concepts) In this case, a set of related seed terms in a certain domain can be identified, then all the concepts in the path from the seed terms to the root of Sensus are included.

Furthermore, Maedche & Staab (2001) distinguished different approaches for developing ontologies from existing data sources based on the type of input. The input can be one of the following: (1) text where the ontology development is carried out by applying natural language analysis techniques to texts; (2) dictionary where the relevant concepts and relations of an ontology is extracted from a machine readable dictionary; (3) knowledge base; is used an existing source for building an ontology; (4) semi-structured data is used for eliciting an ontology from sources which have any predefined structure; (5) relational schema aims to extract relevant concepts, properties, relations from databases schema or relations.

2.2 Knowledge based system & knowledge discovery

Knowledge based systems can be considered as a special type of database "that holds information representing the expertise of a particular domain [Milton, 2008]". Rule based systems are one of knowledge based systems where the each rules can be expressed by *If-Then* statement. The *if*-part is the Left Hand Side (LHS), which is also called the antecedent. It consists of one or more of condition elements. The representation of the conditions may be categorized for simple problems, integer/real intervals or combination of these for more complex problems. The *then*-part -which is called the Right Hand Side (RHS), consequent or action- consists of number of actions. However, in this chapter a rule has only one action. Usually, each rule is associated with some characteristics or features that strengthen or weaken the rule.

Developing and creating rule-based systems is carried out by knowledge discovery techniques which may vary from simple to complicated algorithms. Knowledge discovery is the broader process of turning low level data into high level knowledge which includes data mining with other essential steps; pre-processing and post-processing [Freitas, 2003]. All techniques have different capabilities and limitations; therefore, combining more than one technique is a beneficial way to enhance their capabilities and overcome their limitations. Many approaches tend to combine with evolutionary algorithms in order to make use of their search capability in complex spaces. This chapter uses the learning classifier systems (LCS) [Holland, 1986], which are considered as an evolution-based learning system [Peña-Reyes & Sipper, 2000]. The main advantage of using LCS is its extraction of comprehensible knowledge that provides higher level of readability which is not found in sub-symbolic approaches. LCS has been used in [Kharbat, 2006] to investigate generating readable, interpretable, and organised rules so as to extract high quality knowledge that can be utilised in understanding the real-domain problem.

3. Ontology development engine architecture

Fig. 2 illustrates the general framework to construct and develop an ontology based on the ruleset generated from previous discovery process. The architecture of the ontology development engine consists of the following phases.

1. Phase 1-Knowledge discovery and rules preparation

This phase is concerned with the extraction of patterns from the selected dataset over which a learning system, learning classifier system in particular, is applied. The generated rules are prepared in a suitable form to match the engine requirements.

2. Phase 2-Ontology development engine algorithm

This phase proposes a new algorithm to develop domain ontology from the generated ruleset. In this step, the ontology development engine considers a given ***domain ontology*** as a set of <u>concepts</u> used to describe a <u>specific domain</u>. The concepts are structured by the means of two types of properties namely, *subsumption and domain properties*. The subsumption property represents the subtype relation in which one concept is more general than another whereas the domain property represents the relationships between domain concepts.

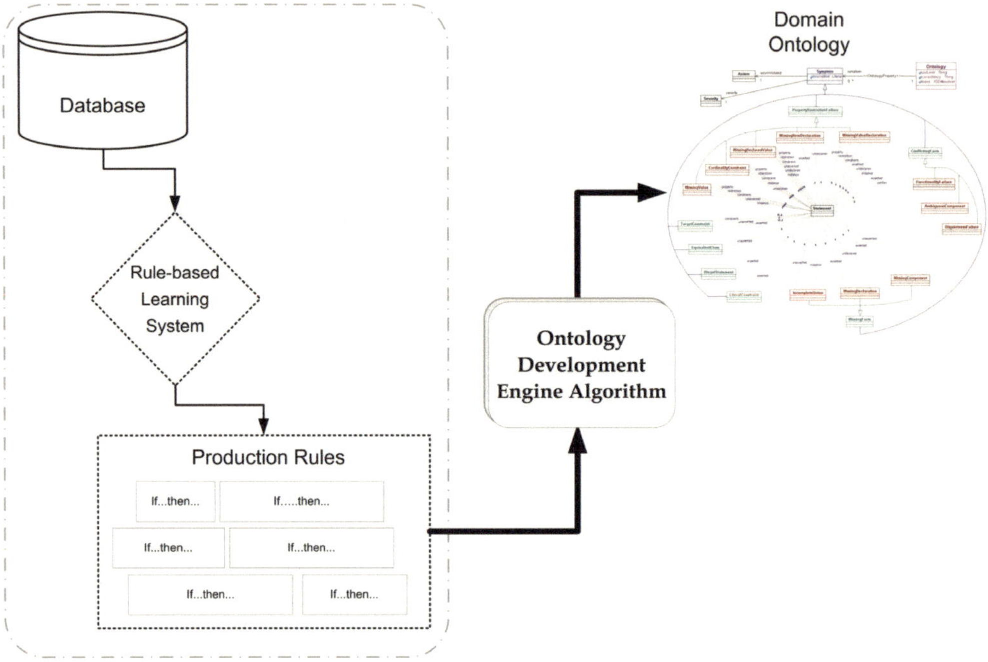

Fig. 2. A general framework.

3.2 Knowledge discovery and rule preparation

In this phase, the initial data exploration is performed to verify the dataset completeness and missing attributes. Moreover, a technical preparation of the dataset in which pre-processing and reformatting mechanisms is performed to meet the requirements of the data mining techniques used within the investigation.

Preparing the original dataset is followed by applying a learning system, learning classifier system in this chapter, over the dataset. This allows the creation of a new knowledge base system which it is able to discover compacted, organised, and representative knowledge and to build a prediction model in order to predict future cases, and to deal with generating a readable human-interpretable output to describe the problem effectively.

The final step in this phase is to prepare the generated ruleset to suit the ontology development engine in the next phase. Firstly, weak rules from the ruleset are identified and removed based on their ***low experience*** or ***high prediction error***. The low experience of rules indicates that they either match a very small fraction of the dataset, which obviously could be matched by other rules, or by those that were generated late in the training process, which implies that the learning system did not have enough time to decide whether to delete them or approve their fitness. Moreover, the high prediction error of a rule indicates its inaccuracy and/or that it has very significant missing information.

Secondly, any integer interval antecedent is converted to a categorical one to minimize the scope of the rules and to group the antecedent into fewer clusters. For example, figure ** shows a rule illustrating its parts as follows:

If X=4 and 5>Y>10 then consequence = action

Antecedent 1 Antecedent 2 Action part

Each integer-interval antecedent (i.e., X=4 and 5>Y>10) is converted to a categorical antecedent based on a determined scale. The scale may vary from one application to another, but this research suggests the following procedure to assist in describing new concepts related to the underlying domain:

- Assign category="Low" for each interval between 1 and 3.
- Assign category="Mid" for each interval between 4 and 6.
- Assign category="High" for each interval between 7 and 10.
- If the interval joins more than one category, then it will be described by an OR operator.

For example, the above rule is transformed using the suggested procedure as follows:

- The first antecedent X=4 falls in the "Mid" category, therefore, it will be replaced by: X=Mid
- The second antecedent 5>Y>10 falls in two categories, that is, Y joins two categories, i.e., "Mid" and "High". Therefore, this antecedent can be replaced by: Y=Mid OR Y=High.

3.3 Ontology development engine algorithm

This section illustrates the second phase of the general framework in figure 2. In this phase, a new ontology development engine algorithm is proposed to accept the generated discovered ruleset as an input to develop a domain ontology that describes representative concepts of the underlying domain. The proposed algorithm is described as follows:

Ontology development Engine

Input : Set of rules (RS) in the form of if antecedent(s) Then Consequent

Output : Suggested domain ontology

Algorithm:

Define Ontology concepts set (OCS) =∅

For every $rule_i \in RS$

Begin-for

1. Map $consequent_i$ to a concept C_i.
2. if $Ci \notin OCS$ then
   Add Ci to OCS
   End-if
3. Define Description Set (DS)=∅
4. for every antecedent of the form ($antecedent_x$ =$category_y$)
   Begin-for
   a. Map $antecedent_x$ to a concept C_x .
   b. Map $antecedent_x$_$category_y$ to a concept C_{xy}.
   c. Attach a subsumption relation between C_x and C_{xy}.
   d. Add C_{xy} to DS.
   End-for
5. Describe concept C_i using the intersection logical operator between elements of DS.

6. Map $Rule_i$ To a concept $RuleC_i$.
7. Attach a subsumption relation between $RuleC_i$ and C_i

End-for.

4. Wisconsin Breast Cancer (WBC) ontology: a case study

4.1 Breast cancer & wisconsin breast cancer datasets

According to the statistics that Breast Cancer Care [2004] has recently presented, 41,700 women are diagnosed each year with breast cancer in the UK, which equals 25% of the total number of cancer diagnoses. Although breast cancer seems to primarily affect women, 1% of the cases are men. Cancer Research UK [online], defines cancer to be "a disease where cells grow out of control and invade, erode and destroy normal tissue". Breast cancer is defined as "a *malignant* growth that begins in the tissues of the breast" [Matsui & Hopkins, 2002].

Briefly, the breast is composed of lobules, ducts, and lymph vessels. The lobules produce milk, and are connected by the ducts that carry the milk to the nipple. Lymph vessels, which are part of the body's immune system, drain and filter fluids from breast tissues by carrying lymph to lymph nodes, which are located under the arm, above the collarbone, and beneath the breast, as well as in many other parts of the body [Highnam & Brady, 1999]. There are many types of breast cancer depending on the tumour's properties, location, and/or size. However, the main challenge in breast cancer treatment is to find the cancer before it starts to cause symptoms; the earlier the cancer is detected, the better chances cancer patients have for cure and treatment. One of the problems is the limitation of human observations: 10-30% of the cases are missed during routine screening [Cheng et al., 2003]. With the advances in data mining algorithms, radiologists and specialists have the opportunity to improve their diagnosis for current cases, and prognosis of the new ones. And thus, scientists have a chance to gain a better understanding of both cancer's behaviour and development.

Wisconsin Datasets are three well-known breast cancer datasets from the UCI Machine Learning Repository [Blake & Merz, 1998]: (1) Wisconsin Breast Cancer Dataset (WBC) which has the description of histological images taken from fine needle biopsies of breast masses, (2) Wisconsin Diagnostic Breast Cancer Dataset (WDBC) where 30 characteristics of the cell nuclei present in each image are described, and (3) Wisconsin Prognostic Breast Cancer Dataset (WPBC) which contains follow-up data on breast cancer cases.

Development of the WBC dataset started in 1989 in Wisconsin University Hospitals by Dr. William Wolberg, and since then it has been heavily used as a test bed for machine learning techniques as a medical dataset [Mangasarian & Wolberg, 1990]. It consists of 699 test cases, in which every case has nine integer attributes associated with the diagnosis. Also, each attribute ranges between 1 and 10 where 1 indicates the normal state of the attribute and 10 indicates the most abnormal state. The diagnostic parameter (action) has binary possibility as either *malignant* or *benign*. The nine attributes are: *Clump Thickness, Uniformity of Cell Size, Uniformity of Cell Shape, Marginal Adhesion, Single Epithelial Cell Size, Bare Nuclei, Bland Chromatin, Normal Nucleoli* and *Mitoses*.

4.2 Knowledge discovery over the wisconsin datasets

Table 1 shows the classification accuracy of LCS (XCS in particular) over the WBC (average and standard deviation) compared to other popular learning algorithms. The experiments were performed using the well-known and traditional classification techniques namely, C4.5

[Quinlan, 1993] and XCS [Wilson, 1995]. C4.5 is a well known decision tree induction learning technique which has been used heavily in the machine learning and data mining communities. The output of the algorithm is a decision tree, which can be represented as a set of symbolic rules in the form of if-then. For the current dataset, results showed that the C4.5 technique achieved using the Weka software [Witten & Frank, 2005] are $95.4_{(1.6)}$ classification accuracy.

The Learning Classifier System (LCS) [Holland, 1976] is a rule-based system which uses evolutionary algorithms to facilitate rule discovery. It has been applied to different data mining problems and shown effectiveness in both predicting and describing evolving phenomenon (e.g., [Holmes *et al.*, 2002]). The vast majority of LCS research has made a shift away from Holland's original formalism after Wilson introduced XCS [Wilson, 1995]. XCS uses the accuracy of rules' predictions of expected payoff as their fitness. In addition, XCS uses a genetic algorithm (GA) [Holland, 1975] to evolve generalizations over the space of possible state-action pairs of a reinforcement learning task. XCS has been shown to perform well in a number of domains (e.g., [Bull, 2004]). For the current dataset, results showed that the XCS technique achieved $96.4_{(2.5)}$ classification accuracy.

	C4.5	XCS
WBC	$95.4_{(1.6)}$	$96.4_{(2.5)}$
WDBC	$92.61_{(1.98)}$	$96.13_{(2.48)}$

Table 1. Accuracy of XCS and C4.5 on the WBC and WDBC averaged over 10 trials, one standard deviation shown in parentheses

It can be seen from table 1 that XCS achieved the highest classification accuracy showing the efficiency and ability of XCS to tackle real complex problems; therefore, the generated rules (knowledge) from XCS are to be applied in the next step for ontology development. Appendix A illustrates the generated ruleset from Wilson (2001) which contains 25 rules all of which considered as strong and efficient patterns that assist in describing breast cancer domain.

Before implementing the Ontology Development Engine over the ruleset, a preparation phase will be performed as explained in the section 3.2.

Example 1:

Rule#1 in Appendix A states:

If ***1>Uniformity of Cell Shape>4 and***
1>Bare Nuclei>4 and
1>Bland Chromatin>3 and
Normal Nucleoli= 1 and
Then ***the diagnosis=benign***

The preparation of this rule converts all the antecedents in the rule to categorized antecedents. Thus, Rule#1 is prepared as follows:

If ***Uniformity of Cell Shape=Low or Mid***
Bare Nuclei=Low or Mid and
Bland Chromatin=Low and
Normal Nucleoli= Low and
Then ***the diagnosis=benign***

4.2 Applying ontology development engine to WBC-ruleset

Applying the ontology development engine algorithm begins after preparing the ruleset which is considered as a source input knowledge for developing the WBC ontology. In what follows, the process of applying the proposed algorithm to WBC ruleset is described by a walked-through example to a specific rule.

Example 2:

Having prepared Rule#1 that describes *benign* diagnosis in example 1, the algorithm of ontology development starts as follows:

1. Figure 3 shows the mapping of the consequent of Rule#1 to a ***benign*** concept using Step-1 since it is not included in the ontology concepts set (ODC).

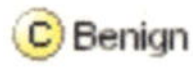

Fig. 3. mapping a consequent to a concept

2. The new concept of a ***benign*** is added to **OCS** using Step-2.
3. A new description set (**DS**) is defined as an empty set to accumulate the rule antecedents' definitions using Step-3.
4. The four antecedents in Rule#1, will be transformed using Step-4 as follows:
   i. The first antecedent of Rule#1 is mapped to a concept of ***Uniformity-of –Cell-Shape.***
   ii. The antecedent of Uniformity of Cell Shape=Low or Mid is mapped to a concept of Low-Uniformity-of-Cell-Shape and to a concept of Mid- Uniformity-of-Cell-Shape.
   iii. A subsumption relation is attached between the concept of ***Uniformity-of Cell-Shape*** and the sub-concepts ***of*** (***Low-Uniformity-of-Cell-Shape*** and Mid-***Uniformity-of-Cell-Shape)*** as shown in Fig. 4.

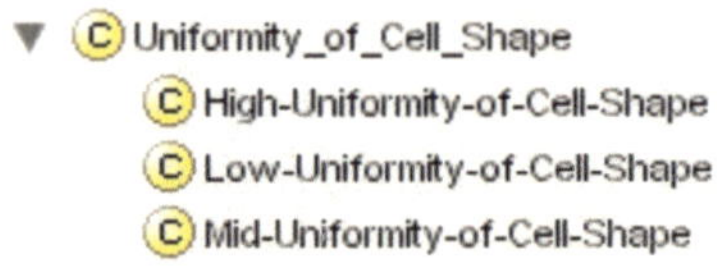

Fig. 4. mapping the subsumption relation between *Uniformity of Cell Shape* and all its antecedent_categories

   iv. Add the concepts of Low-Uniformity-of-Cell-Shape and Mid-Uniformity-of-Cell-Shape to the Description Set (DS) using the union logical operator. i.e., DS contains: Low-Uniformity-of-Cell-Shape ⊔ Mid-Uniformity-of-Cell-Shape.

The sub-steps of Step-4 will be repeated for the following antecedents:

Bare Nuclei=<u>Low or Mid</u>
Bland Chromatin=<u>Low</u>
Normal Nucleoli= <u>Low</u>

Thus, the following concepts and properties will be generated:

   i. The concepts of Bare-Nuclei, Bland-Chromatin, and Normal-Nucleoli..
   ii. The concepts of Low-Bare-Nuclei, Mid-Bare-Nuclei, Low-Bland-Chromatin, and Low-Normal-Nucleoli.
   iii. A subsumption relation are attached between (1) the concept of ***Bare-Nuclei*** and the sub-concepts of (***Low-Bare-Nuclei*** and ***Mid-Bare-Nuclei);*** (2) the concept of ***Bland-Chromatin*** and the sub-concept of ***Low-Bland-Chromatin***; (3) the concept of ***Normal-Nucleoli*** and the sub-concept of ***Low-Normal–Nucleoli.***
   iv. DS contains: (Low-Uniformity-of-Cell-Shape ⊔ Mid-Uniformity-of-Cell-Shape), (Low-Bare-Nuclei ⊔ Mid-Bare-Nuclei), Low-Bland-Chromatin, and Low-Normal-Nucleoli.

5. The concept of ***benign*** is described using the intersection logical operator between elements of DS as follows:

(Low-Uniformity-of-Cell-Shape ⊔ Mid-Uniformity-of-Cell-Shape) ⊓ (Low-Bare-Nuclei ⊔ Mid-Bare-Nuclei) ⊓ Low-Bland-Chromatin ⊓ Low-Normal-Nucleoli

6. Rule#1 is mapped to a concept as shown in Fig. 5.

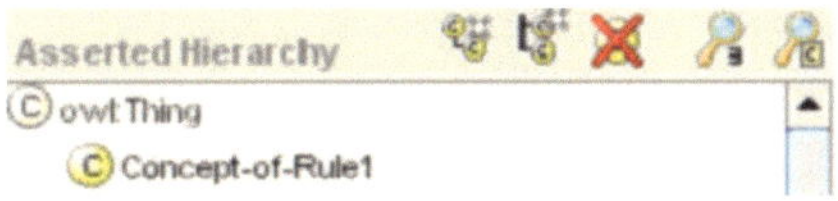

Fig. 5. mapping Rule#1 to a concept

7. A subsumption relation is attached between Rule#1 and the concept of a ***benign*** as illustrated in Fig. 6.

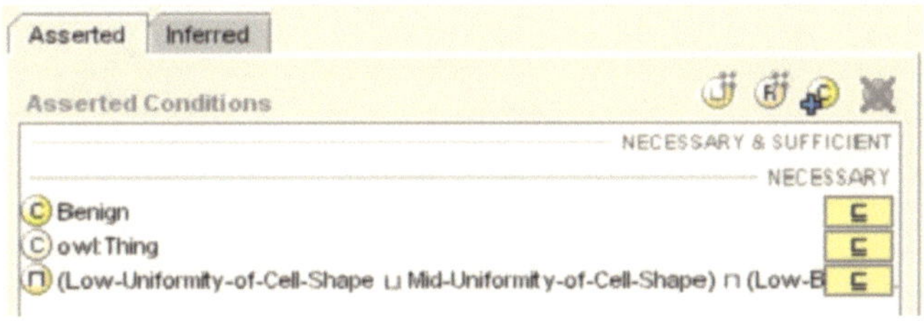

Fig. 6. Rule#1 is a sub-concept from the benign concept and has an intersection concept

This process proceeds for the 25 rules generated from the first-phase of the approach where the WBC ontology is illustrated from different snapshots in Figures 7, 8 and 9.

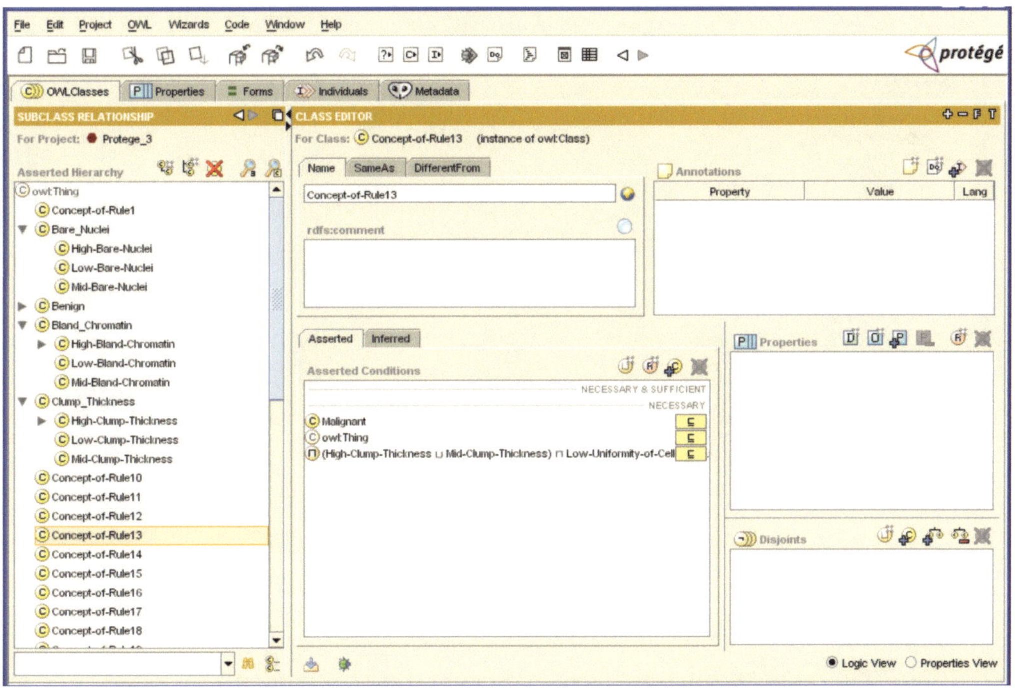

Fig. 7. A snapshot of the generated WBC ontology for rule#13 concept

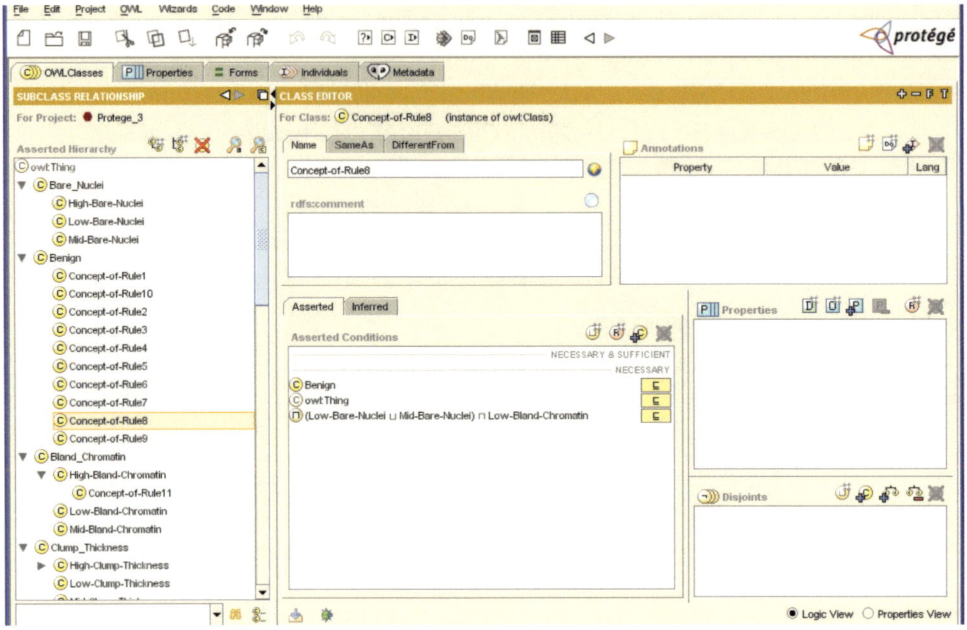

Fig. 8. A snapshot of the generated WBC ontology for Benign concept

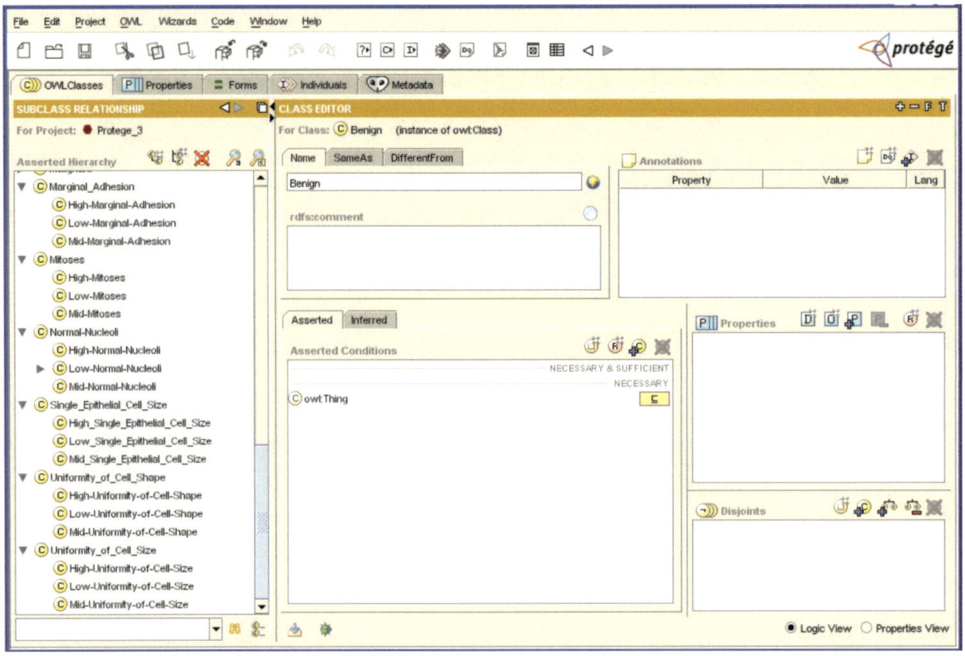

Fig. 9. A snapshot for some of the WBC ontology concepts

5. Conclusion

This chapter has presented a new approach to develop certain domain ontology. The proposed approach has integrated different data mining techniques to assist in developing a

set of representative consensual concepts of the underlying domain. The ontology development algorithm is proposed to transform a generated discovered ruleset to domain ontology. Learning classifier system has been used to generate a representative ruleset, and the Wisconsin Breast Cancer Dataset (WBC) has been selected as a test case. After applying the first phase of the proposed approach to WBC, the generated rulset from XCS contains 25 rules that mainly describe two concepts (Benign and Malignant). The results from phase two have produced WBC ontology with the description of more than concepts using subsumption relations, and the logical operators (and/or) without any human interaction.
While, this research has been focused on exploring the main concepts of the underlying domain, future work needs to consider the possibility of exploring the intrinsic and mutual properties of that domain. This may suggest enriching the process of ontology development and alleviating the complexity in understanding a shared and consensual domain knowledge agreed by a community.

6. References

Baker, P., Goble, C., Bechhofer, S., Paton, N., Stevens, R., and Brass, A. (1999). An ontology for bioinformatics applications. *Bioinformatics,* 15(6), pp. 510-520.

Bernaras, A., Laresgoiti, I. , and Corera, J. (1996). Building and reusing ontologies for electrical network applications, in: Proc. European Conference on Artificial Intelligence (ECAI'96), Budapest, Hungary, pp. 298-302.

Blake, C., & Merz, C. (1998). UCI Repository of Machine Learning Databases [online]. Irvine, CA: University of California, Department of Information and Computer Science. Available from: http://www.ics.uci.edu/~mlearn/MLRepository.html

Breast Cancer Care. (2004). Breast Cancer Facts and Statistics [online]. Available from: http://www.breastcancercare.org.uk/content.php?page_id=1730

Bull, L. (2004)(ed) *Applications of Learning Classifier Systems.* Springer.

Cancer Research. UK, What Is Cancer? [Online]. Available from: http://www.cancerresearchuk.org /aboutcancer/whatiscancer/

Cheng, H., Cai, X., Chen, X., Hu, L., & Lou, X. (2003). Computer-Aided Detection and Classification of Micro-calcifications in Mammograms: *A Survey Pattern Recognition,* 36 (12), pp 2967-2991.

Corcho, O., Fernández-López, M., and Gómez-Pérez, A. (2003). Methodologies, tools and languages for building ontologies. Where is their meeting point? *Data and Knowledge Engineering,* 46(1), pp. 41–64.

Freitas, A. (2003). A survey of evolutionary algorithms for data mining and knowledge discovery. *Advances in Evolutionary Computing: Theory and Applications.* In: A. Ghosh and S. Tsutsui (eds). Natural Computing Series. Springer-Verlag, pp 819-845.

Gómez-Pérez, A., Fernández-López, M., de Vicente, A. (1996). Towards a Method to Conceptualize Domain Ontologies, in: ECAI96 Workshop on Ontological Engineering, Budapest, pp. 41-51.

Gómez-Pérez, A., Fernandez-Lopez, M., and Corcho, O. eds. (2004). *Ontological engineering: with examples from the areas of knowledge management, e-Commerce and the semantic web.* London: Springer-Verlag.

Gruber, T. (1993). A translation approach to portable ontologies. *Knowledge Acquisition,* 5(2), pp. 199-220.

Grüninger, M. , Fox, M.S. (1995)., Methodology for the design and evaluation of ontologies, in: Workshop on Basic Ontological Issues in Knowledge Sharing, Montreal.

Guarino, N. (1998). Formal ontology and information systems. *In:* N. Guarino, ed. *Formal Ontology in Information Systems.* Amsterdam, Netherlands: IOS Press, pp. 3-15.

Hendler, J. (2001). Agents and the semantic web. *IEEE Intelligent Systems*, 16(2), pp. 30-36.
Highnam, R., & Brady, M. (1999). *Mammographic Image Analysis*. Kluwer Academic.
Holland J., (1976). Adaptation *in* R. Rosen and F. Snell *Progress in Theoretical Biology IV* Academic Press, pp.263-93.
Holland, J. (1975) Adaptation in Natural and Artificial Systems. University of Michigan Press.
Holland, J. (1986). Escaping Brittleness: The Possibility of General-Purpose Learning Algorithms Applied to Rule-Based Systems. In: R.S.Mishalski, J.G. Carbonell, and T.M. Mitchell (eds). Machine Learning II. Kaufman, pp 593-623.
Holmes, J., Lanzi, P., Stolzmann, W., & Wilson, S., (2002). Learning Classifier Systems: New Models, Successful Applications. *Information Processing Letters,* 82 (1), pp. 23-30.
Jurisica, I., Mylopoulos, J., and Yu, E. (2004). Ontologies for knowledge management: An information systems perspective. *Knowledge and Information Systems-Springer-Verlag,* 6 (4), pp. 380-401.
Kharbat, F., (2006) *Learning Classifier Systems for Knowledge Discovery in Breast Cancer*, PhD thesis, University of the west of England, UK.
Lacroix, Z. and Critchlow, T. eds. (2003). *Bioinformatics: Managing scientific data.* Los Altos: Morgan Kaufmann.
Maedche A, Staab S. (2001). Ontology Learning for the Semantic Web. IEEE Intelligent Systems, Special Issue on the Semantic Web, 16(2).
Mangasarian, O., & Wolberg, H. (1990). Cancer Diagnosis via Linear-Programming *SIAM News,* 23 (5), pp 1-18.
Matsui, W., & Hopkins, J. (reviewers) (2002). Breast Cancer [online]. Available from: http://health.allrefer.com/health/breast-cancer.html
Milton, N., (2008*) Knowledge Technologies*. Polimetrica.
Noy, N. and McGuinness, D. (2001). *Ontology development 101: A guide to creating your first ontology*. Technical Report No. KSL-01-05, Stanford University.
Peńa-Reyes, C., & Sipper, M. (2000). Evolutionary Computation in Medicine: An Overview, *Artificial Intelligence in Medicine,* 19 (1), pp 1-23.
Pinto, H. S. and Martins, J. P. (2004). Ontologies: How can They be Built? Knowledge Information Systems. 6, 4,, pp. 441-464.
Quinlan, J. (1993). *C4.5: Programs for Machine Learning*. Morgan Kaufmann, San Mateo, CA.
Studer, R., Benjamins, V., and Fensel, D. (1998). Knowledge engineering: principles and methods. *Data and Knowledge Engineering,* 25, pp. 161-197.
Swartout, B., Ramesh, P., Knight, K., Russ, T.(1997). Toward Distributed Use of Large-Scale Ontologies, AAAI Symposium on Ontological Engineering, Stanford.
Uschold, M. and Grüninger, M. (1996). Ontologies: Principles, methods and applications. *The Knowledge Engineering Review,* 11(2), pp. 93-155.
Uschold, M. and Jasper, R. (1999). A framework for understanding and classifying ontology applications. *In: Proceedings of the IJCAI99 Workshop on Ontologies and Problem-Solving Methods (KRR5),* August 1999, Stockholm, Sweden. Available from http://sunsite.informatik.rwthaachen.de/Publications/CEUR-WS/Vol-18/.
Uschold, M., King, M. (1995). Towards a Methodology for Building Ontologies, in: IJCAI95 Workshop on Basic Ontological Issues in Knowledge Sharing, Montreal.
Van Heijst, G., Schreiber, A., and Wielinga, B. (1997). Using explicit ontologies in KBS development. *International Journal of Human-Computer Studies,* 46(2/3), pp. 183-292.
Wilson, S. (2001). Mining Oblique Data with XCS. In: Lanzi. P, Stolzmann. W, and S. Wilson (eds). *Advances in Learning Classifier Systems. Third International Workshop (IWLCS-2000),* pp 253-272, Berlin, Springer-Verlag .
Wilson, S., (1995). Classifier Fitness Based on Accuracy. *Evolutionary Computing,* 3, pp 149-175.

5

Building Clinical Trust in Automated Knowledge Acquisition

Anna Shillabeer
Carnegie Mellon University
Australia

1. Overview

The aim of this chapter is to describe the process of medical knowledge acquisition from a historical context and to define the requirements for producing knowledge which is able to be trusted and applied in a clinical setting. This is related to modern data mining approaches which do not yet adequately address these requirements. This is believed to be the most critical issue in the acceptance of data mining in the medical domain. The chapter will discuss how data mining *can* address these needs and will provide discussion of a technical solution to the stated issues. Overall this chapter aims to demonstrate that the individual needs of all medical professionals can be addressed and that data mining can be a valuable tool in the diagnostic and decision making toolkit. It will also empower medical professionals to take a greater role in the development of such systems by providing a checklist of features to include and pitfalls to avoid, thus ensuring greater success in future systems.

2. Introduction

2.1 Clinical data mining context

While acceptance of data mining technologies is growing, progress has been slow and it is not yet an integrated part of the medical data analysis toolkit. Many reasons have been documented for this but the primary issues are two fold; the decision making and knowledge acquisition processes of the medical domain are not adequately reflected in the technologies available and the systems are too often built to suit the specific analytical needs of an individual user. Whilst this has enabled the application of the technology in specific scenarios, it has resulted in the development of tools which cannot be utilised outside of the specific purpose for which they were built. These issues serve to limit the exposure, applicability and trust of data mining systems to the medical domain.

Data mining researchers have long been concerned with the application of tools to facilitate and improve data analysis on large, complex data sets for the purpose of knowledge acquisition. The current challenge is to make data mining and knowledge discovery systems applicable to a wider range of domains, among them medicine. Early work was performed over transactional, retail based data sets, but the attraction of finding previously unknown knowledge from the increasing volume of data collected from the medical domain is an emerging area of interest and specialisation. This chapter is primarily concerned with defining the manner in which new knowledge is acquired, what constitutes acceptability in new knowledge for the medical domain and how this can be measured and automated through the application of data mining technologies. There is a growing body of work which aims to qualify and define a process for the discovery of new knowledge accross a range of domains, however this work has not focused on the unique needs of the medical domain and hence the domain has remained relatively untouched by the advances in data mining and knowledge discovery technology.

The primary challenge presented by medicine is to develop a technology that can apply a trusted knowledge acquisition process to reveal data patterns in the form of hypotheses which are based on measures that can be relied upon in medical health research and tested in a clinical environment (Ashby & Smith 2002). Due to the broad nature of medical informatics and the diversity of professional roles in medicine, the requirement is to find a solution that is both flexible enough to address the unique and varied data management and analysis requirements within the domain, whilst being specific enough to address the individual needs of an equally broad range of users. To date, automated data analysis systems have been developed for a particular role or field of investigation using a specific and relatively homogenous data set and are not transferable to other professional roles, fields or data sets within the domain. The primary requirements are therefore the provision of a methodology and system to facilitate the acquisition of knowledge which conforms to the requirements of the domain and, the production of statistically valid hypotheses which are appropriately targeted to the role of an individual user and which can provide a sound foundation for further research or clinical trials.

Data mining in medicine is most often used to complement and expand the work of the clinician and researcher by qualifying or expanding knowledge rather than providing new knowledge as is the trend in other domains. Very little health data mining is purely exploratory and hence the technology is generally not applied to provide novel knowledge i.e. to identify previously unknown patterns hidden within the data. One of the difficulties in providing new knowledge in the health domain is the need to sufficiently cross reference and validate the results. It is not sufficient to provide a standard rule in the form of A gives B in the presence of C without substantiating the information held therein. This information could already be known, may be contrary to known medical facts, incomplete due to missing attributes, may not be statistically valid by trusted measures or may simply not relate to the specialisation of the user and is therefore contextually irrelevant.

The barriers to the application of data mining to medical data can be generalised as follows:

1. The low level of flexibility in data mining systems and the need for medical analytical processes to adapt to data mining methodologies rather than data mining adapting to the needs of medicine,
2. The lack of opportunity for incorporating subjectivity when mining medical data,
3. The production of patterns in a technical language and format that are often not understandable or applicable in a clinical setting,
4. The broad range of users and analytical variance in medicine,
5. The production of too many irrelevant results, requiring a high level of user interpretation to discriminate those that are truly useful.

This chapter presents a flexible solution to these issues through discussion of a novel process to more closely reflect clinical medical processes in the technical data mining process. This is achieved through the development of two complementary systems; a hypothesis engine and an Automated DAta Pattern Translator (ADAPT) that provide a mechanism for the translation of technical data mining outputs into a language which can be better understood and accepted by medical professionals. As an integrated unit, the hypothesis engine and ADAPT are able to facilitate greater access to mining technologies, and the ability to apply some of the more complex mining technologies by all medical users without the risk of producing irrelevant or incomprehensible outputs.

The health domain is a myriad of complexity and standardised data mining techniques are often not applicable (Cios, 2002, Imberman & Domanski 2002; Hagland, 2004) hence the need for a deeper analysis of the potential for data mining in the medical domain which in turn requires knowledge of the process of medical knowledge acquisition and how the data mining technologies can facilitate this process. The remainder of this chapter aims to reduce this knowledge gap through a discussion of the processes of knowledge acquisition and diagnostic decision making in the medical domain and of the potential for novel data pattern evaluation methods to augment and automate these processes. Discussion of a collaborative two part solution developed through a merging of theories from data mining, medicine and information retrieval theory will be presented, together with experimental results to demonstrate the application of these solutions to the issues identified in this section.

2.2 The history of medical knowledge acquisition

History has taught us that standardised scientific processes have been followed for centuries to ensure that only trusted, proven knowledge is applied in a clinical setting. The process for defining what and how new medical knowledge is trusted does not readily correlate with current data mining processes. However where the two are combined the rate of acceptance of outputs is higher than in those where data mining process alone is enforced upon the medical knowledge acquisition process. To understand the similarities and differences between the two processes both processes must first be defined.

Throughout recorded history there has been debate over what constitutes knowledge and therefore what constitutes proof of knowledge. Early practitioners of medical science, such as Hippocrates, based their knowledge development in philosophy and their ability "to see with the eye of the mind what was hidden from their eyes" (Hanson, 2006) . By the first century A.D. physicians, such as Galen, were beginning to question the validity and contradictions of Hippocrates work which had stood mostly unopposed since the 5th Century B.C. It is not clear if there was any agreement or understanding of the methods applied by physicians to develop their knowledge base at this time as there was no empirical proof or scientific process documented. Galen was one of the first to suggest that there should be a process for the provision of substantiated evidence to convince others of the value of long held medical beliefs and hence raised the notion of a practical clinical method of knowledge acquisition which combined the Hippocratic concept of hypothesis development through considered thought and a priori knowledge, with clinical observation to evaluate and hence provide proof or otherwise of the hypothesis. This general methodology has survived to the present day and is reflected not only in the provision and acceptance of new knowledge but also in the process of clinical diagnosis.

The historical debate on knowledge acquisition methodologies has primarily focused on three philosophical groups; Methodists, Empiricists and Rationalists. Whilst these three groups are most frequently discussed in a Graeco-Roman context, they were either being applied or paralleled in various other cultural contexts including India and Islam. All three of these cultural contexts are discussed here briefly to demonstrate the extent and foundations of medical knowledge acquisition debate in the ancient world.

2.2.1 The Graeco-Roman context

- Methodists

The first prominent physician practicing according to the Methodist philosophy was Hippocrates of Cos (460-380 B.C.) who is still referred to as the "Father of Medicine" (Hanson, 2006). It is believed by many that he initiated the production of over 60 medical treatises known as the Hippocratic Corpus. The corpus was written over a period of 200 years and hence had more than one author which is reflected in the sometimes contradictory material contained therein. The body of work was however consistent in its reliance on defining a natural basis for the treatment of illnesses without the incorporation or attribution of magic or other spiritual or supernatural means as had occurred previously. Methodists were defined as those whom attributed disease etiology and treatment primarily to an imbalance in bodily discharges. Illnesses were categorised by whether they represented a withholding of fluids, for example a blister holds water, or an excessive releasing of fluids, for example a weeping eye. This group founded its knowledge on an understanding of the nature of bodily fluids and developed methods for the restoration of fluid levels. They were not concerned with the cause of the imbalance or the effect on the body of the imbalance, only in recognising whether it was an excess or lack of fluid and the method for treating that observation.

- Rationalists

Rationalists believed that to understand the workings of the human body it was necessary to understand the mechanism of illness in terms of where and how it affected the body's functioning (Brieger, 1978). They were not interested in the treatment or diagnosis of illness but focused on understanding and recording the functioning of the living system. Two works are of prominence in this group (Corsans, 1997); the Timaeus by Plato which systematically described the anatomical organisation of the human body and; Historia animalium by Aristotle which discussed further both human and animal anatomy and the links between such entities as the heart and blood circulation. This method of knowledge acquisition was criticised as it effectively removed medicine from the grasp of the average man and moved it into a more knowledge based field where philosophical debate or an observational experiential approach was not deemed sufficient (Brieger, 1978). Essentially Rationalists did not believe in a theory unless it was accompanied by reason. They espoused the requirement for knowledge to be founded on understanding both cause and effect of physical change in the body (Horton, 2000).

- Empiricists

The Empiricists believed that it was not enough to understand how the body works and reacts to illness. They pursued a philosophy which stated that it was necessary to demonstrate the efficacy of treatments and provide proof that a treatment is directly responsible for the recovery of a patient rather than providing academic argument regarding why it should result in recovery. Galen is considered to be one of the earliest empiricists (Brieger, 1978). He was both a medical practitioner and a prolific scholarly writer and is certainly one of the best known and more frequently quoted empiricists. He was particularly interested in testing the theories proposed in the Hippocratic Corpus, especially given its frequent contradictions. His work was also produced at a time when medicine as a science was evolving from its previous status as a branch of philosophy. In his work Galen argues that "medicine, understood correctly, can have the same epistemological certainty, linguistic clarity, and intellectual status that philosophy enjoyed" (Pearcy, 1985). Empiricists were the first to concentrate on the acquisition of knowledge through demonstrated clinical proof developed through scientific methodologies which provided conclusive statements of cause and effect.

2.2.2 The islamic context

- The Empiricists (Ashab al-Tajarib).

Dr. Mahdi Muhaqqiq was an early 20th century Iranian scholar who wrote texts on many subjects including medical knowledge acquisition throughout the history of Iran. He recorded that the early Empiricists believed that medical knowledge was derived from experience obtained through the use of the senses and that the knowledge is comprised of four types; "incident (ittifaq), intention (iradah), comparison (tashbih) and the adoption of a treatment that was used in another similar case (naql min shay' iki shabihihi)" (Muhaqqiq, 2007).

- Incident - this can either describe a natural event such as a sweat or headache, or an accidental event such as a cut or a broken limb.
- Intention - denotes an event experienced by choice for example taking a cool bath to reduce a fever.
- Comparison - A technique employed by a practitioner whereby he notes that one of the above techniques results in a useful effect which can be applied to other similar presentations. For example applying cold water to reduce localised burning of the skin following the observation that a cool bath can reduce generalised fever or body heat.
- Naql - A technique whereby the physician applies a treatment for a similar presentation in the instance of a presentation which has not been encountered before. An example might be the prescribing of a medication for a previously unencountered infected tooth where that medication had only previously been used for an infection elsewhere in the body.

The empiricists treated a patient through knowledge of that patient's demographics and therefore all patients of a certain age and sex with some similar complaint were treated the same whereas patients of the opposite sex may have been treated differently even though the condition was the same. Their knowledge was based on patient characteristics rather than a specific condition or set of symptoms. Whilst this seems to differ from the Graeco-Roman definition of empiricism, both groups believed that knowledge acquisition occurred through observing or testing the effect of a treatment and producing rules based on what is considered reliable empirical proof rather than conjecture and debate.

- The Dogmatists (Ashab al-Qiyas).

The Dogmatists believed that while scientific belief and knowledge should be derived from experience and observation this should be tempered by the use of thought and considered evaluation (Mohaghegh, 1988). They believed that changes in the bodily functions must be precipitated by some event and that it is necessary to not only understand what these changes are but also what the specific causes of those changes are in order to correctly diagnose and treat any condition. Changes are defined as being of two types (Muhaqqiq, 2007):

- Necessary change - drink reducing thirst. This is a change which is required for normal bodily functioning.
- Unnecessary change - dog bite causing bleeding. This change is not a requirement to aid or enhance bodily wellbeing.

Dogmatists based their treatments upon the nature of the condition rather than the type of patient as seen with the empiricists. The treatments were therefore selected through knowledge of the causes of illness and the effects of those treatments upon the illness or symptoms. This required an understanding of the physical body and the changes that result from illness in a similar manner to that of the Graeco-Roman Rationalists.

- The Methodists (Ashab al-Hiyal).

This group believed in a generalist view of illness and treatment and categorised conditions in terms of the extent to which bodily fluids and wastes are either retained and/or expelled. Treatments were generally natural remedies based upon adjusting the balance between such aspects of life as food and drink, rest and activity, etc. Methodists were not interested in the type of patient or cause and effect of illness and were hence considered to be more prone to error (Muhaqqiq, 2007). This is in direct parallel to the Methodist philosophy discussed in Section 2.2.1.

It has been suggested that in general, Islamic physicians relied primarily upon analogy which reflects their focus on logic in other scholarly areas (Mohaghegh 1988). This has resulted in widespread support for the Dogmatist methods of knowledge acquisition through research and understanding of cause and effect in the human system. However there is still debate between scholars with some believing that Dogmatism alone is the only method of ensuring progress in medical diagnosis and treatment as it is the only method which tries to seek new understanding rather than relying upon past experience or a closed assumption that there is a single cause for all illness (Mohaghegh, 1988). Others prefer to adhere to the Graeco-Roman perspective (developed by Plato) that a combination of experience and analogy is required if a holistic, 'correct' practice of medicine is to be achieved (Muhaqqiq, 2007).

2.2.3 The Indian context

India is not well known for its scientific contributions or texts, however it has a long history in the development of medical knowledge. In the 11th century a Spanish scholar, Said Al-Andalusi, stated that he believed that the Indian people were "the most learned in the science of medicine and thoroughly informed about the properties of drugs, the nature of composite elements and the peculiarities of the existing things" (al-Andalusí, 1991). The reasons for this apparent invisibility of Indian scientific progress may be due to religious debate in India which has frequently negated the influence of scientific explanation instead preferring to rely upon mystical or spiritual beliefs. There are however documented scientific approaches to the development of a body of knowledge regarding medicine from centuries before the texts of Hippocrates and which, although often earlier, discuss similar theories to those presented in the Graeco-Roman texts.

- The Rationalist schools

One of the earliest groups to produce texts concerning the acquisition of knowledge regarding the human state were the Upanishads which were believed to have been written between 1500 and 600B.C. and were concerned with knowledge regarding the spirit, soul and god (Tripod, 2002, Kaul & Thadani 2000). Although these texts were embedded in mysticism and spirituality they used natural analogy to explain the notion of the soul and god and allowed the expression of scientific and mathematical thought and argument which formed the basis for the emergence of the rationalist period. Early rationalists included the Lokyata, Vaisheshika school and the Nyaya school. These groups espoused a scientific basis for human existence and a non-mystical relationship between the human body and mind. They also developed primitive scientific methodologies to provide "valid knowledge" (Tripod, 2002, Kaul & Thadani 2000).

The Lokyata were widely maligned by Buddhist and Hindu evangelicals as being heretics and unbelievers due to their refusal to ``make artificial distinctions between body and soul'' (Kaul & Thadani 2000). They saw all things in terms of their physical properties and reactions and gave little attention to metaphysical or philosophical argument, preferring to believe only what could be seen and understood. They developed a detailed understanding of chemistry, chemical interactions and relationships between entities. They are also believed to be the first group to document the properties of plants and their uses, this provided an elementary foundation for all pharmaceutical knowledge which followed.

The primary input of the Vaisheshika school toward the progression of human knowledge was their development of a process for classification of entities in the natural world and in their hypothesis that all matter is composed of very small particles with differing characteristics (Tripod, 2002). Their theory stated that particles, when combined, give rise to the wide variety of compounds found upon the earth and allowed them to be classified by the nature of the particles from which they were formed. This school also introduced the notion of cause and effect through monitoring and understanding temporal changes in entities. The importance of this work lay in the application of a methodology for identification and classification of relationships between previously unconnected entities. This early recognition of the need for a documented scientific process provided a mechanism for the schools which followed to present substantiated proof of evidence for theories in the sciences including physics, chemistry and medicine.

The Nyaya school further developed the work of the Vaisheshika school by continuing to document and elaborate a process for acquiring valid scientific knowledge and determining what is true. They documented a methodology consisting of four steps (Tripod, 2002):

- Uddesa was a process of defining a hypothesis.
- Laksan was the determination of required facts "through perception, inference or deduction".
- Pariksa detailed the scientific examination of facts.
- Nirnaya was the final step which involved verification of the facts.

This process would result in a conclusive finding which would either support or refute the original hypothesis.

The Nyaya school also developed definitions for three non scientific pursuits or arguments which were contrary to the determination of scientific truth but which were often applied by others to provide apparent evidence for theories or knowledge (Tripod, 2002, Kaul & Thadani, 2000). These included jalpa to describe an argument which contained exaggerated or rhetorical statements or truths aimed at proving a point rather than seeking evidence for or against a point; vitanda which aimed to lower the credibility of another person and their theories generally through specious arguments; and finally chal, the use of language to confuse or divert the argument.

Further to this again a set of five 'logical fallacies' were developed:

- savyabhichara - denotes the situation where a single conclusion is drawn where there could be several possible conclusions,
- viruddha - where contradictory reasoning was applied to produce proof of the hypothesis,
- kalatita - where the result was not presented in a timely manner and could therefore be invalidated,
- sadhyasama - where proof of a hypothesis was based upon the application of another unproven theory, and
- prakaranasama - where the process simply leads to a restating of the question.

These concepts were unique in their time but many remain applicable in modern scientific research.

This section has demonstrated that the quest for new medical knowledge and a deeper understanding of the human system is not a recent initiative but in fact one which has its foundations up to four centuries B.C. While there were several distinct cultural groups all were primarily concerned with defining the most reliable methodology for evaluating what knowledge could be trusted and applied clinically. The Graeco-Roman and Islamic practitioners were concerned with the means by which evidence was obtained and the Indians were more concerned with methods for proving the validity of knowledge after it had been discovered. Both of these foci remain topics of debate in the 21st century and as late as 1997 a report was published by the International Humanist and Ethical union regarding trusted versus untrusted clinical practices and the requirement for proof of the benefits of medical treatments. The opening of a Mantra Healing Centre at the Maulana Azad Medical College in New Delhi was described as "ridiculing the spirit of inquiry and science" through its application of "sorcery and superstition in their rudest form" (Gopal, 1997). The report did not however argue that there was no worth in mantra healing but that there was no proof of worth as per the requirements of the still flourishing rationalist opinion. The debate on what is trusted and clinically applicable knowledge forms the focus of this chapter as it investigates the application of new knowledge acquisition tools and aims to identify best practice procedures for automating the acquisition of new medical knowledge.

2.3 Non-scientific knowledge acquisition

History has shown that the acquisition of much currently accepted medical knowledge was based on serendipity or chance accompanied by a strong personal belief in an unproven hypothesis. Further to this, much knowledge was acquired through a process which directly contradicts accepted scientific practice. Whilst there was usually a scientific basis to the subsequent development of proof this was often produced through a non traditional or untrusted application of scientific processes. Unfortunately this frequently resulted in lengthy delays in acceptance of the work. The following list provides a range of such breakthroughs over the past 250 years which can be attributed to little more than chance, tenaciousness and the application of often radical methods to obtain proof.

1. James Lind (1716-1794) (Katch, 1997). Based upon an unsubstantiated personal belief that diet played a role in the development of scurvy on naval vessels, Dr Lind performed limited randomised trials to provide proof and then published his Treatise on the Scurvy which is still relevant to this day.
2. Edward Jenner (1749-1823) (Sprang, 2002). During his apprenticeship Dr Jenner overheard a milkmaid suggest that those who have had cowpox can not contract

smallpox. He then tested the theory by infecting a young boy sequentially with each pathogen and as a result created the concept of a vaccine and initiated the global eradication of smallpox.

3. John Snow (1813-1854) (Ucla, 2002, BBC, 2004). Dr Snow believed, without any direct evidence, that the transmission of viral agents was possible through contaminated water. In 1854 he applied the theory and provided an answer to the cholera epidemic.
4. Alexander Fleming (1881-1955) (Page, 2002). Dr Fleming stumbled upon a discarded culture plate containing a mould which was demonstrated to destroy staphylococcus. The mould was isolated and became the active ingredient in penicillin based antibiotics.
5. Henri Laborit (1914-1995) (Pollard, 2006). During his ward visits Dr Laborit noticed that patients given an antihistamine named promethazine to treat shock not only slept but reported pain relief and displayed a calm and relaxed disposition leading to the development of medications to treat mental disorders including schizophrenia.
6. Robert Edwards and Patrick Steptoe (1925 - , 1913-1988) (Swan, 2005, Fauser & Edwards, 2005). These doctors were the first men to deliver a baby through in-vitro fertilisation after 20 failed attempts and great ethical debate following a lack of proof in animal subjects.
7. Barry J Marshall (1951-) (Marshall, 1998). Dr Marshall worked against accepted medical knowledge to provide proof of the bacterial agent, Heliobacter Pylori, as the cause of stomach and duodenal ulcers. So strong was the opposition to initial clinical testing of the theory he resorted to using himself as the test subject.

Whilst each of these examples provided wide reaching benefits to human health and contributed significantly to the body of medical knowledge in some cases, they would not have been possible if only standardised scientific methodologies had been applied using only trusted traditional processes. This demonstrates that there is often a need to do things differently and not only apply what is comfortable and safe to enable the acquisition of knowledge, although there is always a requirement to provide substantiated proof and an argument based upon scientific principles. The applicability of this notion is particularly relevant to this chapter which focuses on the application of new techniques and technologies which have demonstrated an ability to provide an important impetus to the acquisition of knowledge in other domains and which have not been demonstrated to be detrimental to the process in the medical domain. However, the same proof of hypothesis hurdles must be overcome and an equally strong argument and testing methodology must be provided for the resulting knowledge to be accepted. Throughout history the same quality of evidence has been required and the omission of this evidence has often resulted in decades of latency between hypothesis statement and the generation of conclusive evidence in support (or otherwise) of that hypothesis.

Regardless of the methodology for producing the evidence required for knowledge acquisition, the above examples all had to fulfil a number of further requirements prior to the acquired knowledge being accepted. These requirements are summarised following:

1. Replication of results.
2. Non contradictory results.
3. Scientifically justified theories and hypotheses.
4. Ethical methodologies and measures.
5. Results demonstrated to be representative of the population.
6. Results derived from sufficient numbers of cases.
7. Publicly documented processes and results.

2.4 The application of data mining

Medical history has recorded many instances of the manual use of data mining techniques resulting in medical breakthroughs crucial to the preservation of thousands of human lives if not entire populations. Over centuries medical professionals have (often unknowingly) employed the same scientific analytical methods to data as are applied during data mining in order to develop hypotheses or to validate beliefs. Whilst these techniques have been applied in a simplistic form they clearly demonstrate the applicability of the founding principles of data mining to medical inquiry and knowledge acquisition. A number of the examples discussed in Section 2.3 are used to demonstrate this.

- Data sampling - James Lind (Katch, 1997). Dr Lind performed small randomised trials to provide proof of the cause of scurvy. In his position as Naval doctor he was able to test his theories on the crews of the vessels he sailed on, however without documented proof it was not possible to test the entire navy en mass. Developing sufficient proof in this manner was a lengthy process and it was 50 years before the British Admiralty accepted and applied his theories, a delay which cost the lives of many sailors. Lind's process shows the use of examining subsets of the population, being able to clearly identify the variant in the knowledge gained and then substantiating that knowledge by testing on similar populations to ensure the finding is representative is a suitable technique for hypothesis testing and knowledge substantiation.
- Association rules and support and confidence heuristics - Edward Jenner (Sprang, 2002). Following development of a hypothesis from the knowledge that milkmaids were less likely than members of the general population to develop small pox due to their increased contact with cow pox, Jenner conducted further tests over a period of 25 years to validate the relationship and publish his findings. This work demonstrates the use of the concept of support through Jenner's realisation that there was a frequently occurring and previously unknown pattern in a data set or population. That pattern was subsequently tested to provide confidence levels by showing that contracting cowpox almost always results in an inability to contract smallpox.
- Clustering - John Snow (Ucla, 2002, BBC, 2004). In his investigation of the cholera outbreak of 1854 Dr John Snow applied a meticulous process of interviewing to collect data. He used the information collected to develop a statistical map which clustered interview responses based upon the water pump which supplied water to the individual. This revealed that every victim had used a single supply of water and no non-sufferers had used that supply. Further investigation showed that this pump was in fact contaminated by a nearby cracked sewage pipe. This shows not only the power of the use of medical data for statistical purposes, but the benefits that can result from applying clustering techniques to that data.
- Association rules and classification - Henri Laboit (Pollard, 2006). Laboit extended the use of promethazine to treat mental disorders including schizophrenia by realising patterns in side effects from administering the drug during surgery on non mentally ill patients. This was achieved through identifying association rule style patterns to describe associations between focal and non focal attributes, for example combinations of relationships between diagnosis, treatment, symptoms, side effects and medications. Analytical techniques were employed to classify conditions exhibiting similar patterns of presentation and clinical testing was utilised to demonstrate the effect of applying an identified drug to control those classes of symptoms.

These techniques until recently were employed manually and hence were on a much smaller scale than we see today through the application of automated data mining systems, however they demonstrate the impressive potential for automated data analysis techniques to be applied with greater benefits and applicability than ever thought possible. There is a belief by some that the rate of medical breakthroughs of the calibre of those listed above has slowed dramatically since the 1970s (Horton, 2000). This could be attributed to the inability of the human mind to manage the volume of data available (Biedl et al., 2001, Lavrak et al., 2000) and that most if not all patterns in data which may reveal knowledge and which occur frequently enough to be noticed by the human analyst are now known. This adds significant weight to the argument for the application of more effective and efficient automated technologies to uncover the less visible knowledge or less frequent but equally important patterns in the data. We must however learn from history and ensure that the validation requirements for knowledge acquisition, as discussed previously, are adhered to by any automated process as for all other methods of knowledge acquisition even though this has been described as "the hardest part of the expert system development task" (Lavrak et al., 2000). Too often in recent work there has been a focus on developing new methods for determining the quality and value of outputs which does not take into consideration the many lessons we can learn from history, and is often little more than a process of reinventing an already rolling wheel (Ordonez et al., 2001).

3. The automation of medical knowledge acquisition

To automate it is not sufficient to simply understand how the process has occurred manually or how that process developed, although this is important in ensuring the results can be trusted. There is also a requirement to develop a seemless transfer from the clinical application of the process to the technical automated application of the same process and to provide accountability so that the results are trusted, justified and actionable in a clinical environment. In data mining systems, these accountability values are often measured through a concept termed 'interestingness' which essentially aims to measure the level of interest a user may have in the outputs provided by a system

3.1 What is interesting?

The term 'interest' is one which is widely accepted and used within data mining to denote output which has value on some level. This section is concerned with how we might define interest or value in clinical terms. The work discussed in this chapter began with the naive idea that interest can be measured and quantified for medicine as a homogenous entity as occurs in many other domains. This notion is now considered laughable at best. Medicine is not a homogenous entity and is not even a single entity in any contextual argument. Whilst it is defined generally (Oxford, 2007) as the science of studying, diagnosing, treating, or preventing disease and other damage to the body or mind, or treatment of illness by the ingestion of drugs, modification of diet or exercise, or other non-surgical means. The means by which those engaged in the practice of medicine achieve this outcome or engage in this activity varies widely depending upon individual needs, experience and data. If we are developing an automated system to assist or guide in this activity then the system must also be able to perform according to individual needs, experience and data. As discussed in the chapter introduction, data mining systems are able to manage a broad range of data types and analytical processes, but they are usually tailored to a user and hence are designed to work with their individual technical proficiency and analytical requirements. Whilst work is ongoing in this area, uncertainty remains regarding the ability of automated systems to address the varied and fluid requirements of the user population. There are therefore two questions posed:

1. How can we identify the varied individual requirements of the user body?
2. Can we automate these requirements into a system which caters to a range of users?

To overcome this issue it is necessary to define what is interesting and what makes one thing more or less interesting than another and further to develop an algorithm to measure the extent to which the outputs of data mining conform to the user definition of interesting. As each of us finds different things interesting it is not possible to define a single specification for what is interesting to any group of people. Within the context of the focus of this chapter however, we can say that the degree to which something is deemed interesting can be quantified through the application of statistical methods. This method of value measurement is one which is applied in clinical testing where such measures as those shown in Table 1 are frequently used as a basis for determining which trial or trial arm has provided evidence that is clinically applicable or worthy of progression to the next level of testing (Gebeski & Keech 2003, Moser et al., 1999, Hilderman & Hamilton 2001, Geng & Hamilton 2006). Many of the same statistical methods are also applied within data mining systems but the provision of individual methods or combinations of methods are fixed and provide an inflexible analytical toolbox unlike in the clinical setting where any method can be chosen and applied. The requirement is therefore to provide a more flexible approach and not 'invent' another formula to determine the level of interest but to allow the user to determine how to define interest for each run or data set as occurs in clinical analysis. An added benefit in this is the ability to reinforce and support medical professionals control of their domain and the processes they apply to an analysis task. It should not be acceptable for technology to dictate how a medical professional (or any other) should practice.

Measure	Type	Application	Domain
P	Statistical	Determine degree of difference in results	Medicine
chi2	Statistical	Determine degree of difference in results	Medicine
chi2	Statistical	Result comparison	Medicine
Pearson's Correlation	Comparative	Measure of difference	Bio-inf
Euclidian Distance	Comparative	Measure of difference	Bio-inf
Cosine Similarity	Comparative	Measure of similarity of text	Linguistics
Support	Statistical	Probability, Frequency	Retail
Confidence	Statistical	Probability, Frequency	Retail
Accuracy	Domain	Determination of class membership	Medicine
Sensitivity	Domain	Measure of ability to find true positives	Medicine
Specificity	Domain	Measure of ability to reject true negatives	Medicine

Table 1. Some of the more commonly applied statistical tests.

In essence if the results of analysis are to be deemed interesting they must fall within defined thresholds as measured by one of more statistical method. The selection of appropriate methods is both objective and subjective. Objectively, certain qualities must be present in an interesting result and methods will be selected to provide evidence of this quality. For example if the result must be indicative of an accurate prediction of disease classification then such measures as sensitivity and specificity could be chosen as they are designed to measure this quality. Subjectively an analyst may place greater trust in one method over another due to experience or availability even though they both provide a method for measuring a particular quality. An example here may be the choice between using a p-value or chi^2 which can both provide similar quantified evidence. There is a long list of statistical methods which can be applied and they are selected based upon a combination of user objectivity and subjectivity which will potentially be different for each user. Although the provision of a fixed subset of available statistical methods represents the commonly applied data mining technique for evaluating interest, for the reasons discussed herein, it is not an appropriate methodology for the medical domain where there is no fixed notion of what is interesting or of how to measure the qualities which define interest. Whilst the process would be vastly simplified by ignoring the concept of individual interest it is necessary to overcome a number of issues with the application of data mining to medical data. The most important issue is that of non acceptence of the technology even though its benefits are many. Non acceptance is due to a defined set of factors:

- The complexity of medical data frequently results in a huge number of results; too many to be evaluated by the human user and a method for reducing the results to only those of greatest interest is necessary (Roddick et al., 2003; Ordonez et al., 2001)
- Each user has a trusted set of methods which are applied during clinical analysis and which are rarely seen in a system that is not purpose built for that user or their analytical requirements; this increases the cost of providing the technology, the frustration in trying to use the technology and allows the technology to dictate the analytical process rather than the other way around. Being able to facilitate and apply a range of interest definitions in a single system would open up the technology to a greater audience.
- Many users are not technically adept and do not trust something they do not understand; the provision of a recognised process which offers a personalised perspective within a generalised framework provides comfort and security.

To overcome these barriers to the technology it is neccesary to move away from a user focussed approach, which has in fact created many of the issues presented here, and towards an interest based approach which is guided by individual needs as it is the level of interest to each user that primarily determines the acceptability of results. If we can develop a generic approach to interest that can be individually adapted then we can apply this to develop data mining systems which can be similarly founded upon a generic principle that can be personalised for individual use. The provision of such a solution is the focus of the remainder of this chapter.

3.2 A role based approach

The issue of developing a flexible data mining system with the intention of enabling the generic production of results with an acceptable level of interest for each individual user has been the focus of recent work by the author. The approach has been to investigate the concept of a role in various forms and its relationship to the concept of interest as defined above.

Each of us plays many roles in our daily lives as a student, doctor, nurse, teacher, parent, guitar player, amateur photographer etc. etc. Each of these roles will define a level of interest in the world around us, which will be determined by how relevant to each role the world is at any specific time. As each of us has a unique set of roles then each individual will have a corresponding unique set of interests or interest triggers, and different information will appeal to us at different times. Our role is therefore defined by how we measure the value of our interest in information that is presented to us. For example an Oncologist would most likely have been interested in an article on new cancer treatments in a Weekend Australian newspaper entitled "Hype or Hope?" (Cornwell, 2005), as it relates to their professional role and, even an evaluation of keywords contained in the article, would have revealed many matches to a similar evaluation of keywords in their set of interests. In contrast an Electrical Engineer would most likely not have had the same level of interest unless they also held the role of cancer sufferer or carer of a cancer sufferer for example. Therefore we can define a role as being a collection of quantifiable interests. The focus of work presented here has been to develop a system that will allow the identification of these interest sets and develop a method for determining how to measure and evaluate how strongly the information is able to trigger interest. To achieve this it was necessary to provide a quantitative evaluation of interest by evaluating the requirements of an interest set and measuring the applicability of the information or data mining results to that unique set.

3.2.1 The application of role

The application of a role in determining which data mining outputs are of relevance is more complex than simply looking for the presence of keywords. In the field of epidemiology for example the simple presence of the word 'flu' is not sufficient to trigger interest, there needs to be statistical augmentation to the information. In particular it needs to be shown that the incidence of the condition is sufficiently different to that expected for a population at a defined time. The difficulty is in determining which heuristics will give an acceptable measure by which we can include or exclude results for each role. A role based result evaluation engine has been designed in preference to other options including new heuristics and new heuristic combinations as these fixed solutions can not provide a generic answer to the issue of evaluating the level of interest for the health domain as a whole given the complexities noted above. It was necessary for an evolution in current thinking in the area and for single-user solutions to be discarded. A generalised solution to the issue of result reduction for this domain cannot be achieved due to the broad range of roles and requirements to be addressed. Early work has since evolved into developing a system that can incorporate the range of roles without the need for a separate system for each. As it is the role that determines how the strength of general interest is measured, it was a natural step to discriminate the analysis by the role of the current user as defined by a set of measurable interests. Users should be able to analyse and focus their data mining outputs using a single system regardless of their speciality or analytical requirements. Whilst the needs of each role are unique there is also considerable overlap and the heuristics required to determine interest strength varies from role to role and also within each user role depending upon the nature of the analysis being undertaken (Kuonen, 2003; Bresnahan,

1997; Tan et al., 2002). A system with a high level of flexibility and methods to facilitate user definition was deemed to provide the best use of resources to accommodate this.

Role based access models have been successfully implemented in a wide range of domains and have demonstrated an ability to overcome issues such as those seen in health including a need for careful management of sensitive information and the need to provide enterprise level security policies which discriminate on a local level based on the role of the user (Cabri et al., 2004; Ferrailo & Kuhn, 1995). Role based access models have provided a fixed framework from which to apply highly flexible system definition and this concept was the major attraction in the creation of a role based results evaluation process for data mining applications in the health domain.

The following features of role based systems have been adapted and incorporated into a hypothesis engine as discussed in Section 4.

- The accommodation of roles that allow for overlapping requirements and measures.
- The ability for a user to have more than one role at a time.
- The ability to enforce constraints on data access where required to accommodate ethical sensitivities.
- The ease of modifying the role of a group of users to accommodate new technologies or methodologies.
- The ability to constrain at a global level and provide flexibility at a local level.

Whilst the choice of interest strength heuristics will often fluctuate little across mining runs, some vary greatly, become redundant or require supplementation by new or existing measures. This high level of flexibility is not currently available in documented data mining systems. Algorithms and selected heuristics are applied singly or in a fixed combination with others within a specific system designed for a specific use. The ability to utilise the interest role as a means of selecting and applying a significant number of the range of measures in a unique combination as required has not been documented and is believed to be a novel approach to the issues presented here. Support for such an approach has been provided by health domain professionals and domain based publications including the Medical Journal of Australia (MJA) which stated that appropriate statistical methods for analysing trial data are critical and suggested that the statistical methods used in each trial should be specifically tailored to each analysis (Gebski & Keech, 2003). Each specialist field and role has its own requirements and hence the level of flexibility in data mining software packages must be equally flexible, open to adaptation and tailored for the user role at run time.

As discussed in the previous section, there are many methods which can be applied to measure the strength of interest a user may feel towards any information. An initial aim was to group these measures based on the role that uses them, this was rejected due to the overlaps discussed earlier. The aim was thus modified to group the measures into classes based upon their type and the characteristic of interest they are able to quantify, thus allowing each role to select and apply them as required. While there is no fixed notion of what defines interest strength for a particular role in each instance, there is agreement on the characteristics that indicate strength and these can be grouped and measured to quantify their level of expression in results presented. These classes were verified in discussion with a range of medical professionals during a work in progress seminar (Workshop in population health, 2005) presented to by the author. In attendance were medical specialists from several fields including cardiology, epidemiology, biostatistics, nursing, clinical research and government and all agreed that the proposed classes defined the qualities they looked for during hypothesis development and results testing. It was noted that whilst most of those present could not adequately describe what determined a strong interest in a result for the domain generally, it was felt that the classes presented would provide an acceptable quantification for any role within the domain if applied uniquely for each role or field. It was also proffered that each test result was considered individually depending upon their needs at the time often the heuristics employed were often not selected until the time of evaluation thus strengthening the argument away from a generalised approach. This, in fact, emphasised the need to utilise traditional measures but in a flexible combination for each evaluation.

By allowing a subjective selection of heuristics and evaluating their application objectively it is possible to take the outputs of data mining and measure their value uniquely and flexibly for each role rather than utilising a unique but fixed sub set of heuristics for each system. Based upon the values achieved by each heuristic, unqualified mining outputs can be eliminated from presentation thus providing only those outputs which meet the requirements of the role and adequately contain the desired characteristics to be of interest.

Six classes or criteria are provided for interest strength measurement and each of these may require a number of statistical, comparative or other tests to determine the overall strength for each criterion. The individual values are then combined to provide a comprehensive measure of interest strength for a mining output based on the total requirements for the user role. A greater strength suggests an output that is more likely to be of value to the role that defined the heuristics and their scopes. The criteria for measuring interest and hence strength of new information or knowledge patterns produced through data mining are discussed following.

- Novelty - Is it unknown in the body of domain knowledge? This is more complex than simply not duplicating existing knowledge or presenting expected patterns. New patterns based upon existing knowledge may still be of interest if the strength or content of the new knowledge differs sufficiently from that which is expected. For example, medical professionals would reject as new a pattern which states that 3.6% of pregnant women develop gestational diabetes mellitus (GDM) as this is known and expected knowledge even though it would have sufficient strength by some traditional measures to warrant further investigation (Stone et al., 2002). However if a pattern were to report that the incidence rate of GDM in a data set primarily for a North Asian population was 3.6% then the interest in this may be greater as the rate would be expected to be higher. Hence it is the pattern novelty as a whole which is being evaluated and which thus determines the strength of interest. There are a number of measures that can be applied to quantify the expectedness or similarity of hypotheses to existing knowledge and it may be necessary to test this criterion using several classes of tests to adequately assess the novelty of a pattern.
- Applicability – Is it relevant to the current user? This infers that either some contextual information is required, or that previous patterns are tagged as interesting (or not) so that the system can learn and reference. The definition of applicability (or relevance) is context based and should be maintained on an individual level. An outlier that is strong in every aspect except for prevalence may not be relevant to an epidemiologist as it is not representative of the population but still may potentially be of interest to a clinical specialist or medical researcher and should be tagged for reference by that role. The implication is that any derived pattern produced from a medical data store is

potentially valuable to some role in the medical domain. If accepted, this suggests the importance of strength determination at a role based level to ensure that each role sees only patterns they are most likely to have an interest in and be able to act upon but that no strong pattern is omitted completely from consideration.

- Relativity - Is it valid relative to the data from which it originated or a class of object that it describes? Once again the applicability of this criterion is determined by the context within which it is measured. Within epidemiology it is important for pattern to be shown to be applicable for a generalised population. Results therefore need be demonstrated to apply across the human race or a definable sub section of it. A recent study published in the MJA discussed a potential but low correlation between passive smoking and breast cancer (Smith & Ebrahim, 2004). Whilst the link was biologically plausible in 1999 it was not deemed to be representative of the female population in an epidemiological sense and hence was not deemed interesting. Further work was done which focussed on the effect of environmental tobacco smoke across the age variable specifically. It is now accepted that there is enough evidence to suggest that passive smoking specifically in the early years of a females' life has a measurable impact upon the incidence of breast cancer later in life. Investigation at a finer granularity resulted in a hypothesis that is accepted as representative of a defined sub section of the population. This suggests that strength should be measured for all applicable classes, not only the most obvious or highest ranking. Patterns also need to be shown to be representative of the data set from which it came and there are standardised checklists such as that provided by CONSORT (Consolidated Standards of Reporting Trials) (Lord et al., 2004, Gebeski & Keech 2003, Altman et al., 2001) which are widely used within medical research and should be incorporated into the planning of data mining systems.
- Provability - Can it be proven through clinical testing? This reflects the actionability of the outcomes of data mining and incorporates the need to adhere to guidelines such as CONSORT discussed earlier. Whilst there are perceived difficulties in automatically determining what could be tested clinically, there are several requirements which define what the foundations of a clinical hypothesis should be and these should be present in hypotheses in the form of patterns derived through data mining also (Lord et al., 2004) . For organisations that adhere to research guidelines, it is important that the pre-requisites are met for further work so that the potential for follow up clinical testing is not prevented. This criterion aims to ensure that potential hypotheses are not rendered inactionable due to the methodology employed for their derivation rather than trying to determine what will be actionable.
- Understandability - Can it be understood through appropriate presentation? New knowledge that cannot be described easily or accurately is of little use. The inability for the human brain to assimilate and perform functions upon large amounts of complex data is the very foundation upon which the field of data mining was based. When presenting patterns, this must be given due consideration. An overly complex or lengthy pattern may be overlooked in favour of those that can be read and understood quickly. Consideration must also be given to domain specific terminology and semantic hierarchies (Ashby & Smith, 2002). This will ensure that patterns are presented using uniform, accurate and appropriate terminology (Bojarczuk et al., 2001, Lavrak et al., 2000). Results should also be presented via a medium that is accepted as standard by each role or domain and there is a body of work in the fields of visualisation and linguistics that is attempting to address some of these issues.

- Validity - Is it statistically valid according to trusted domain measures? There are a wide range of statistical measures available to test these classes and each user role should be able to apply measures to each analysis based on the nature of the analysis and personal experience. The authors work argues for the use of role based metrics which are manipulated and utilised according to the individual needs of each user and suggests that pre-defining specific heuristics for statistical validity is redundant and archaic.

3.2.2 Concept formalisation

Whilst it is not possible to give a single definition to what is interesting it is possible to formalise the nature of interest as described in this chapter. As discussed, interest can be determined by a variety of objective and subjective criteria which in combination can provide an indication of the degree to which this output can be trusted. We can therefore formalise interest as following:

I = { m1 ... mn} where I is Interest which is defined by a set of statistical methods or other heuristics (m).

Furthermore the applied heuristic or method (m) can be denoted in the following form:

m = { metric, Tmin, Tmax, var1 ... varn} where Tmin is the minimum acceptable threshold for the metric and Tmax is the maximum acceptable threshold for the metric and var is any other variable which may affect the application of the metric. A var example may be 'sex' and the metric 'weight', therefore there would be different Tmin and Tmax for weight thresholds for men and women. Thus the method is described as an object which has a number of qualities through which it can be defined or represented. All qualities except for metric name would be optional.

By applying the definition of interest (I) we can determine that the outcomes of data mining are likely to be trusted as they apply trusted metrics and are likely to be understood as again they are qualified using known metrics whose outputs are in a standardised form. The selection of these metrics, thresholds and variables should be done by each user at run time to allow for a measure of subjectivity to be applied to the definition of interest.

Further to this, it is necessary to determine how interesting an outcome might be, as one pattern may not adhere to all parts of the definition but should not necessarily be excluded on that basis. Many things are interesting not because they adhere to our schema but because they 'almost' adhere to the schema or in contrast because they do not at all adhere to the schema (RoddickRice 2000). It was therefore deemed useful to give some indication of how close to the interest schema the pattern is as defined by the metric set. This binary classification is formalised as:

PI = { m1r ... mnr} where r denotes that this is the result of applying metric m to a pattern P. m1r to mnr were coded as either 1 or 0 depending upon whether or not they fell within the thresholds with (1) denoting within and (0) denoting the result was outside of the threshold for that method. PI is an expression of the likely interest strength in a pattern based upon consideration of all applied metrics.

Whilst this was a satisfactory representation for results which had to absolutely comply with the stated thresholds and are hence critical to acceptance, it provided no indication of where results were outside of, but close enough to, the required thresholds as determined again by a user measure of acceptable flexibility. There are numerous statistical measures and methods available to test a pattern (Imberman & Domanski, 2002; Beals et al., 1999), however they may not be critical measures of pattern interest strength to a particular user.

Hence there is a need to define both needs and wants and be able to discriminate on that basis. For example, a confidence of between 80 and 95% may be wanted, however patterns with a lower confidence may still be of interest if other heuristics achieve acceptable levels, hence confidence would be considered a flexible measure. Conversely in an epidemiological context the incidence of a condition would need to be greater than background levels to be of interest, and anything less than or equal to background levels will not be interesting regardless of other factors. These heuristics are deemed to be critical measures as the scope for acceptance is inflexible.

For those methods that could be applied flexibly a fuzzy logic was applied to allow for a more considered pattern evaluation to occur. This fuzziness allowed for a result to be described in terms of four classes; far from interesting (f); close but lower (cl); close but higher (ch); and within thresholds (wt) thereby providing for a range of interest outcomes as follows:

f...cl...wt...ch...f

f appears at both ends of the scale as it can be uninteresting because it is too far above the stated thresholds or because it is too far below the stated threshold, however in some cases for example in pathogen monitoring it may be that both f's and/or values for cl and ch may not be applicable as a user may not have defined both a Tmin and Tmax.

By applying all of these constructs it may be possible to provide a meta description of a pattern as an array in the form of A and B appear in the presence of C {(M1 (metric, Tmin, Tmax, var1 ... varn)(wt)), (M2(metric, Tmin, Tmax, var1 ... varn)(1)), Mn(metric, Tmin, Tmax, var1 ... varn)(result))}

4. A flexible solution

4.1 The hypothesis engine

Human intuition often plays a strong role in determining what is interesting in a health context and many breakthroughs are born out of a serendipitous discovery that is subsequently validated through further research not by statistical validity (Bresnahan, 1997). A final decision on what is interesting may be based on little more than gut feeling and hence the need for flexibility in determining the metrics for inclusion and exclusion of a pattern that becomes a hypothesis for clinical testing is required to mirror the natural process. The foundation for applying the theories presented here is the development of a hypothesis engine. The engine provides a flexible means to discriminate data mining patterns and therefore hypotheses based upon individual role based requirements. The engine provides a system that allows the following functionality:

1. The flexible application of a wide range of heuristics through the provision of a wide range of heuristics for user selection,
2. The run time selection and scoping of heuristics provided through an interface which allows the selection of any combination of heuristics and thresholds for each,
3. A role based default heuristic selection developed through analysis of the most commonly applied heuristics and thresholds for the user,
4. A means of discriminating hypotheses based on critical and non-critical requirements by applying the selected heuristical methods and developing an interest array as described in Section 3.2.2
5. A measurement of information strength based on trusted classes of heuristics through combining heuristic values in hypotheses of interest.

This functionality provides for a two phase hypothesis culling process as shown in Figure 1. The hypotheses are systematically culled as they attempt to propagate upwards through the evaluation phases from individual heuristics to a quantified information strength for the pattern. Any individual heuristic achieving within the role defined thresholds would automatically propagate to the next level. A metric that does not achieve a level within the thresholds would be filtered through a switch. If the metric is critical (needed) to determine strength then the switch would cull that hypothesis. If the metric is not critical (only wanted) then the switch would not be activated resulting in that heuristic value and the hypothesis being included in the next level providing no other critical heuristics fail for that hypothesis. The switches have the dual purpose of reducing the numbers and increasing the validity of hypotheses presented.

The hypothesis engine allows for patterns to be produced at the broadest level and then evaluated to allow the provision of only those which match a pre-defined interest role as defined by a user designed schema at run time. This addresses a number of the major barriers to the acceptance and application of data mining in the medical domain described earlier in this chapter;

1. The low level of flexibility in data mining systems requiring medical analytical processes to adapt to data mining methodologies rather than vice versa.
2. The lack of opportunity for incorporating subjectivity when mining medical data,
3. The broad range of users and analytical variance in medicine,
4. The production of too many irrelevant results, requiring a high level of user interpretation to discriminate those that are truly useful.

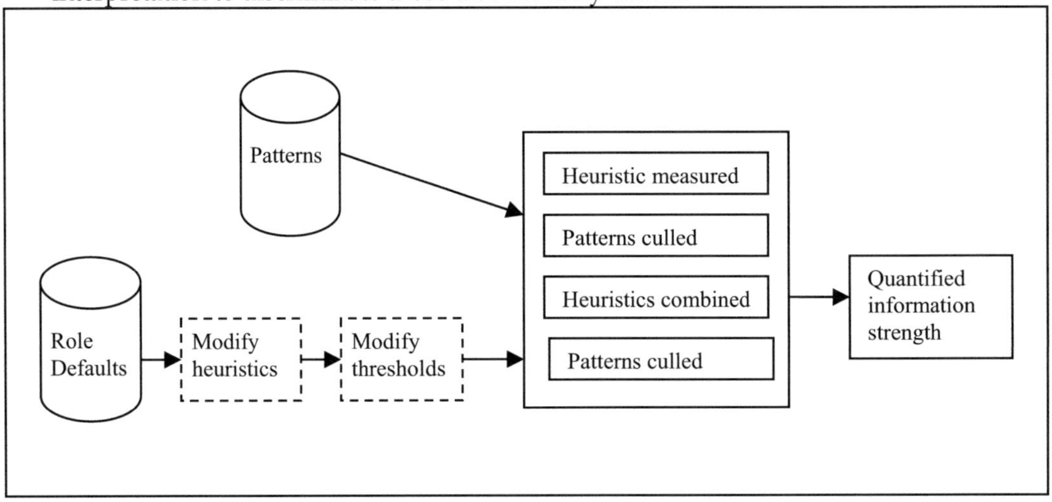

Fig. 1. Hypothesis Engine Overview

4.2 Medical diagnostic decision making

The process of interdisciplinary research and analysis discussed in this chapter has resulted in a methodology for identifying knowledge which is interesting in a clinical context and has facilitated the definition of a mechanism for evaluating the level of interest an individual user may have in the knowledge or rules produced as a result of mining medical data. This mechanism was built into a hypothesis engine as described in the previous section. However, whilst useful as a standalone adjunct to the data mining process, the engine does not address all of the issues identified in Section 2. To achieve this end a demonstration system named ADAPT (Automated DAta Pattern Translator) has been built. This system aims to facilitate greater access to mining technologies for all medical users, and to provide an ability to apply some of the more complex mining technologies to acquire new medical knowledge without the risk of producing incomprehensible outputs. It also adds weight to the solutions provided by the hypothesis engine, and addresses the issues not able to be solved by the engine. The development of ADAPT grew primarily out of an understanding of the issues with applying data mining technologies in the medical domain and an aim to create a solution to those issues. It required not only an understanding of the medical knowledge acquisition process but also an understanding of the more common clinical processes. One of the most frequently performed processes of a practicing clinician is that of diagnosis. This process is briefly described here and forms the basis for gaining a deeper understanding of the requirements in an automated knowledge application and decision making system. The decision making process of medical practitioners usually if not always occurs at a subjective level following an objective information gathering process. This information is collected and interrogated during the consultation phase of the patient episode and generally includes all or some of the following artefacts;

- The symptoms as described by the patient
- The findings of the physical examination
- The results of tests
- Diagnostic imaging
- Clinical referrals
- Historical reports.

Once collated this information is generally evaluated through either of two common diagnostic methodologies; by exclusion or by pattern categorisation (Frenster, 1989; Merck, 2003; Elstein & Schwartz, 2002):

1. The exclusion method is considered the safer but more expensive of the two options. Here a doctor will reach a decision on the most likely diagnosis and treatment pattern for a set of stated symptoms exclusively through a series of objective and often invasive tests. These tests allow the doctor to reach a decision based upon an ability to exclude potential diagnoses based upon the results of the tests. A final diagnosis is usually not made until the results of all required tests are known. The potential disadvantages of this option are that it results in a lengthy and costly process which can yield an unacceptable level of false negatives or positives and cause psychological stress for the patient during the wait; especially if the tests are for a condition for which the outcome is potentially life threatening, for example cancer, meningococcal infection or HIV.

2. Pattern categorisation is the preferred option in the medical community as it is more cost and time effective than diagnosis by exclusion, however it is generally only applied by more experienced doctors and specialists. In this scenario a doctor will reach a diagnosis by comparing the presenting patient's pattern of symptoms and test results to known patterns of condition diagnosis, progression and treatment. It is often the case that rather than making a single diagnosis the practitioner will develop a cluster of potential diagnoses based upon the similarity of the potential diagnoses to the pattern of the patient's condition that initiated the medical consultation as shown in Figure 2. Probabilistic pattern completion is often required and the diagnosis and treatment patterns are derived from a comparison to all others in the practitioner's body of knowledge and those sufficiently similar to the

patients' pattern are selected. The diagnosis is therefore more holistically targeted to the patient and case rather than the cause or effect exclusively. A drawback of this is that a rare case or combination may mean the most suitable pattern is missed or incorrectly identified and errors can be made.
With experience, doctors become efficient at recognising what's expected in a pattern and which patient or condition characteristics are most influential or critical when forming a diagnosis. The speed of pattern recognition may be increased by fuzzy matching which takes into account only matches between critical attributes or attribute values which fall within a range. Attributes or values which occur frequently cannot be applied to discriminate between patterns, but knowing which attributes to focus on and which to eliminate from the comparison is a skill developed through years of experience. Given the importance of the ability to recognise which pattern elements or attributes are important in the clinical diagnostic process, it is a logical step to move towards an automated process of identifying the important elements of patterns derived from the application of data mining technologies.

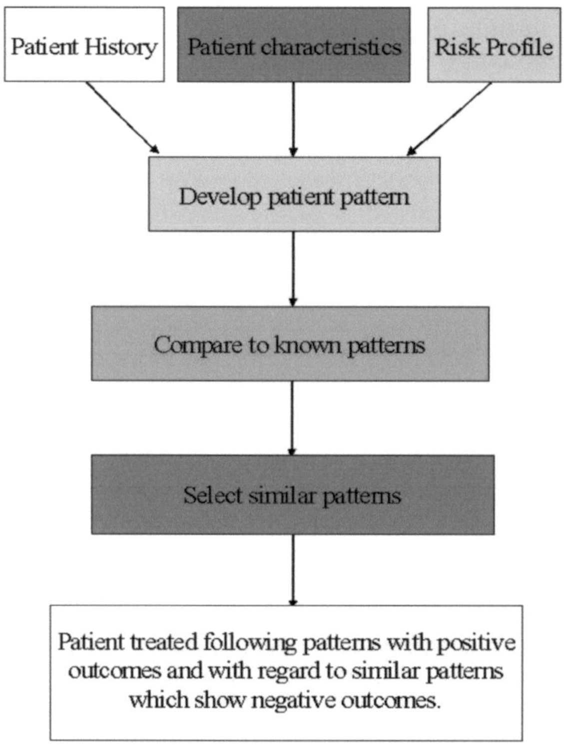

Fig. 2. Diagnostic process model. Note: Darker shading denotes higher level of subjective input.

For automated processes to be applied and accepted it is important that they are able to mirror or facilitate current practices. This requires the provision of knowledge which is able to be trusted, descriptive from an objective viewpoint and informative in a way which assists in the subjective appraisal of a patient. Unfortunately many data mining outputs (patterns) are presented in a non-intuitive and frequently opaquely coded form. The above diagnostic methods suggest that there is a requirement for heuristic triggers and substantiated hypotheses which can suggest rather than dictate a course of action based upon pattern similarity and a need to be able to deconstruct the pattern into more and less influencing pattern elements upon which to base the diagnosis or treatment. If we accept these requirements, it is a logical step to move towards an automated process of identifying and describing the important elements of patterns derived from the application of data mining technologies and it is this precept that has defined the development of ADAPT.

For brevity and to ensure understanding of the system at an algorithmic level several definitions are provided here:

- Data mining is essentially an automated data analysis process, however there are almost as many formal definitions of data mining as there are data miners. One of the more commonly quoted definitions is that it is a "non-trivial process of identifying valid, novel, potentially useful and ultimately understandable patterns in data" (Fayyad et al., 1996). These patterns are often described through the standard heuristics of support and confidence.
- Support essentially quantifies the frequency with which a pattern occurs within the original data source, expressed as a percentage. The minimum support threshold is generally set by the user at runtime. A pattern is defined as a set of attribute values produced through a process of association rule mining, which occur equal to, or greater than, the minimum support required by the user. Patterns take a general format as shown in the following example; Condition 'A' + Treatment 'B' lead to an outcome of 'Recovery Time C' with support of 20%.
- Confidence quantifies as a percentage the degree to which we can rely on the presence of part of a pattern given another part of the same pattern. For example, given Condition 'A', the confidence states how often we could expect Treatment 'B' to also occur in the same pattern.
- A pattern element is a part of a pattern. In the example above, Condition 'A', Treatment 'B' and Recovery Time 'C' are the three elements of the pattern. Treatment 'B' leads to a Recovery Time 'C' is also an element, as it represents only a part of the pattern.
- Elemental support is the support for a pattern element. This concept is explained in further detail in foundation work by the author (Shillabeer & Roddick 2006).

4.3 ADAPT

Data mining outputs are currently deficient in their application to the medical domain as they are not able to identify which pattern elements directly affect the medical outcome or which have no effect and are therefore little more than confounders, although as explained earlier, this is necessary if patterns derived from medical data are to assist in processes such as diagnosis.

The ADAPT system aims to provide guidance and structure to the application of translating technical outputs into clinically relevant patterns of diagnosis or treatment, and presents a novel approach to post-mining pattern evaluation. There are six steps identified in the process:

1. Identify a set of interesting patterns,
2. Calculate the representative pattern element weightings,
3. Deconstruct the support for each pattern and determine its elemental supports,

4. Determine the positive, negative and inert elements,
5. Order patterns by their degree of representation,
6. Present patterns with their associated heuristics.

Data mining processes that have attempted to evaluate the patterns presented have focussed primarily on step 1, however approaches taken have often been unsuitable for the medical domain due to the wide range of user types and definitions of interest. Medically focussed solutions have been developed but have generally provided a user specific solution. This chapter has described a hypothesis engine developed specifically to address the requirement for flexibility in interest evaluation and quantification. Unfortunately this step alone still presents patterns which are potentially unsuitably formatted, and/or do not inform sufficiently well for direct clinical application. The need to supplement information content to aid understanding of the patterns produced as a result of data mining is the focus of steps 2 to 4. Presentation of patterns in a logical and value driven order is the focus of steps 5 and 6. Steps 2 to 4 are described following.

4.3.1 The argument for elemental support

The concept of elemental support arose out of an understanding of the need to determine which pattern elements are important in medical decision making as raised in the previous section, and the realisation that not all elements of a pattern necessarily carry the same importance. Two examples are provided to demonstrate the relevance of the argument.

1. Taking dymadon and lemsip together are unnecessary to control the symptoms of a cold, as they both contain the same active ingredient, but some patients may choose to do so from habit or ignorance. In a mining sense the pattern of dymadon + lemsip = reduction in symptoms, would be viable however we can see that in reality the removal of any one of the treatments would probably not affect the outcome but this information would not be available in traditional reporting of the presented pattern.
2. In the treatment of AIDS many medications were prescribed singularly and in combination before the specific combinations were found that made a genuine contribution to the well being and longevity of the patient. The individual medications may have demonstrated sufficient mining support for their ability to associate with a positive outcome which would have therefore been suggestive of an ability to facilitate a positive outcome alone, as demonstrated in Figure 3. However, if in fact their efficacy were true only when combined with specific other medications this should be evidenced through the metadata or heuristics provided to describe the pattern. It should be that as the single medication does not achieve sufficient support in isolation it is therefore not reported unless combined with the other medications in a pattern that can be substantiated statistically and medically.

Through considering these issues it was identified that data mining may not be able to ensure completeness, soundness and medical accuracy of results in the medical domain and a method for determining the importance of pattern elements rather than whole patterns is deemed necessary. As shown in figure 3, traditional support does not provide sufficiently granular information and may in fact be misleading although it is a frequently applied determinate. In the example, treatment A and procedure B are both quantified as strong using the support metric and this could suggest that their individual implementation would lead to a positive outcome for the patient. However as the value for the pattern element includes instances of that element in all other patterns also, and does not isolate to the prevalence of that specific pattern no conclusions should be drawn. It is necessary to be able to discriminate and differentiate by knowing the support for treatment A or procedure B in isolation rather than only as an element in a longer pattern as shown in Figure 4. This more clearly denotes that applying either element alone will not necessarily lead to a positive outcome but when applied together there is a far greater chance of a positive outcome for the patient.

This understanding resulted in the following requirement list:

- The requirement for mining outcomes to be evaluated with a non-traditional application of the support measure.
- The requirement to discriminate between the overall incidence of an element in any pattern and the incidence of that element in isolation.
- The requirement to provide a clear description of the information held in a pattern to aid subjective judgement.

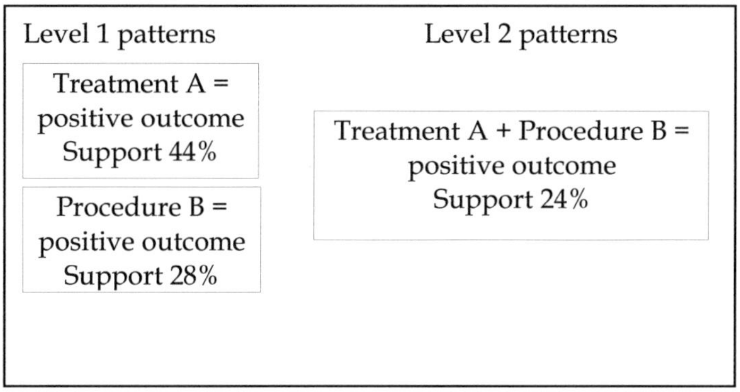

Fig. 3. Traditional support values for a sample data pattern.

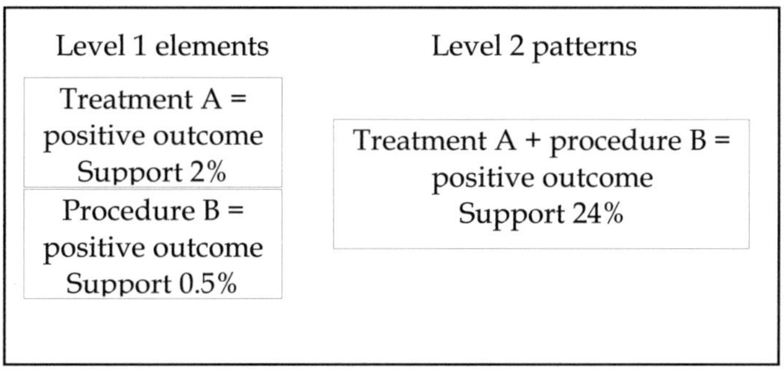

Fig. 4. Elemental support values for the sample data pattern.

Two methods were developed to address these requirements. These methods have been termed support deconstruction and element weighting.

4.3.2 Support deconstruction

Support deconstruction is a novel method which aims to determine the value of each element to a pattern. If 3 element patterns have the same support as 2 element patterns then we can logically deduce that the third element does not add any extra value as the likelihood of achieving the same outcome is equal. In our earlier example of cold medications, the addition of lemsip to the pattern 'dymadon = relief of symptoms' would probably not significantly increase the support for a relief in symptoms. To determine the effect of each element we need to calculate the support for the pattern before and after adding each extra element to the pattern. In effect we need to take the incidence of BC from BCD to determine the effect of D. In a pattern ABCD = a positive outcome, each element appears as often as each other; therefore by applying traditional support metrics, suppA = suppB = suppC = suppD and each element could be considered equally strong. To determine the effect of element 'A' on pattern 'ABCD', its participation in all of the following relationships must be considered:

Level 1		A	
Level 2	AB	AC	AD
Level 3	ABC	ABD	ACD
Level 4		ABCD	

From being a single element (level 1) to being an element of the 4 element pattern (level 4), element 'A' participates in 7 elements or relationships and in this example it would lend part of its traditional support to each of these. Support sharing on any level can be denoted as the sum of supports for all elements on lower levels occurring alone. Whilst this is logical there is further complexity, as traditionally the support for AB has included the instances of ABC, ABD and ABCD and so on, and it is not clear how many times AB occurs in seclusion. To determine this there is a need to reverse engineer or deconstruct the support as demonstrated in Table 2. To reveal the deconstructed elemental support for each element the participation of each element at all levels must be calculated get an accurate value for each element in isolation not simply in those patterns with a direct linear relationship. This can be denoted as:

Esupport(focus element) = Tsupport(focus element) – Esupport for each lower level element in which the focus element occurs. (E denotes elemental and T traditional).

Elements	A	AB	ABC	ABCD	Total
Traditional support %	16	10	5	4	35
Elemental support %	6	5	1	4	16

Table 2. Comparison of traditional and elemental supports.

In the simplified example in Table 2, we can see that the effect of adding element C to element AB is negative in that it has a lower elemental support than AB alone. In contrast adding element D to element ABC increases the elemental support of ABC, and hence denotes an increase of a positive outcome overall using this example. The obvious other comparisons needed here are the elemental supports for ABD, ACD, AC and AD to determine whether C actually adds value in the presence of D or if it is redundant and D is really the differentiator. This method has demonstrated a potential to show how much each element affects the outcome described in the pattern. In a real world example this would, for example, show the most or least effective combinations of medications which would allow for more accurate targeting of medications and potentially a reduction in the number of medications taken.

Through developing a greater knowledge regarding the importance of an element to an overall pattern three types of element can be identified; positive, negative and inert.

- Positive elements are those which increase the elemental support of an element it joins with in a manner which would influence the subjective interest in the resultant pattern.

- Negative elements are those which decrease the elemental support of an element it joins with and again would influence the subjective interest in the resultant pattern.
- Inert elements are those which do not affect the elemental support of an element it joins with. The subjective interest in this element cannot be determined. It could be that the lack of effect would in itself be valuable knowledge and would therefore affect a decision based upon it.

Elemental support can report on how important each element is to each pattern it participates in. A remaining issue is how to determine those pattern elements which have been recorded frequently enough to be eliminated due to the probability that they would already be known. Essentially the more relationships an element is involved in the more likely it is to be uninteresting. By evaluating the overall frequency of the pattern we can determine which are more unique or important and this would also assist in reducing the overall numbers of patterns by facilitating the removal of patterns or pattern elements which contain knowledge encountered frequently. This issue can be addressed by a determination of element weighting.

4.3.3 Element weighting

A frequent criticism of automated data analysis in medicine is that too many rules are produced and they often represent knowledge which is commonly known. For example if an element 'A' participates in only one pattern whereas 'C' is involved in many patterns it could be assumed that the effect of 'C' is more likely to be known, as it has been recorded more frequently. Solutions have been documented which involve the development and referencing of a knowledge base to hold 'known' patterns (Kononenko, 1993; Lucas, 1996; Perner, 1996; Moser, 1999). Whilst this has been demonstrated to be a valuable tool for reducing the numbers of known patterns presented, there are potential issues with this approach:

- The human resource time required to build and maintain a sufficiently complete knowledge base for practical use;
- The need to apply the knowledge subjectively to prevent exclusion of unusual or marginally different patterns and inclusion of different but non-informative patterns, and;
- The need to be sure that the knowledge base was developed from a sufficiently similar data set so that a comparison can be confidently made

This section presents a solution that begins to address these issues through a method of evaluating patterns based on pattern element weightings. ADAPT uses element weightings to compare the importance of elements within patterns, and combined element weights to compare patterns within levels. In this way element weights allow for subjective judgements to be made from original data rather than from comparison to external sources which may have been developed using different heuristics and/or from data with different characteristics, and/or origins. Pattern element weightings also facilitate subjective pattern evaluation through an understanding that the patterns and elements are representative of the data set from which they were derived and the rate of occurrence in the patterns can be compared with the occurrence in the data source to ensure that what seems frequent or rare is actually so. As suggested above, an element which participates in many relationships is more likely to be known and cannot effectively be used as a discriminator, but elements which participate in few relationships can be considered a discriminating participant and the application of element weightings will allow for accurate quantification of this quality.

As a first step toward automating the determination of element representation, a technique commonly used in the field of Information Retrieval (IR) that finds its origins in Information Theory (IT) has been utilised. IR is concerned with the classification of text and text based documents and offers a valuable perspective on the evaluation of worth for individual text elements of a set in the context of document classification, indexing and searching. Modern applications have included the evaluation of internet search results to quantify the relevance of a document to the user supplied search terms. Results containing a higher frequency of terms or a greater number of terms would be classified as more relevant. Researchers in the field suggest that rather than having a binary weighting, a non-binary measure should be used to determine the degree of similarity between sets of terms in a document or query (Baeza-Yates & Ribeiro-Neto, 1999). This would be applied to rank results even if they only partially matched the requirements. Fuzzy set theory is applied to allow for consideration of partial membership of a set and gives a measure of closeness to ideal membership i.e. how similar each set of terms is to each other. Seminal work in this area was published in 1988 by Salton and Buckley (Salton & Buckley, 1988) which described the use of a formula named tf.idf (TFIDF) to quantify the similarity between the contents of a document and user requirements as defined through a set of query terms.

TFIDF's ability to represent the amount of information value contained in a word in a sequence or document suggests a similar approach may be useful in determining element and/or pattern relevance. TFIDF is a weighting comprised of the two functions Term Frequency (TF) & Inverse Document Frequency (IDF). Term frequency is the frequency of a specific term in a document which indicates the importance of a term t_i to that document. It is formally described as;

$$TF = \frac{n_i}{\sum_k n_k} \tag{1}$$

where n_i is the number of occurrences of the specific term in a document and $\sum_k n_k$ the number of occurrences of all terms in the document.

Inverse document frequency indicates a terms importance with regard to the corpus. Based in part on information theory it is the logarithm of all the documents divided by the number of documents containing a specific term. Formally it is;

$$IDF = \log\left(\frac{|D|}{|(d_i \supset t_i)|}\right) \tag{2}$$

where $|D|$ is the total number of documents in the corpus and $|(d_i \supset t_i)|$ is the number of document within which term t_i occurs assuming $n_i \neq 0$.

TFIDF quantifies word frequency in a document such that the more frequently a word appears in a document (e.g., its TF, term frequency is high) the more it is estimated to be significant in that document while IDF measures how infrequent a word is in the collection and accordingly if a word is very frequent in the corpus (collection of documents), it is considered to be non-representative of this document (since it occurs in most documents). In contrast, if the word is infrequent in the text collection, it is suggested to be very relevant for the document. This characteristic facilitates the filtering out of common terms due to their lower ranking scores/weights.

This approach can be translated to the evaluation of medical patterns by simply re-stating the concepts and substituting comparable terms as follows:
TF can be applied to determine the frequency with which a pattern element occurs within a particular pattern sub-set at the same level or cardinality for a given support e.g. all 4 element patterns with a minimum support of 40%. This is given the assumption that patterns of the same cardinality and support are contextually similar enough to be associated/chunked much like that of the sentences of a document and thus form a pseudo document. IDF can be applied to determine the frequency with which a pattern element occurs within the original data set. When brought together in the TFIDF calculation, the information represented by patterns at an equal level can be compared to the total set to derive an entropic measure at the element, pattern and sub-set levels. This is useful for the subjective analysis of medical patterns as it allows for the recognition of the amount of intra and inter-pattern importance (information value) of individual elements.
In data-mining terms TF can be seen as comparable to the traditional support of the pattern as it could be applied to determine the frequency of the pattern within the total pattern set or data. The novelty of the solution becomes apparent through the application of IDF. In pattern analysis this could be defined as either the frequency of the pattern against all patterns in the present set or data source or the frequency of the element in all patterns in the set or data source. As the focus is on the value of an element within a pattern, the second definition was applied. By combining both of these into a value for TFIDF the frequency of element ABC within the pattern set is calculated and multiplied by the log of inverse frequency of element ABC in the data source. This will show us if that element participates in many or few other patterns and whether the element frequency is representative of the data source. If we achieve a low value this will show that the occurrence of the element in the pattern set is dissimilar to that in data source. If we have a high value then this is indicative of an inert element for example the gender element in the gender = female and condition = pregnancy pattern which would occur with high frequently in both the data source and the pattern set.
Traditional metrics have not been documented in such an application, but for the reasons discussed above it is an important issue in medical pattern analysis.

5. Experimental results

5.1 Methodology

ADAPT was tested using data collected from the Royal Australasian College of Surgeons National Breast Cancer Audit[1,2].
Association rule patterns were produced from these data to demonstrate that ADAPT is able to perform well on the most problematic mining algorithm for medical data due to the potential for a large number of patterns to be presented. It is hence the area which stands to benefit most from ADAPT.

---

[1] The supplied data has since been superseded and hence results detailed herein may or may not accurately reflect current data or practices within the management of breast cancer in Australia or New Zealand and hence should not be relied upon in a clinical setting.
[2] Acknowledgement and thanks are hereby given to the ASERNIP-S Adelaide team for their permission to use this data.

The original source data held 23,259 patient records, 53,950 separate surgical procedure records for those patients and 82 attributes with an average of 5 potential values per attribute across three tables. After combining patient records with their surgical procedures, allowing for multiple procedures performed together, then removing duplicate columns and extraneous data including dates, 42,705 records with 39 columns were mined using a simple association rule mining tool with support set at 1%.

ADAPT was applied to test the validity of four theories, and provide information relating to one area of interest described in the data dictionary provided with the data. The 5 cases analysed were:

1. "Some treatment recommendations differ by menopausal status, e.g. Ovarian ablation is not indicated after the menopause."
2. "The omission of axillary dissection should be considered only in the case of small primary tumours and is least desirable in pre-menopausal women but is standard in cases of DCIS"
3. "The presence of a significant amount of DCIS in or adjacent to an invasive tumour is a predictor of high relapse rates following wide local excision and radiotherapy.
4. "For DCIS, 'clear margins' as defined by no tumour within 1mm of any inked margins are associated with a high rate of recurrence."
5. It was also suggested that "correlations between excision technique and cosmetic result may be useful."

Interesting patterns were defined as those which contained the particular attribute values required to test the cases - as described in the results section.

5.2 Results

Association rules were developed to provide patterns relating to the five cases listed above using the attributes and values detailed in Table 5. For some cases it was necessary to apply different sets of attributes and develop more than one set of patterns for analysis to test each part of a more complex theory in isolation.

The results of the five test cases are detailed in Table 6 which shows elemental supports and TFIDF values. TFIDF was categorised on whether it fell in the upper or lower values for representativeness. Positive elements are shown in bold, negative in italic and inert in standard text and were classified as described earlier. One is denoted as both positive and negative based upon the elements which preceded it. Table 7 shows the descriptive potential of ADAPT based on these heuristics. Overall, only one of the theories was fully supported by the data and two were fully discounted with one gaining partial support. The TFIDF value was able to indicate if this result is generally representative. Where the theory pattern was in the lower level of representativeness it suggests that the theory should not be depended upon and its foundation should be investigated further.

5.3 Discussion

Data mining has many documented benefits for the medical domain and much work is being done to provide medicine specific solutions to data analysis problems. However this work has focussed on the adaptation of technologies to manage the complexities and non-uniform nature of medical data and while the management of input is being addressed, research by the author has been unable to find evidence of a similar effort in the management and translation of outputs. This is an issue when non statisticians or computer scientists are attempting to make sense of the technology and its products. It has been reported that medical practitioners in general have little experience in statistical analysis and as a result are unable to apply or comprehend results which do not match their sphere of knowledge and understanding and as such they need assistance in translating or deciphering the meaning or content of statistical analysis which is beyond the complexity of a 0.05 p-value or confidence interval of 95% (Shillabeer & Pfitzner, 2007, Link & Marz, 2006). This has a

Case	Focal Element A	Element B	Element C	Element D
1	Menopause Status 1	Ovarian ablation 1	NA	NA
2.1	Ax Dis. 3	DCIS 2	NA	NA
2.2	Ax Dis. 3	Menopause Status 1	NA	NA
2.3	Size > 15	Aux Dis. 0	NA	NA
3.1	Relapse 2	EIC 1	Surgery 2	Radio 1
3.2	Relapse 1	EIC 1	Surgery 2	Radio 1
4	Relapse 2	DCIS 2	Clear mar.	NA
5.1	Surgery	Symmetry3	NA	NA
5.2	Surgery	Symmetry1	NA	NA

Table 5. Pattern attributes and values for each case

Case	A	AB	AC	AD	ABC	ACD	ABD	ABCD	TF/IDF	Theory proven/ Representative
1	59.85	0							NA	Yes/NA
2.1	10.01	*4.61*							0.1975	No/upper - generally applicable
2.2	12.88	**13.04**							0.1421	Yes/lower - conditionally applicable
2.3	18.04	0							0.1837	Yes/upper - generally applicable
3.1	2.27	0	0	0					NA	No/NA
3.2	12.62	*2.27*	2.44	**4.18**	*0.53*	**2.04**	**9.91**	*1.46*	0.0704	No/lower - conditionally applicable
4	0.22	**1.03**	0						NA	No/NA
5.1	30.98	*1.02*							0.1488	NA/lower - conditionally applicable
5.2	13.59	*7.2*							0.1510	NA/lower - conditionally applicable

Table 6. Elemental supports and TFIDF heuristics

Case	Traditionally formatted data mining patterns for each case	ADAPT description
1	"Meno_Status":2.00, "Ovarian_Ablation":2.00 (49.48%) "Meno_Status":2.00, "Ovarian_Ablation":9.00 (9.83%)	No post-menopausal patients received an ovarian ablation.
2.1	"Insitu_Necrosed":2.00 (14.62%) "Insitu_Necrosed":2.00, "Ax_Type":3.00 (4.61%)	Axillary Dissection is equally applied and omitted in DCIS cases.
2.2	"Meno_Status":1.00 (25.92%) "Meno_Status":1.00, "Ax_Type":3.00 (13.04%)	Half of all pre-menopausal women have axillary dissection and there was no level of omission.
2.3	"Tumor_Size":20.00, "Ax_Type":3.00 (3.10%) "Tumor_Size":0.00, "Ax_Type":0.00 (10.35%)	No cases of larger tumours avoid axillary dissection.
3.1	None	Relapse is not paired with relevant attributes.
3.2	"Surgical_Event":2.00, "Status":1.00, "EIC_Status":1.00, "Radiotherapy":1.00 (1.46%)	Non relapse is paired with the theoretical pattern.
4	None	Clear margins with DCIS are not an indicator of relapse.
5.1 5.2	"Surgical_Event":5.00, "Symmetry":1.00 (1.49%) "Surgical_Event":4.00, "Symmetry":3.00 (1.02%) "Surgical_Event":4.00, "Symmetry":1.00 (15.44%) "Surgical_Event":3.00, "Symmetry":1.00 (3.53%) "Surgical_Event":2.00, "Symmetry":1.00 (24.44%) "Surgical_Event":1.00, "Symmetry":1.00 (7.20%)	Only total mastectomy was associated with a poor result. Open biopsy has ranked highest for good results >50%

Table 7. Comparison of data mining pattern output and ADAPT description output

potential two pronged effect, it puts data mining technologies and the like out of the reach of many medical practitioners and, it necessitates the application of only the most basic analytical tools thus negating the potential of the more powerful tools.

The contribution of the work presented here is in its ability to broaden the applicability and marketability for the technology by making outputs approachable to all user types and levels without minimising the complexity or range of processes available. It does not attempt to modify the data mining process as the algorithms and statistical methods available currently are generally applicable and effective for the medical domain and have been used successfully by many medical teams. However these projects are often undertaken by specialists who understand the tools and technologies or they have required manual post mining translation or interpretation of outputs by domain specialists (Imberman & Domanski 2002; Moser et al., 1999). The results presented here show that ADAPT is able to facilitate the ordering and presentation of complex outputs in a more intuitive language and provide the knowledge items required for decision making as described earlier. It is also able to overcome some of the more potent criticisms of the technology, for example the belief that the results of data mining are not always representative of the data set from which they were created and they are often misreported as a result (Milloy, 1995; Raju, 2003; Smith & Ebrahim, 2002). Whilst ADAPT pattern interpretations are currently manually created, a future challenge will be to create an automated natural language description of patterns based on the heuristics provided by the process.

5.4 Conclusion

Results have been developed from patterns which are far simpler that the technology is capable of providing; however the theories were often binary and did not require the production of multi-faceted patterns. Data mining would not generally be applied to develop such simple patterns but it has proved to be a suitable demonstration of the process in a realistic application. Also, the focus here was on the application of the ADAPT process rather than on the application of data mining technologies and the simplistic patterns provided an unambiguous and non-complex platform from which to work. ADAPT has demonstrated an ability to mirror the earlier identified trusted process of medical knowledge acquisition thereby facilitating the application of data mining technologies into clinical decision making, theory validation and hypothesis generation. Of particular relevance is the ability to apply both objective and subjective measures of interest to guide the knowledge aquisition process. The novelty and power of the solution is demonstrated through its ability to provide individualised case based knowledge reflecting the growth in personalised, evidence based clinical care. The logical next step is to process the results of more complex association rule mining through ADAPT and validate the output through empirical testing. This work tested and demonstrated the potential for ADAPT on essentially one tailed tests, but the real power of the methodology and its parts will become evident when applied to purely exploratory data mining.

The primary areas of contribution are in its ability to respond to the following issues;

1. The low level of flexibility in data mining systems and the need for medical analytical processes to adapt to data mining methodologies rather than data mining adapting to the needs of medicine,
2. The production of patterns in a technical language and format that are often not understandable or applicable in a clinical setting,
3. The production of results that require a high level of user interpretation to discriminate those that are truly useful.

The functionality and process flow of the system was designed to reflect the process of medical diagnostic decision making and is demonstrated through its ability to discriminate and translate the technical outputs of data mining into a clinically understandable and applicable form. Both the hypothesis engine and ADAPT are able to manage any data mining outputs but testing has been performed on the most problematic form of mining output; association rules. It is in this use of the technology that we see the greatest problem with large numbers of uninteresting or irrelevant results that require intensive user evaluation and interpretation. It is believed that by addressing the area of greatest issue the power of the solution has most clearly been demonstrated.

There are many applications of data mining technologies in medicine with some being more successful than others as discussed in this chapter.

Specific applications and benefits of the work presented in this chapter include:

- providing a more approachable interface to data mining technologies
- provision of a more medicine specific format for outputs both in terms of user needs and technical knowledge
- ability to reduce pharmaceutical costs through the ability to identify most beneficial or effective combinations of medications for particular conditions or sub sets of the population
- Ability to enhance the knowledge base of the practicing clinician as required and in a real time context
- Ability to provide an automated solution which can mirror trusted methodologies
- provision of a system which can apply trusted metrics for the measurement of validity and applicability of outcomes
- provision of a system which can provide statistically valid and trustworthy hypothesis
- provision of an automated system that can assimilate the subjective and objective needs of any medical professional
- provision of a system which incorporates current technologies and provides knowledge in an understandable format and language
- provision of a system which is developed through an understanding of the unique needs of the medical profession and is based upon the application of methodologies developed over centuries of medical research
- development of solutions to the documented impediments to the acceptance and utilisation of data mining in the medical field
- development of solutions to address many of the documented issues in medical data mining

5.7 Future research

The need now is to build systems which allow for changes and improvements without the need to rebuild systems and carry the burden of lost productivity due to development time and cost, neither of which are insubstantial. Also it will become increasingly important in the future to consider a wider range of users as patients themselves become more empowered and willing to collaborate with their treating professionals in regard to their own treatment. There is an increasing thirst for personalised knowledge and information and an increasing expectation that this thirst will be quenched in real time thus necessitating a tool such as that discussed in this chapter. It was estimated in 2001 that up to one third of all Internet surfing was related to the search for health information (Kapur, 2001). Increasing use of the Internet has empowered the general public but this empowerment has not always been embraced by medical professionals. The environment in which medicine is practiced has changed dramatically through history although the founding principles have remained relatively static. The biggest change has been in the informedness and hence power of the people to influence and engage in their diagnosis and treatment, thus requiring a greater breadth and depth of knowledge in the treating specialist.

Whilst the discussion presented in this chapter has clearly demonstrated the potential benefits of the application of automated data analysis techniques such as data mining in the search for new, clinically applicable knowledge in the medical domain, the following issues remain;

- The lack of perceived trust in automated systems
- Lack of computer literacy across the medical profession making the application of technical solutions to data analysis needs currently unfeasible.
- The lack of uniform data standards within and across jurisdictions.
- The difficulty in sourcing suitable datasets for the development and testing of automated systems
- Lack of data sharing protocols for data sharing between health providers.

Although this is a leading edge area of research and the building blocks of solutions to address the changing needs of medicine have already been built and tested, work must now continue to perfect solutions to these issues before automated knowledge acquisition becomes integrated as a natural part of standard medical data analysis practice.

6. References

Said al-Andalusí, Science in the Medieval World: "Book of the Categories of Nations" (trans. Sema'an I. Salem and Alok Kumar, 1991, University of Texas Press.

Ashby, D., Smith, A.: The best medicine? Plus magazine - living mathematics (2002)

BBC. :John Snow (1813-1854). Accessed 15/05/04 at www.ph.ucla.edu/epi/snow.html

Beals, M., Gross, L., Harrell, S.: Diversity indices: Shannon's H and E (1999)

Beals, M., Gross, L., Harrell, S.: Diversity indices: Simpsons (1999)

Baeza-Yates, R. & Ribeiro-Neto, B., (1999), "Modern Information Retrieval", Addison-Wesley, Sydney

Biedl, T., Brejova, B., Demaine, E. D., Hamel, A. M., Vinar, T. Optimal Arrangement of Leaves in the Tree Representing Heirarchical Clustering of Gene Expression Data. Technical Report 2001-14. University of Waterloo, ON, Canada.

Bojarczuk C. C., Lopes H. S., Freitas A. A., Data mining with constrained-syntax genetic programming: applications in medical data sets. In proc. Intelligent Data Analysis in Medicine and Pharmacology (IDAMAP-2001)

Bresnahan, J.: Data mining - a delicate operation. CIO Magazine (1997)

Brieger, G. H. (1977), 'H 1 coulter. divided legacy: A history of the schism in medical thought.', Isis 69(1), 103--105.

Cabri, G., Ferrari, L., Leonardi, L., Zambonelli, F. Role based approaches for Agent Development. AAMAS'04. July 19-23 2004. New York U.S.A.

Cios, K.J., Moore, G.W. Uniqueness of Medical Data Mining. Artificial Intelligence in Medicine Journal. Vol26. No. 1-2, September-October 2002 1-24.

Cornwell, J. Hype or Hope? The Weekend Australian Magazine. Aug 27-28 2005. 36-41.

Cosans, C. E. (1997), 'Galen's critique of rationalist and empiricist anatomy', Journal of the History of Biology 30, 35--54.

Elstein AS, and Schwartz A. Evidence Base of Clinical Diagnosis. BMJ March 2002: Vol. 324: 729-732.

Fauser, B. C. & Edwards, R. G. (2005), 'The early days of IVF', Human Reproduction Update 11(5), 437--438.

Fayyad U.M, Piatetsky-Shapiro G, and Smyth P. From Data Mining to Knowledge Discovery in Databases. AI Magazine. 1996: Vol 7 Issue 3: 37-54.

Ferrailo, D., Kuhn, R. An Introduction to Role-Based Access Control. NIST/ITL Bulletin December 1995.

Frenster JH. Matrix Cognition in Medical Decision Making. In: Proceedings of the AAMSI Congress on Medical Informatics. San Fransisco: Volume 7 1989; pp 131-134.

Gebski V, and Keech A. Statistical methods in clinical trials. Medical Journal of Australia. 2003: 178: 182–184.

Geng L, and Hamilton HJ. Interestingness Measures for Data Mining: A Survey. ACM Computing Surveys 2006; Vol.38(3): Article 9.

Gopal, K. (1997), Rationalist victory, Technical report, Online at http://www.iheu.org/node/668.

Hagland M. Data mining. Healthcare Informatics Online 2004: 21:33-6. Accessed 28/3/2005.

Hanson, A. E. (2006), Hippocrates: The "greek miracle" in medicine, Technical report, Online at www.medicineantiqua.org.uk/sa_hippint.html.

Hilderman, R.J., Hamilton, H.J.: Evaluation of interestingness measures for ranking discovered knowledge. In 5th PAKDD 2001. Volume 2035 of LNCS., Hong Kong, China, Springer (2001) 247–259

Horton, R. (2000), 'How sick is modern medicine?', The New York Review of Books 47(17).

Imberman SP, and Domanski B. Using dependancy/association rules to find indications for computerised tomography in a head trauma dataset. Artificial Intelligence in Medicine. September 2002: Vol. 26: 55-68.

Katch, F. I. (1997), History makers, Technical report, Online at www.sportsci.org/news/history/lind/lind_sp.html.

Kaul, M. & Thadani, S. Development of philosophical thought and scientific method in ancient India, Technical report, Online at http://members.tripod.com/INDIA_RESOURCE/scienceh.htm.

Kononenko I. Inductive and Bayesian Learning in Medical datasets. Journal of Applied Artificial Intelligence. (1993) 317-337.

Kuonen, D.: Challenges in bioinformatics for statistical data miners. Bulletin of the Swiss Statistical Society (2003) 10–17

Lavrac N., Keravnou E., Zupan B. Intelligent data analysis in medicine. Encyclopaedia of Library and Information Science. Vol. 68 Supplement 31. (2000) 209-254.

Link TM, and Marz R. Computer literacy and attitudes towards e-learning among first year medical students. BMC Medical Education. June 2006: 6:34.

Lord, S., Gebski, V., Keech, A.: Multiple analyses in clinical trials: sound science or data dredging? MJA 181 (2004) 452–454

Lucas P. Enhancement of Learning by Declarative Expert-based Models. In proc. Intelligent data analysis in biomedicine and pharmacology. Budapest, Hungary. (1996)

Marshall, B. J. (1998), Peptic ulcers, stomach cancer and the bacteria which are responsible, Accessed 15/03/06 from www.knaw.nl/heinekenprizes/pdf/37.pdf.

Merck & Co. Medical Decision Tests. www.merck.com/mmhe/print /sec25/ch300/ch300.html Accessed 14/09/2006.

Milloy S. Science Without Sense. The Risky Business of public health, Cato Institute, Washington DC.

Mohaghegh, M. (1988), 'Miftah al-tibb wa minhaj altullab (a summary translation)', Medical Journal of the Islamic Republic of Iran 2(1), 61--63.

Moser SA, Jones WT, and Brossette SE. Application of Data Mining to Intensive Care Unit Microbiological Data. Emerging Infectious Diseases. 1999:5:3: 454-457.

Muhaqqiq, M. (n.d.), 'Medical sects in islam', al-Tawhid Islamic Journal 8(2).

Ordonez, C., Omiecinski, E., deBraal, L., Santana, C., Ezquerra, N., Taboada, J.,Cooke, C., Krawczynska, E., Garcia, E.: Mining constrained association rules to predict heart disease. In: ICDM'01, San Jose. California. (2001) 433–440

Page Wise. The History of Penecillin. Accessed 15/05/04 from http://oh.essortment.com/historyofpen_pnd.htm

Pearcy, L. (1985), 'Galen: a biographical sketch', Archaeology 38(6 (Nov/Dec)), 33--39.

Perner P. Mining Knowledge in X-Ray Images for Lung Cancer Diagnosis. In proc. Intelligent data analysis in biomedicine and pharmacology. Budapest, Hungary. (1996).

Pollard, R. (2006), Fortuitous discovery led to a revolution in treatment, Technical report, Online at http://www.smh.com.au/news/science/fortuitous-discovery-led-to-a-revolution-in-treatment/2006/10/11/1160246197925.html.

Raju S. Data Flaws. American Council on Science & Health. www.healthfactsandfears.com/high_priorities/vs/2003/data072303.html Accessed 23/9/2003.

Roddick, J.F., Fule, P., Graco, W.J.: Exploratory medical knowledge discovery : Experiences and issues. SigKDD Explorations 5 (2003) 94–99

Roddick, J.F., Rice, S.P.: What's interesting about cricket? - on thresholds and anticipation in discovered rules. SIGKDD Explorations 3 (2001) 1–5

Salton, G. and Buckley, C., (1988), "Term-Weighting Approaches in Automatic Text Retrieval", Information Processing Management, Vol. 24, No. 5, pp.513-523.

Shillabeer A, and Pfitzner D. Determining pattern element contribution in medical datasets. In: ACSC, Vol.29. No.7. ACSW Frontiers 2007; pp 209-216.

Shillabeer A, and Roddick JF. Towards Role Based Hypothesis Evaluation for Health Data Mining. Electronic Journal of Health Informatics 2006:1(1):1-8.

Smith GD, and Ebrahim S. Data dredging - bias or confounding. BMJ Dec. 2002: Vol.325:1437-1438.

Sprang, K. (2002), Dr. Edward Jenner and the smallpox vaccination, Technical report, Online at http://scsc.essortment.com/edwardjennersm_ rmfk.htm.

Stone, C., McLachlan, K., Halliday, J., Wein, P., Tippett, C.: Gestational diabetes in victoria in 1996: incidence, risk factors and outcomes. MJA 177 (2002) 486–491

Swan N. IVF Pioneers. Radio National Australia. Accessed 25/04/2005 from www.abc.net.au/rn/talks/8.30/helthrpt/stories/s1349685.htm

Tan P. N., Kumar V., Srivastava J. Selecting the right interestingness measure for association patterns. SIGKDD. Alberta, Canada. (2002)

Tripod South Asian History Project (2002), Philosophical development from Upanishadic metaphysics to scientific realism, Technical report, Online at http://india_resource.tripod.com/upanishad.html.

Work In progress workshop in population health. May 19th 2005. Flinders Medical Centre.

6

Radiology Data Mining Applications using Imaging Informatics

Richard Chen MD, MBA[1], Pattanasak Mongkolwat PhD[2] and David Channin MD[2]
[1]*Ohio State University College of Medicine, Columbus, OH*
[2]*Northwestern University Feinberg School of Medicine, Chicago, IL*
USA

1. Introduction

The radiology department is a unique department within the healthcare enterprise. It has its roots within technology and is a naturally information-rich area within which data can be mined, analyzed and used to improve departmental operations. The recent migration of many healthcare enterprises to PACS (picture archiving and communication systems) helps to facilitate this trend. This chapter will provide an overview of the various technologies in the radiology department that allow for data-mining. Case-examples utilizing these technologies are then discussed in detail.

2. PACS and DICOM

PACS are computer distribution networks that are dedicated to the storage and retrieval of medical images. The systems started as simple image management systems which have currently involved to include images, voice, text, medical records, and video recordings (Huang et al, 2005). Numerous studies have reported productivity gains associated with PACS implementations (Mackinnon et al., 2008). Fundamental to PACS is the display of images using Digital Imaging and Communications in Medicine (DICOM) headers.
DICOM is a universally used format for medical image storage. The standard was originally created by the National Electrical Manufacturers Association (NEMA) and the American College of Radiology (ACR) for medical image archiving and communication (NEMA, 2008, Horii et al., 1992). It is currently maintained by the DICOM Standards Committee. It is important as it guarantees a minimum level of compatibility between hardware and software publishers from a number of different manufacturers. DICOM encapsulates datasets objects which accompany the image. These dataset objects contain much information about the associated image(s). DICOM files contain a header which specify information related to patient name, medical record number, image type (x-ray, CT scan, MRI, ultrasound, etc), and image dimension. The files then also contain all of the image data. This differs from other formats which store the header and image data in separate files. DICOM also allows storage space for more elaborate data constructions, from which an innumerable amount of information may be gleaned. This includes information such as

image transit information across the PACS system marked with timestamps, or radiologist view and dictation times (NEMA DICOM, 2008).

3. Health level 7 and integrating the healthcare enterprise

In addition to DICOM standardization for PACS platforms, there are multiple efforts underway to standardize and improve the way with which information is exchanged within the healthcare industry. The goal is to develop semantic language structures to meet the demands and challenges of inter-operability between existing and future generations of health information systems (Lopez et al., 2008, Blobel et al., 2006). One such initiative is Health Level 7 (HL7), a volunteer, not-for-profit organization which provides a framework to share electronic health information (HL7, 2008). The scope of HL7 includes standards for the exchange of clinical data in all settings – it allows the exchange of information through a generalized reference informational model, via various data types, and through the use of decision support trees. It includes provisions for security, XML data exchange, and general electronic health record use (Hammond, 2003). Derivations of the reference informational model also allow inclusion of clinical documents, such as the ANSI-approved Clinical Document Architecture (CDA), a document markup standard that specifies the structure and semantics of clinical documentation (Dolin et al., 2001).

Another initiative to facilitate healthcare data exchange is that of the IHE (Integrating the Healthcare Enterprise), a collaboration between healthcare professionals and industry members to improve data interoperability, focusing on the development of global integration profiles and a clear implementation path using existing medical standards such as DICOM and HL7, while encouraging members to uphold compatibility (IHE, 2008). IHE is important because it approaches tasks at a much higher level, taking care not to specify specific roles for specific applications, but rather defining a set of generic "actors" and a set of roles that these actors much play to successfully accomplish a given task (Channin, 2000). Systems supporting IHE have been shown to enable healthcare providers to use information more effectively in providing better and more-informed care when managing patients ((Lian et al., 2006). Its success lies in its adoption by industry professional organizations representing both buyers and vendors (Hussein et al., 2004).

4. Case example: RadMonitor

4.1 Introduction.

This section describes a case example, RadMonitor. The tool was designed within our department as a platform-independent web application designed to help manage the complexity of information flow within a healthcare enterprise. The system eavesdrops on HL7 traffic and parses statistical operational information into a database. The information is then presented to the user as a treemap – a graphical visualization scheme that simplifies the display of hierarchical information. While RadMonitor has been implemented for the purpose of analyzing radiology operations, its XML backend allows it to be reused for virtually any other hierarchical dataset.

4.2 Technologies.

The RadMonitor design involves a traditional three-tier architecture consisting of the database, server and client (Figure 1). Radiology operations information flows from an HL7 data feed to a MySQL relational database. Clients then interact with this data through a JavaScript enabled web browser and a server-side processing script.

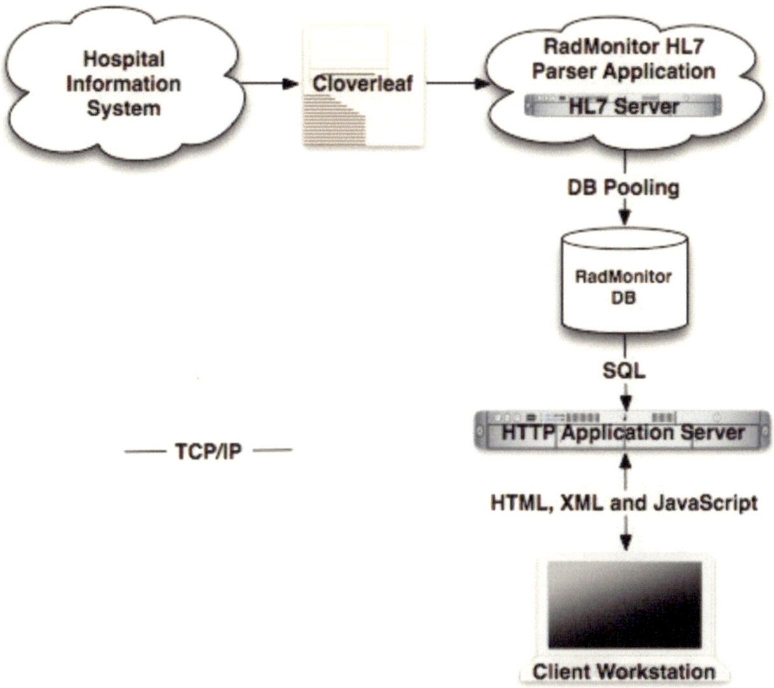

Fig. 1. RadMonitor implementation design.

In the backend, an HL7 application on the server receives order message (ORM) and result message (ORU) data feeds from Quovadx, formerly known as Cloverleaf. It is used to parse the HL7 messages, and allows us to map, route and extract data from the hospital information system. Statistical information relevant to radiology operations management is stored in the RadMonitor database. Database entries include fields that represent order status changes, and start and stop dictation and transcription time events.

The information in the database is available to the client to query and retrieve. This is done through a server-side processing script written in PHP. All of the exchanges between the server and client are done using HTML, XML and JavaScript. While these technologies have been around for some time, RadMonitor makes extensive use of a relatively new twist of the technology - the XmlHttpRequest object.

4.3 Implementation.

RadMonitor was implemented to improve the delivery and utility of the treemap construct through a web platform. Our goal was to build a lightweight, extensible and standards-based solution, complete with the interactivity and responsiveness expected of a desktop application. Application interactivity was a key component in our design, and the use of AJAX allowed us to dramatically improve the user experience by deviating from the traditional web interaction model (Figure 2).

Initially, only HTML is rendered in the client web browser. This acts as an empty layout template, upon which subsequent AJAX queries fill respective sections of the page. The first section to be loaded is the treemap itself.

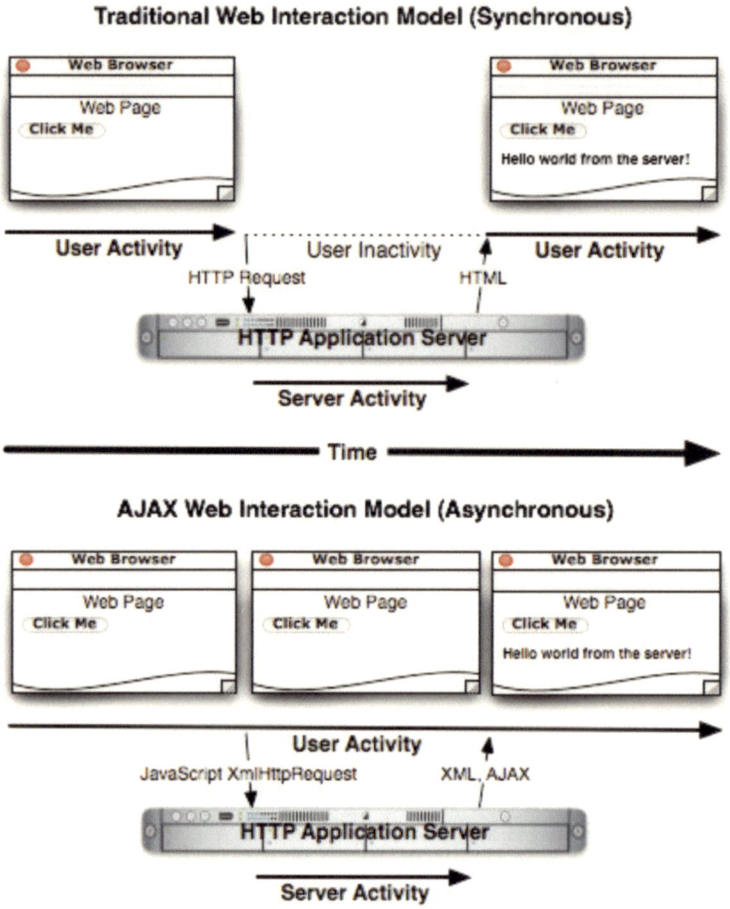

Fig. 2. The asynchronous AJAX user model provides for a user experience that is continuous without user inactivity as a result of time lags associated with page refreshes in a synchronous model.

The treemap is the centerpiece of the application (Figure 3). The three treemaps that RadMonitor currently supports are Orders, Radiologist and Staff. These selections are made using the radioboxes in the upper right corner of the page. The Radiologist treemap is a representation of the radiologists' average dictation time. Information is divided into a hierarchy of modalities, and radiologists within a modality. The size of an individual radiologist's rectangle is related to the number of studies that the radiologist has dictated. Correspondingly, the size of a modality's rectangle is indicative of the total number of studies dictated within that modality. The color and color gradient of a radiologist's rectangle is a measure of the average time that the radiologist has spent dictating exams as compared to the modality average. Green represents an average dictation time faster than the modality average, and red indicates times slower than the average. A similar hierarchical breakdown is applied to the Staff treemap, which displays information based on the staffs' average transcription time.

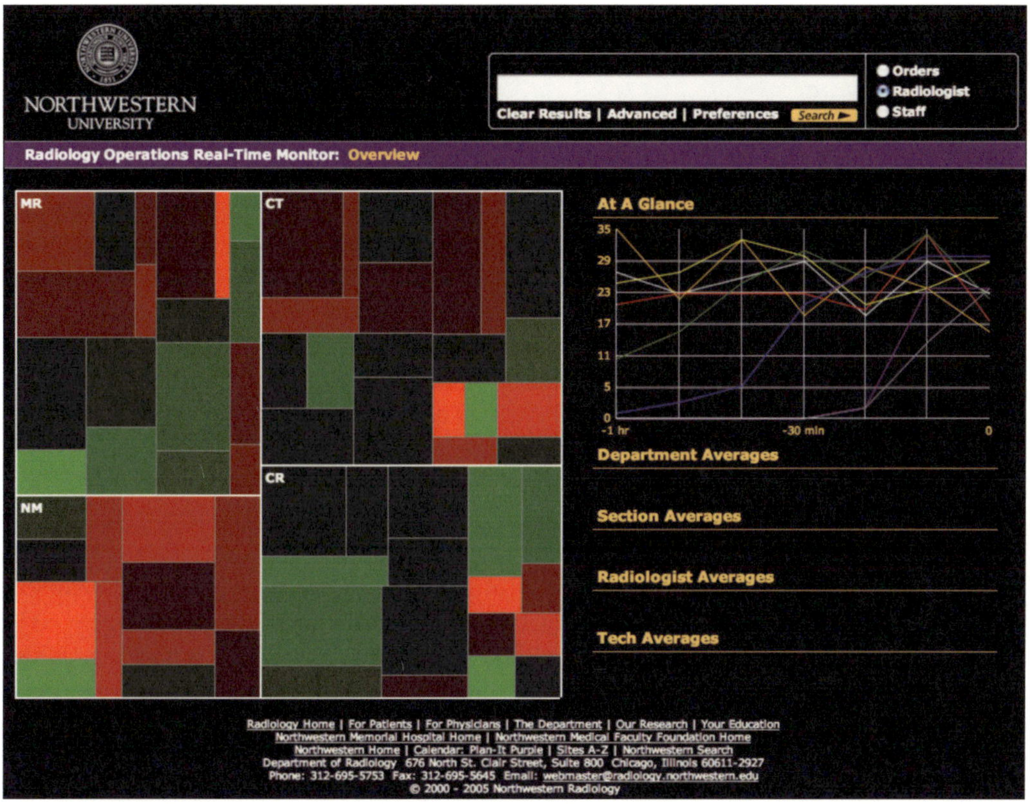

Fig. 3. RadMonitor application showing treemap with radiologists' comparative average dictation time represented by color and films read represented by size.

4.4 Discussion.

The use of these parameters results in a treemap that conveys information about the real-time operational statistics of the radiology department. This information is intuitively represented, and allows us to readily answer questions such as: Which modality reads the most number of exams? The least? How are the dictation times different between modalities? How about within a modality?

Information is the lifeblood of any business and healthcare is no exception. No single information system can manage the entirety of a healthcare enterprise of any significant size. RadMonitor is a tool designed to help manage the complexity of information flow within the hospital network. As with the dashboard concept, its utility lies in its use of proprietary or open data standards to interact and interface with other hospital information systems.

HL7 and DICOM standards are critical to this process. Specifically, the data feeds are instrumental for the communication of non-image and image based information, respectively. Furthermore, both HL7 and DICOM data feeds can serve as a source of valuable information about the status of operations in a department. A surprising amount of analytical information is contained within these messages. In addition to being vital to clinical and research activities, this information can be monitored, in real-time, to provide immediate decision support for administrative and management activities.

5. Case example: PACSMonitor

5.1 Introduction.

PACSMonitor is a tool designed to help manage the complexity of radiology information flow within the hospital network. As with the dashboard concept, its utility lies in its use of proprietary or open data standards to interact and interface with other hospital information systems. As with the above example, PACSMonitor mines HL7 and DICOM data for valuable information about the status of operations in the department. This information can be monitored, in real-time, to provide immediate decision support for administrative and management activities.

5.2 Technologies.

The PACSMonitor implementation involves a traditional three-tier architecture consisting of the database, server and client. The software was built to seamlessly interface with typical commercial PACS distributions. The stability of a PACS system with minimal unexpected PACS downtime is a fundamental concern for all hospitals. In order to maximize server load and minimize downtime and instability without adversely impacting system performance, PACSMonitor mines PACS information related to patient studies, examination acquisition studies and so forth during a daily off-peak cycle and stores this information in a separate pre-parsed database exclusively dedicated to PACSMonitor. In the backend, an HL7 application on the server receives order message (ORM) and result message (ORU, RAD-28) data feeds from Quovadx, formerly known as Cloverleaf. The ORM messages are based on IHE technical framework transactions RAD-1, RAD-2, RAD-3, RAD-4, RAD-6, RAD-7, RAD-10, RAD-13, RAD-20, RAD-21, RAD-42, and RAD49. These HL7 messages are parsed according to our application needs, allowing us to transparently map, route and extract data from the hospital information system. Statistical information relevant to radiology operations management is stored in the PACSMonitor database.
The information in the database is immediately available for clients to query. All client interaction with the web application is done via server-side processing scripts written in PHP. The exchanges between the server and client are all based on web standards using HTML, XML and JavaScript.

5.3 Implementation.

The main screen of PACS monitor is divided into a right frame comprising of various user reports and a left main window which houses both the report builder and the visualizations (Figure 4). Creating a report starts by choosing the database table from which the user wishes to query information. These table names are dynamically populated by inspection of the database and including all tables that are identified as containing statistical data. Next, the user has the option of choosing the type of report he wishes to view, including "Table", "Graph", or "Treemap". Each of these report types include options specific to their display. A table report, for instance, allows users to select which columns that they would like to include. The graph report allows users to specify the x and y axis, specific colors, as well as the type of graph (Figure 5). The treemap visualization allows users to select both the color and size of the data representations. Users are further able to customize the reports that they create using the "Match the following rules" option. This option allows users to fine-tune the data that they query from the database. Creating the report causes the new report to show up in the right frame.

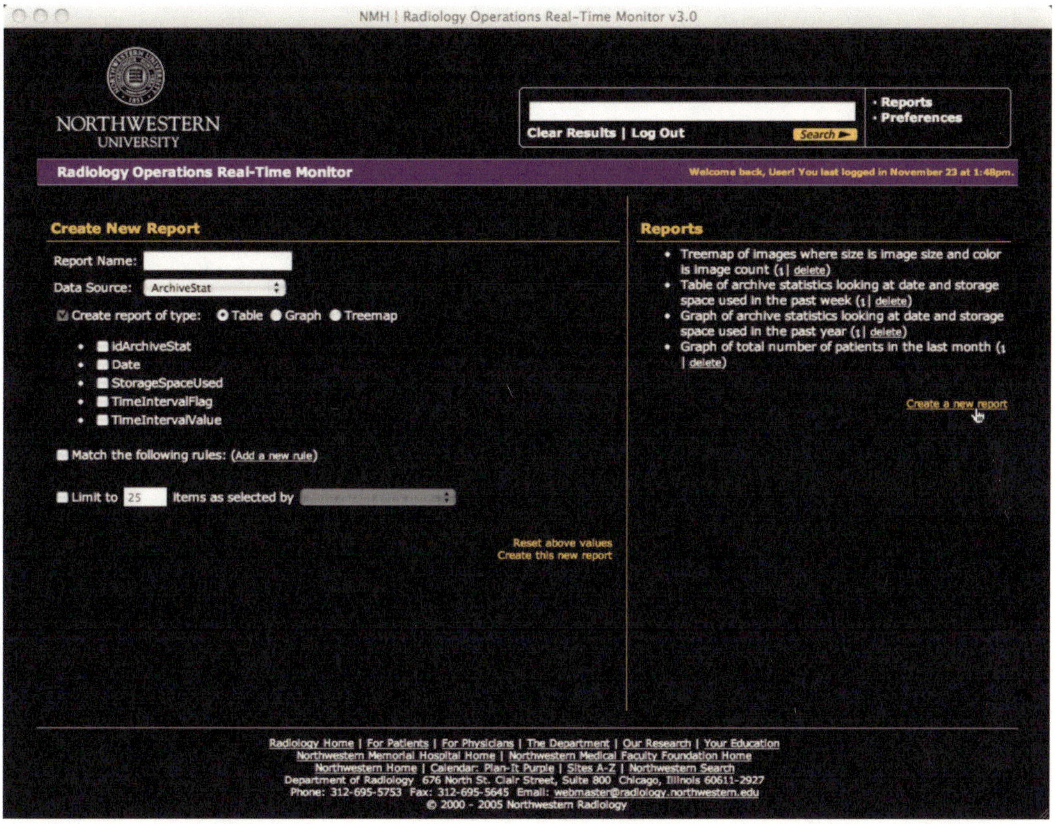

Fig. 4. This is a screenshot of the default view of the application. In the right frame, you can select an existing report to view or create a new report. The left frame shows an example of creating a new report.

The report builder interface simplifies the workflow by which users choose the information that they want to obtain. It offers standardized templates from which to choose and construct reports. Each report is stored on the database as a dynamically constructed SQL query. At the same time, the interface offers flexibility and customization for power users via "smart" selections that allow users to apply selective filters to the data queried from the database (Figure 6). These filters modify the SQL query to include modifiers such as "where", "limit", or "sort by". It is an example of the power of user-specified and user-constrained data, similar to that of the "smart playlist" concept in Apple's iTunes software. Users are thus virtually unlimited in the number of ways by which they can query specific data from the backend servers. Clicking on a report to view triggers the SQL query for the requested information, and the resulting dataset is sent to the report viewer script to render.

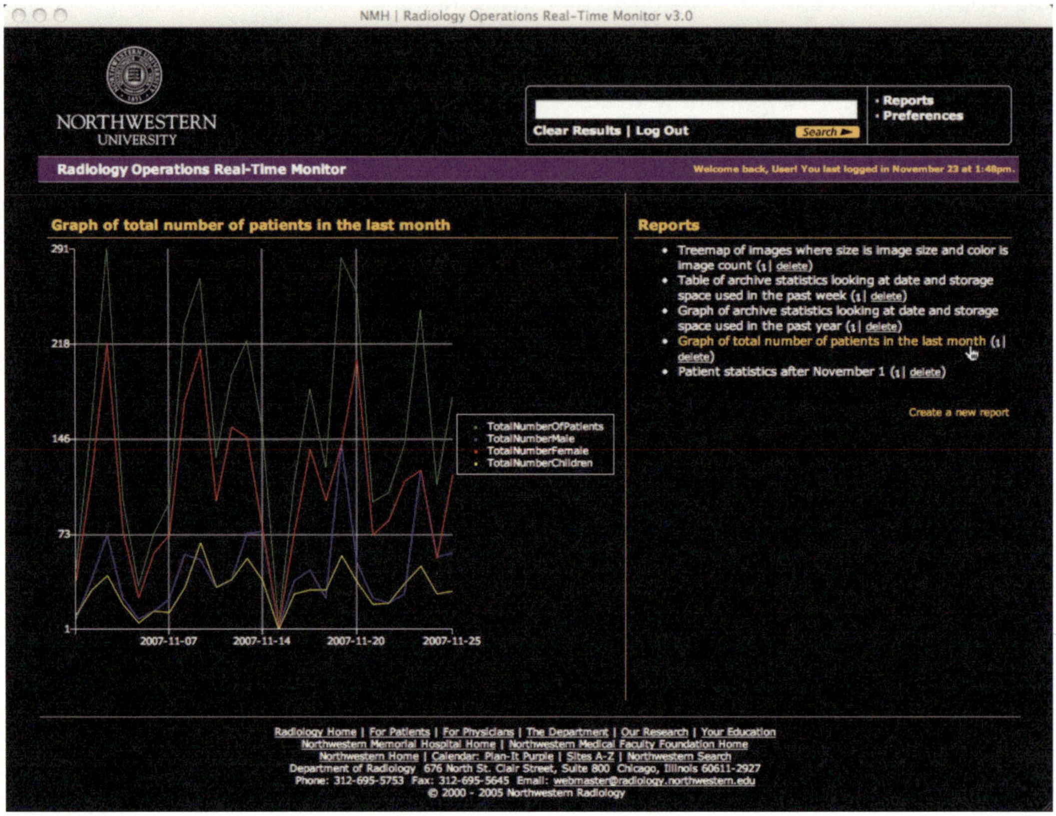

Fig. 5. Many different data combinations are possible. This graph shows the total number of patients within the past month.

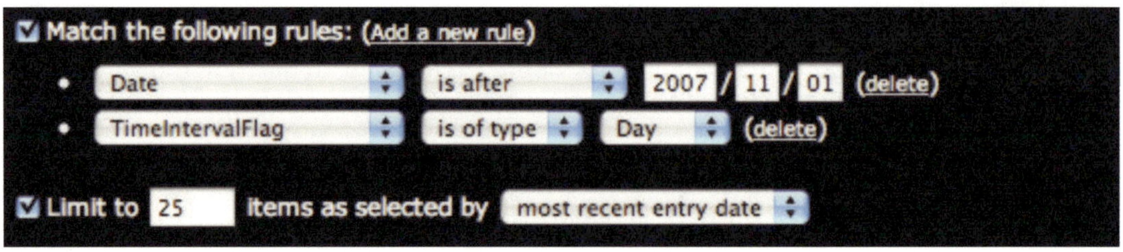

Fig. 6. Users are able to provide precise modifiers on the type of data that they want to see.

5.4 Discussion.

The gigabytes of radiologic imaging information that is transferred daily within a hospital enterprise PACS installation is associated with significant metadata, or data describing data. These bits, flags, dates, and numbers can be obtained by eavesdropping on HL7 traffic. By parsing and running statistical calculations on specific items of interest, this metadata serves as a powerful metric for analyzing and interpreting real-time radiology operational information.

PACSMonitor provides web-based operational reports of underlying PACS metadata. Instead of mining this information directly from the PACS, an activity that could threaten its stability and performance, we make periodic transfers to a separate database and then provide tools to the users to visualize this information. Examples of daily reports include "studies not yet completed within 24 hours" or "cancelled studies containing valid images". Longer-term monthly reports may describe the "rejected image rate" or "examinations without a procedure description". The ease with which users can access these metrics makes this a powerful tool to facilitate interpretation of daily and long-term operations in a data-driven fashion.

6. References

Blobel BG, Engel K, Pharow P. (2006). Semantic interoperability--HL7 Version 3 compared to advanced architecture standards. Methods Inf Med. 2006;45(4):343-53.

Channin DS. (2000). M:I-2 and IHE: integrating the healthcare enterprise, year 2. Radiographics. 2000 Sep-Oct;20(5):1261-2.

Dolin RH, Alschuler L, Boyer S, Beebe C, Behlen FM, Biron PV, Shabo Shvo A. (2006). HL7 Clinical Document Architecture, Release 2. J Am Med Inform Assoc. 2006 Jan-Feb;13(1):30-9. Epub 2005 Oct 12.

Hammond WE. (2003). HL7--more than a communications standard. Stud Health Technol Inform. 2003;96:266-71.

Health Level 7 (HL7). (Last accessed June 2008). http://www.hl7.org

Horii SC, Bidgood WD Jr. (1992). PACS Mini Refresher Course: Network and ACR-NEMA Protocols. Radiographics. 1992 May;12(3):537-48.

Huang HK. (2005). PACS and Imaging Informatics: Basic Principles and Applications. Hoboken, NJ: Wiley, 2004. ISBN 0-471-25123-2.

Hussein R, Engelmann U, Schroeter A, Meinzer HP. (2004). Implementing a full-feature PACS solution in accordance with the IHE technical framework: the CHILI approach. Acad Radiol. 2004 Apr;11(4):439-47.

Integrating the Healthcare Enterprise (IHE). (Last accessed June 2008). http://www.ihe.net

Lian JD, Lin IC, Wu HC. (2006). Case report: Taiwan's experience in adopting IHE technical framework to integrate systems. Stud Health Technol Inform. 2006;122:877.

Lopez DM, Blobel BG. (2008). A development framework for semantically interoperable health information systems. Int J Med Inform. 2008 Jul 11. [Epub ahead of print].

Mackinnon AD, Billington RA, Adam EJ, Dundas DD, Patel U. (2008). Picture archiving and communication systems lead to sustained improvements in reporting times and productivity: results of a 5-year audit. Clin Radiol. 2008 Jul;63(7):796-804. Epub 2008 Mar 25.

National Electrical Manufacturers Association (NEMA). (Last accessed June 2008). http://medical.nema.org/

National Electrical Manufacturers Association DICOM (NEMA DICOM). (Last accessed June 2008). ftp://medical.nema.org/medical/dicom/2008/

7

Application of Data Mining and Text Mining to the Analysis of Medical near Miss Cases

Masaomi Kimura[1], Sho Watabe[1], Toshiharu Hayasaka[1], Kouji Tatsuno[1], Yuta Takahashi[1], Tetsuro Aoto[1], Michiko Ohkura[1] and Fumito Tsuchiya[2]
[1]*Shibaura Institute of Technology,*
[2]*Tokyo Medical and Dental University*
Japan

1. Introduction

Not only the side effects of medicines themselves, but also their abuse, namely the lack of safety in drug usage, can cause serious medical accidents. The latter applies to the case of the mix-up of medicines, double dose or insufficient dose. Medical equipments can also cause accidents because of wrong treatment, such as wrong input to equipments and wrong power-off. In order to avoid such accidents, it is necessary to investigate past cases to identify their causes and work out counter measures.
Medical near-miss cases caused by wrong treatment with the medicines or the medical equipments are strongly related to medical accidents that occur due to the lack in safety of usage. Medical near-miss cases are incidents, which could be medical accidentsavoided owing to certain factors, and happen more frequently than medical accidents. Incorporating Heinrich's law, which shows the tendency of frequency and seriousness of industrial accidents, we estimate that near-miss cases happen three hundred times per one serious medical accident or thirty minor accidents. This can be interpreted as there being many causes of medical accidents, most of which are eliminated by certain suppression factors, which lead to near-miss cases. The rest of the causes lead to medical accidents. From this perspective, we can expect that both medical accidents and near-miss cases originate from the same type of causes, which suggests that the analysis of data on near-miss cases is valid to investigate the cause of medical accidents, since their occurrence frequency is much larger than that of medical accidents.
For the reasons stated above, we analyze the data of medical near-miss cases related to drugs and medical equipments, which have been collected in previous years to determine the root cause of medical accidents caused by the neglect of safety of usage. Though simple aggregation calculations and descriptive statistics have already been applied to them, the analyses are too simple to extract sufficient information such as pairs of medicines that tend to be confused, and the relationships between the contents of incidents and the causes. To realize such analyses, we utilize data mining techniques such as decision-tree and market-basket analysis, and text-mining techniques such as the word linking method.
The related works analyzing medical databy utilizing natural language processing ormachine learningwere introduced by Hripcsak et al (Hripcsak et al., 2003), who suggested the framework todetect events such as medical errors or adverse outcome.Recently,

Tsumoto(Tsumoto& Hirano, 2007) collected incident reports independently of a national project and applied decision tree algorithm, whose results show that errors caused by nurses depend on the part of their working hour and that an uncooperative patient tends to diminish nurses' power of attention and causes medication errors.
We have applied data-mining/text-mining approaches to the nation-wide incident reports collected by Japanese government, which is focused on the use of medicines or medical equipments and show the obtained results (Hayasaka et al., 2006; Hayasaka et al., 2007; Kimura et al., 2007; Takahashi et al., 2004; Takahashi et al., 2005; Tatsuno et al., 2005; Tatsuno et al., 2006; Watabe et al., 2007; Watabe et al., 2008). We introduce the results in this paper.

2. Target data and tools

Our target data are the medical near-miss cases related to medication and the use of medical equipments collected by the Japan Council for Quality Health Care, which is an extra-departmental body of the Japanese Ministry of Health, Labor and Welfare.
As for medication, we analyzed 1341 records included in the results from the 1st to the 11th investigations and 858 records in those from the 12th to the 14th. Since some data items in the latter investigations are added to the former ones, as is shown in Table 1 and Table 2, if we use such added items, we restrict the records having the data items, and if not, we use all records in the target data.
As for the use of medical equipments, we analyzed 500 records whichare obtained from the investigations conducted at the same time of the investigations about medication. The data items used for investigations for medical equipments are similar to those for medication and increase as the investigations proceed, namely, five items for the first investigation and 26 items for the 14th investigation.
In fact, there were some problems with analyzing the data using a computer program. We introduce some of them as follows:

- Data with many levels of abstractness were contained in one data item. For example, though 'misconception' is a concept which should be included in 'human error', this was adopted as a value in the data item 'major cause of the case'. Because of this, we had to redefine the categories and reclassify the data.
- In the Japanese language environment, there are several ways to express English letters and numbers such as single-byte letters (ASCII), double-byte English letters and Japanese Kana. This causes the diversity of expression. For instance, we can express 0.001g not only as '1mg', but also as '１ｍｇ' or '１ミリグラム' (which stand for 1 milligram in Japanese Kana).
- The diversity of drug name expression is also caused by the ambiguity when adding the medicine information, such as dosage form. For example, both 'アダラート' (Adalat) and 'アダラート錠' (Adalat tablet) are used to denote the name of the medicine which is administered in near-miss cases.

The diverse expression has to be standardized to ensure correct analysis. Though it is ideal to control the input data by designing the entry user interface appropriately, since it is difficult to realize such control, we standardized the notation of the resultant data before the application of the data/text-mining method.
The standard unit of contents or density consists of a numerical part and a unit part. In the case of standard unit error, we can know how many times the patient (almost) received an overdose of the medicine from the ratio of numerical parts of the wrong standard unit to

that of the correct unit. Since the target data possessed the standard unit of each medicine in one data item, we had to separate it into two parts, respectively.
There also exist many vacancies in the data, which we can fill if we figure out what is referring to here by reading other data items, such as free-description data.
Applying text-mining to the free-description data in the data items such as 'Contents of the incident', 'Background and cause of the incident' and '(Candidates of) counter measures' required the deletion of characters, such as symbols and unnecessary line feed characters, and the standardization of synonyms.
In order to analyze the data, we used Clementine, which is data-mining software released by SPSS Inc., and its text-mining plug-in software, Text Mining for Clementine.

Major cause	Discussed cause	Name of wrong drug	Dosage form of wrong drug
Medical benefit of wrong drug	Name of right drug	Dosage form of right drug	Medical benefit of right drug
Content of incident	Opinion	Remarks	-

Table 1. Data items in 1st to 11th investigations.

Day of the week	Week day or holiday	Time	Place
Department	Content of incident	Psychosomatic state of the patient	Job title
Experience (year)	Experience (month)	Affiliation (year)	Affiliation (month)
Medical benefit class	Nonproprietary name	Name of wrong drug	Dosage form of wrong drug
Effect of wrong drug	Name of right drug	Dosage form of right drug	Medical benefit of right drug
Discussed cause	Concrete contents of the incident	Background/cause of the incidents	Candidates of counter measure
Comment	-	-	-

Table 2. Data items in 12th to 14th investigations.

3. A brief review of data/text-mining techniques used in this study

We mainly utilized the market-basket analysis technique and decision-tree algorithm to extract the relationships between data and the rules to be followed in them. Market-basket analysis originally identifies combinations of goods bought together in a store and generates rules of the purchase tendency, which tell us which goods customers will also buy if some item is put in his/her basket. By applying this method to the values in the multiple data items, we obtain the information on the relations between the values. There are several algorithms supporting the analysis, among which we employ the Apriori algorithm and Web graph.
The decision-tree algorithm identifies the conditions dividing the data into groups by allowing minimization of entropy or the Gini index, and provides a tree that shows the optimal division of data to classify them. As the decision-tree algorithm, we use C5.0, which is suitable for classifying the categorical data.

In order to perform text-mining, we utilized the Word-linking method (Kimura et al., 2005). It is common to analyze textual data based on the frequency of words obtained by morphological analysis applied to the text. Morphological analysis extracts terms (morphemes) in the text, but loses the relationship information between the terms, which forces us to read the original textual data to interpret the result.

To avoid such inconvenience, it is useful to employ dependency structure analysis, which allows us to obtain the relationship between words in a sentence. If there are many sentences whose contents and structures are similar, we can expect that some particular patterns of word-dependencies will emerge and that such sentences can be reconstructed by rearranging these dependencies correctly. This is the basic idea behind the Word-linking method.

The steps of this method are as follows:

- Derive the dependency relationships between words (morphemes) from each sentence using dependency structure analysis. Let W denote the word which depends on another word W′.
- Create a Web graph of the co-occurrence relation between W and W′, where a link is provided between W and W′. We rotate the link to allow W to sit to the left of the link and W′ to the right.
- If W′ of a link coincides with W of another link, we connect the links by placing W′ and W in the same place.
- Read out the sentences from the rearranged links.

Figure 1 illustrates the results obtained with this method. There are links such as the one connecting'経口薬 (oral drug)' to '数 (number)', which indicates that the dependency '経口薬の数 (the number of oral drugs)' occurs many times. Connecting the links shows us the sentences '経口薬の数が減る (the number of oral drugs can be reduced.)', '経口薬が減る (the oral drugs can be reduced.)', and '経口薬が多い時 (when the patients have to take many medicines.)'.

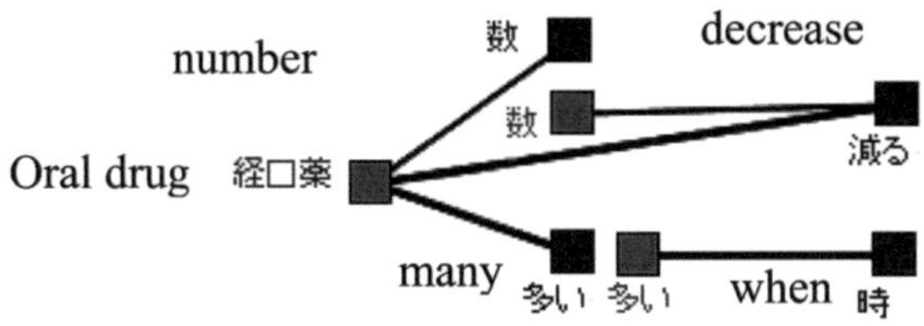

Fig. 1. Word-linking method (example)

4. Resultsonthe analysis on medication

4.1 Relationships between the contents of near-miss cases and their major causes

Incidents occur in various service phases. From the viewpoint of prevention of near-miss cases (and consequently medical accidents), it is important to assess the relationships among the contents of incidents, the service phase in which the incidents take place and their major cause. We therefore applied decision-tree analysis to determine the rules of the reason why the incidents happen, by assigning the data items 'the service phase when the incident occurs' and 'the content of the incident' to explanatory variables, and 'the major cause' to an objective variable.

Figure 2 shows the resultant decision tree. This indicates that the major causes are classified mainly by the contents of incidents, namely medicine error or not.

In the case of medicine error, the major causes mainly consist of resemblance of name and/or external form. This suggests that the source of the problem is the confusing name or shape of the medicines (including their packaging). Moreover, the cases of medicine errors can be classified by the service phases, that is to say, preparation, administration of drug and others (prescription, dispensing and after medication). The result tells us that the major cause is resemblance of external form in the preparation phase, carelessness in the administration phase and name resemblance in the other phase. This suggests that the major cause of medicine errors is different depending on its service phase.

On the other hand, cases other than medicine error mainly stem from carelessness and misconception. The decision tree also shows that they can be classified in more detail, and states that the cases of an error in amount (quantity and/or standard unit) particularly originate in carelessness and misconception and that the errors of route of administration and un-administration of drug are mainly caused by communication errors and unpatency of infusion bags in addition to carelessness. This indicates that, though double checks will have a beneficial effect on the errors in amount, improvement of communication will also be effective to prevent errors related to administration.

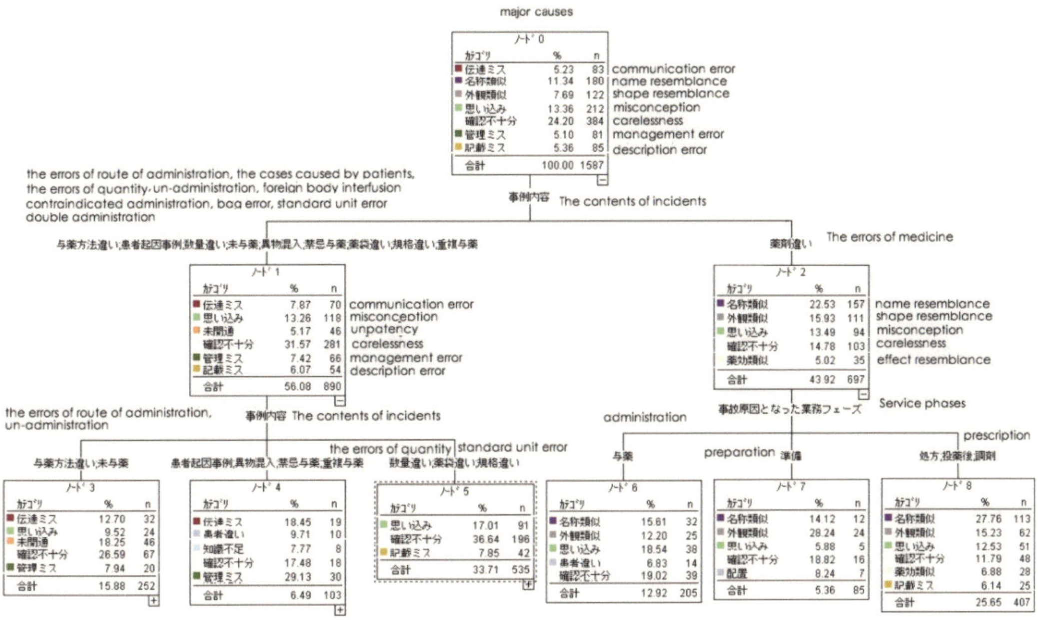

Fig. 2. Decision Tree (major causes versus the contents of incidents and service phases)

4.2 Relationship between Service phases, contents of incidents and Oversight

When a near-miss case occurs, it is crucial to detect the errors by confirmation to prevent it from becoming a medical accident. Moreover, it is also important to determine the rule of occurrences of oversights of errors depending on the circumstance and situation in order to improve counter measures. We, therefore, applied the Apriori algorithm to determine the rules of oversights depending on service phases and contents of incidents. We defined the occurrence of oversight as the difference in the occurrence phase of error and its finding phase. Table 3 shows the result of the analysis, which indicates that an oversight tends to occur:

- if an error happens in the administration phase,
- if a quantity or standard unit error happens,
- if a medicine error happens in the administration phase,
- if the case of un-administration happens.

Support is the ratio of records for which the rule holds. This suggests to us that medical experts have to pay attention at the administration phase and/or with errors related to amount, whose rules have high support value.

Result	Prerequisite	Support	Confidence	Lift
Oversight='yes'	Occurrence phase='administration'	49.052	98.663	1.055
Oversight='yes'	Content of incident='quantity error'	18.732	98.054	1.049
Oversight='yes'	Content of incident='medicine error' and Occurrence phase= 'administration'	13.732	96.825	1.035
Oversight='yes'	Content of incident= 'un-administration'	12.682	96.552	1.032
Oversight='yes'	Content of incident= 'standard unit error'	10.714	95.238	1.018

Table 3. Rules obtained by the Apriori algorithm.

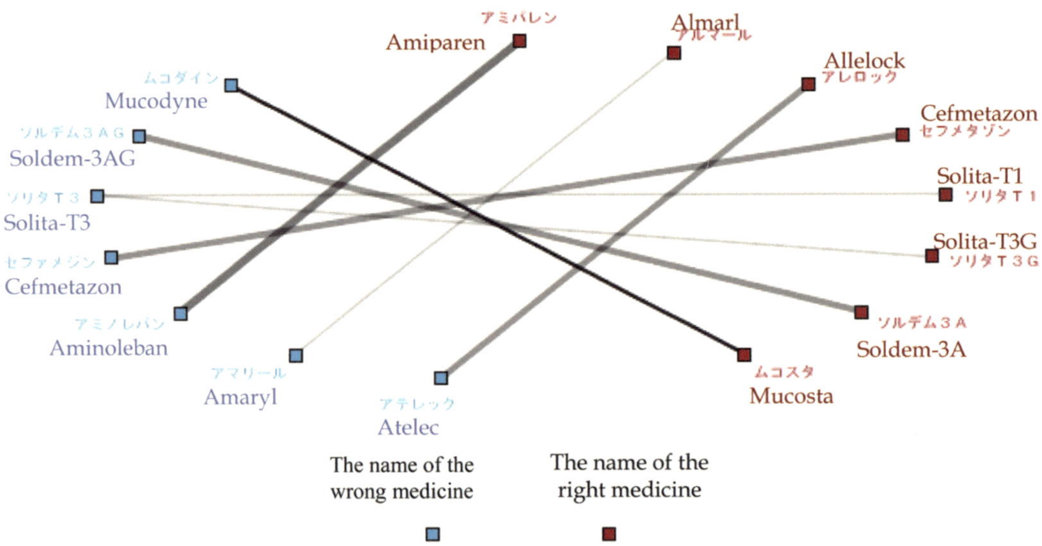

Fig. 3. Combinations of medicines mixed-up by name resemblance.

Shape	Ratio	Degree
similar	83.6%	209
different	16.4%	41

Table 4. Similarity in dosage form of pairs of medicines mixed-up by name resemblance

4.3 The combination of mixed-up medicines

In Section 4.1, we showed that the cause of medicine errors stems from the resemblance of their name. In this section, we identify which medicines are mixed-up because of the name resemblance by means of a Web graph.

Figure 3 shows the pairs of medicines appearing as cases of name resemblance more than five times. We can see that there are two types of name resemblance, one of which is the similar line of letters and the other of which is the same name apart from the last symbol (usually English letter or number). Since most of the paired medicines unfortunately have similar dosage form (both are tablets, etc.) as is listed in Table 2, pharmaceutical companies should keep from naming a medicine with a similar name to one of the existing medicines whose dosage form is also similar, and medical experts should be cautious when they treat people using those medicines.

We propose a similarity index of names of medicines making use of the String Subsequence Kernel, to realize the objective standard of name resemblance which medical experts (especially pharmacists) feels. Using the index is expected to help pharmaceutical companies seeking medicines with similar names.

4.4 Analysis of free description data on the background/cause of the incidents

We applied the Word-linking method to the field 'background/cause of the incidents' in the 12th to 14th investigations, to determine the concrete information on the cause of incidents. Compared with the formatted field 'major cause' in the data, which we deal with in Section 4.1, the field 'The background/cause of the incidents' contains free description data, which gives us more information than the formatted field.

We applied the method by occupation to determine the difference in backgrounds and causes of incidents depending on the job title. Figures 4 and 5 show the result of nurses' and pharmacists' comments, respectively. Though both figures contain the common opinions 'the problem of the checking system of the protocol and the rule' (A) and 'confirmation is insufficient' (B), nurses point out 'the systematic problem of communication' (C) and pharmacists 'the problem of adoption of medicines' (C'). We can see that, though B comes from individual fault, A, C and C' are systematic problems.

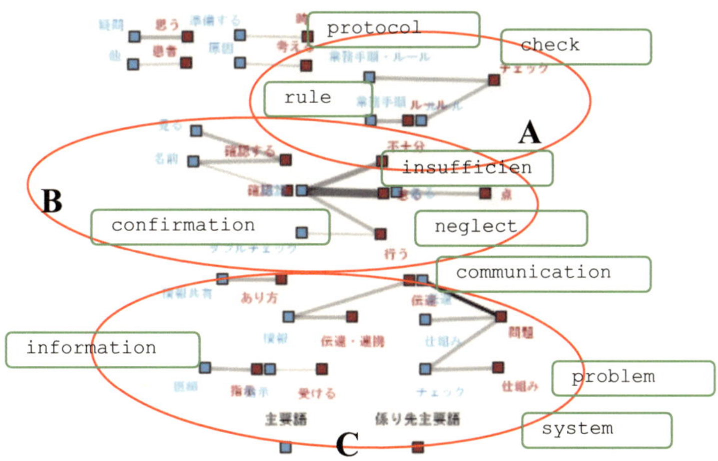

Fig. 4. Backgrounds and causes of incidents (nurse)

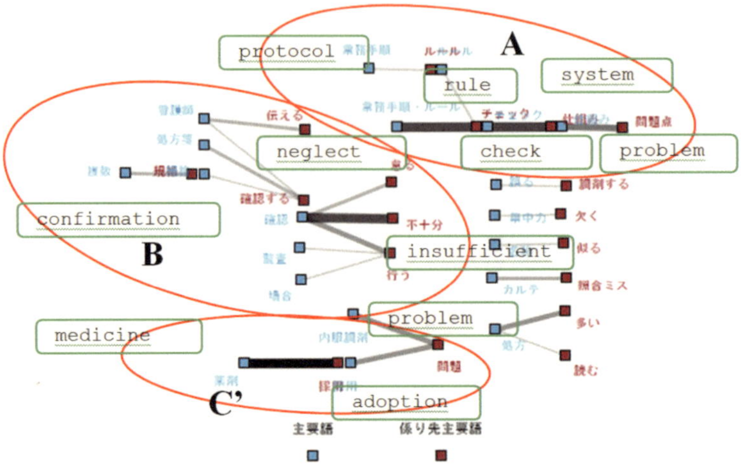

Fig. 5. Backgrounds and causes of incidents (pharmacist)

4.5 Analysis of free description regarding counter measures

We applied the Word-linking method to the field '(Candidates of) counter measures' to summarize the nurses' and the pharmacists' opinions about the counter measures to prevent the incidents. Figure 6 is the summary of the counter measures described by nurses, and suggests that there are many opinions stating '(it is necessary to) instruct to confirm and check', 'make a speech' and 'ensure confirmation'. Figure 7 shows the summary of the counter measures proposed by pharmacists. This says that, besides the confirmation and audit, it is also necessary to invite (pharmacists') attention and to devise ways of displaying medicines such as labels.

Compared with the results in Section 4.4, except for the pharmacists' opinion about the device of labels, there are few opinions on the counter measures related to the system of the medical scenarios pointed out in Section 4.4. This suggests that the medical experts such as nurses and pharmacists tend to try to find the solutions to problems within themselves. To solve the structural problem in medical situations, it is important not only to promote the effort of each medical expert, but also to take measures to improve the organization to which they belong. It is also desirable for them to be aware of the importance of organizational innovation, and to propose measures against the systematic error.

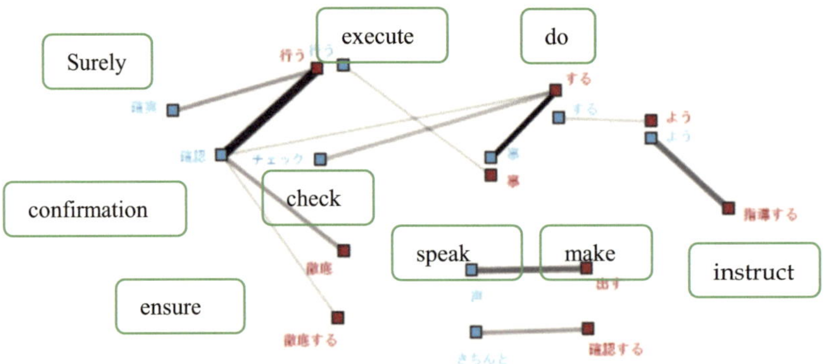

Fig. 6. Counter measures suggested by nurses (with links appearing more than 5 times)

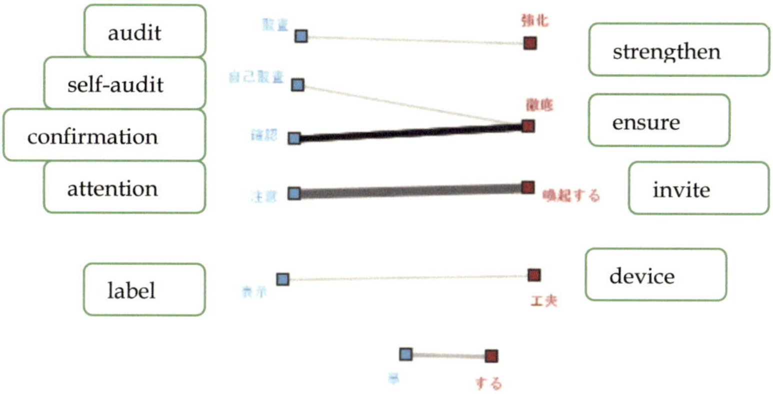

Fig. 7. Counter measure suggested by pharmacists (with links appearing more than 4 times)

5. Results on the analysis on the usage of medical equipments

In order to find the pattern of the relations between the causes of incidents, we visualized the co-occurring relations by use of Web graph(Fig. 8). This shows that the hub node of the graph is 'misuse' and that there is co-occurrence of 'insufficient maintenance', 'failure' and 'malfunction' to no small extent. We can see two groups in Fig. 8, one of whichdenotes the group of 'misuse','inadequate knowledge', 'plural standards', 'hard to handle' and 'an error in connection' related to misuse of operators, and the other of which is the group of 'insufficient maintenance', 'failure' and 'malfunction' related to issues of maintenance of equipments. As to derive these groups from data, we applied TwoStep clustering algorithm to the data and found two clusters (Fig.9), which are clusters corresponding to misuse (Cluster 1) and issues of maintenance(Cluster 2) and are consistent with the groups in Fig.8. Note that the bar charts in Fig.9 denote the ratio of selection (right)/deselection (left) and that some causes, such as'misuse',characterize the clusters, though their selectionsdo not dominate in the cluster.

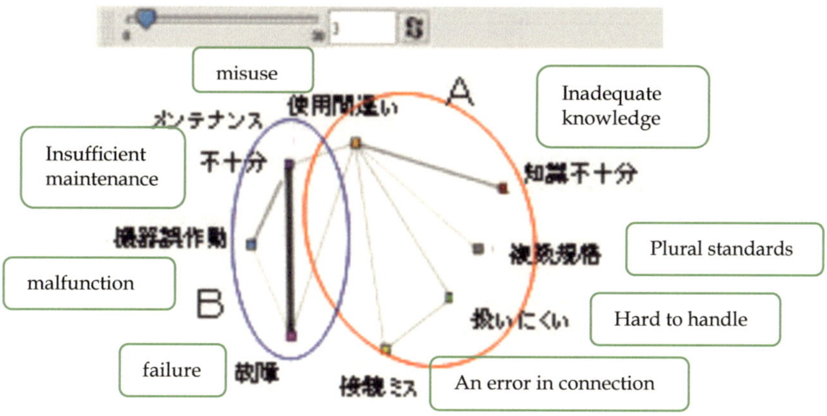

Fig. 8. Co-occurrence relations between the causes of incidents

To understand the condition under which these clusters can be causes of each incident, we applied a decision tree algorithm, where we set the cluster to which the incident belongs as an objective variable and the types of equipments, the time and the location the incident occurs, and the occupation and the period of job experience of the person concernedas explanatory variables. Fig. 10 shows that the main parameterseparating the incident records into the clusters is the type of equipments.This says that the apparatus such as a catheter, a tube, a puncture device is related to Cluster 1 (misuse)and that the incidents associated with the structurally-complex equipmentsuch as a pump set, a mechanical ventilator,a hemodialysis monitor and an X-ray apparatusare mainly caused by the causes in Cluster 2 (issue of maintenance).

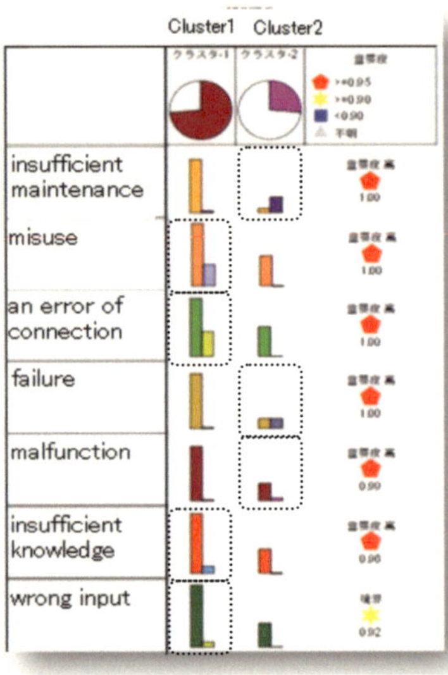

Fig. 9. The clusters of the type of causes based on their co-occurrence relations (main part)

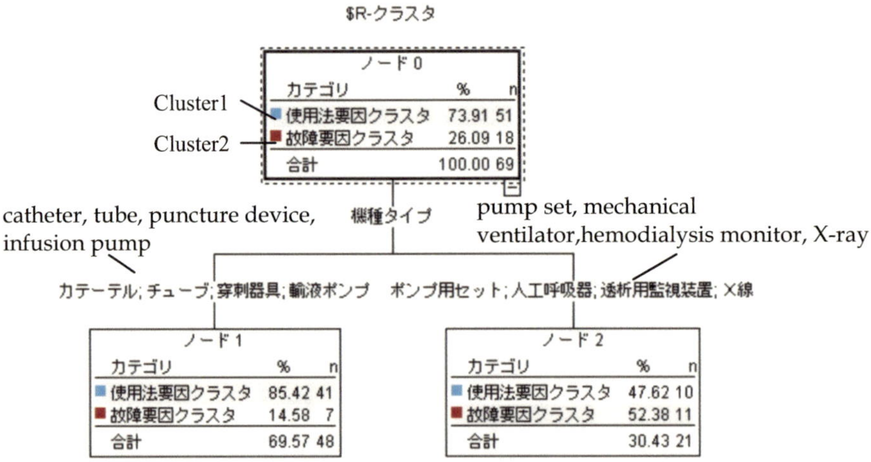

Fig. 10. The decision tree which relates the type of medical equipments and their cause

Notice that Fig. 10 indicates the incidentsassociated withan infusion pump is also caused mainly by misuse (Cluster 1), though it hasrelatively complex structure. In order to clarify the relationships between the type of equipments and the causes of incidents, we again used

Web graph (Fig. 11) and found that the incidents related to an infusion pump are mainly caused by 'wrong input', 'an error of connection', 'misuse' and 'oblivescence of holding down a switch' rather than 'inadequate knowledge' or 'failure'. This suggests that there is a problem of an infusion pump, which itself seducesusers into the wrong use because of its human-machine interface, and that it is necessary to improve the interface to prevent from operation mistake.

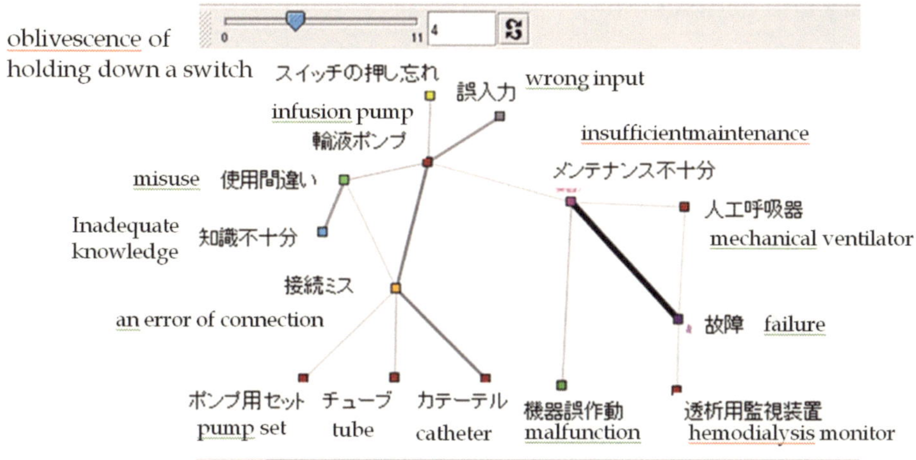

Fig. 11.The relation between the type of equipments and the causes of incidents

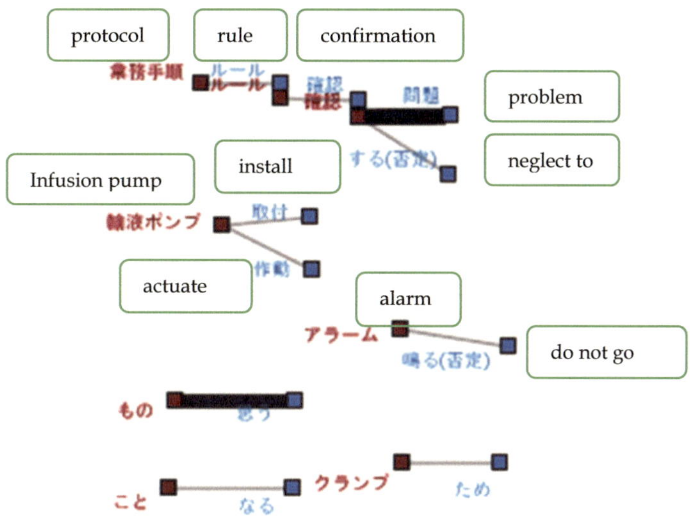

Fig. 12. Backgrounds and causes of incidents related to medical equipments

We applied Word-linking method to the free description data,which describes the background and the causes of incidents (Fig. 12). This indicates that there are major statements such as '(The person concerned) neglects to confirm (based on) a rule and anprotocol','alarm did not go off', 'actuation/installing of the infusion pump'.Comparing this result to the oneon the analysis on medication, it is common thatboth of them focus on the necessity ofconfirmation. Medical equipments, however, leave a room of improvement of a user interface to lead an operator to confirm spontaneously and of mechanism to checkhis/her configuration under the assumption that people may forget to confirm. This is necessary because it is hard to force medical experts to perfectly confirm under the circumstances where interruption of a task frequently occurs.

5. Summary and conclusion

We applied data-mining and text-mining techniques to medical near-miss case data related to medicines and medical equipments, and analyzed the causal relationship of occurrences of the near-miss cases and the opinions on the counter measures against them.

As for medication, the decision tree obtained by the C5.0 algorithm shows that the major causes are classified mainly by the contents of incidents, namely medicine error or not. In the case of medicine error, the major causes mainly consist of resemblance of name and/or external form. The other cases mainly come from carelessness and misconception. This suggests that, as a counter measure of near-miss cases and medical accidents, it is valid to avoid adopting a confusing name or shape of the medicines themselves or their packages, not just to pay attentions.

To prevent oversights of errors, which may become a medical accident, it is also important to determine the rules of the occurrences of the oversights. We, therefore, applied the Apriori algorithm to determine the rules of oversights depending on service phases and contents of incidents. The result indicates that an oversight tends to occur, if the error happens in the administration phase, or the error is related to amount. Especially, the tendency of oversight in the case of medicine error in the administration phase is consistent with the results of the decision tree.

Since the cause of medicine errors stems from the resemblance of their name, we identified which medicines are mixed-up because of the name resemblance using a Web graph. As a result, we found that there are two types of name resemblance, one of which is the similar line of letters and the other of which is the same name apart from the last symbol. Since most of the paired medicines unfortunately have a similar dosage form, pharmaceutical companies should avoid naming a medicine with a similar name to existing medicines whose dosage form is also similar, and medical experts should pay attention to these.

We applied the Word-linking method to the free description data and found concrete information on the backgrounds and the causes of the incidents depending on job titles. Both describe the common statements on the problems of the checking system of the protocol and the rule, and the unsatisfactory confirmation. Nurses point out the systematic problem of communication and pharmacists indicate the problem of adoption of medicines. Those are systematic problems. In spite of such indications, there are few opinions on the counter measures related to the system of medical situations. This suggests that medical experts such as nurses and pharmacists tend to try to find the solutions to problems within themselves.

As for medical equipments, we utilized Web graph and TwoStep clustering algorithmto find the pattern of the co-occurring relations between the causes of incidents, which consist of two clusters corresponding to misuse and issues of maintenance. To understand the condition under which these clusters can be causes of each incident, we applied a decision tree algorithm, where we set the cluster to which the incident belongs as an objective variable and the types of equipments, the time and the location the incident occurs, and the occupation and the period of job experience of the person concerned as explanatory variables. This says that the apparatus with relatively simple structure is related to the cluster of misuse and that the incidents associated with the structurally-complex equipment are mainly caused by the causes in the cluster related to maintenance. The exception is an infusion pump, whose incidents are also caused mainly by misuse, though it has relatively complex structure. This suggests that there is a problem of an infusion pump, which itself seduces users into the wrong use because of its human-machine interface.

To prevent near-miss incidents, it is obviously desired to promote the effort of each medical expert, but it is important to take measures against systematic error, such as the adoption policy of medicines with confusing names, the system of communication, better user interface to prevent from misuse and to prompt user to confirm.

As we showed in this paper, data-mining and text-mining are powerful tools to discover information that cannot be found by simple aggregation calculations and descriptive statistics. This is because these methodologies neglect the information contained in the relationship between data items, which can be extracted by data-mining and text-mining approaches.

In order to find countermeasuresagainst near-miss cases and medical accidents related to medicinesby means of data/text-mining approaches, it is necessary to collect and disclose the near-miss cases continually to find time series patterns and to confirm the validity of our countermeasures.

8. References

Hayasaka, T.; Kimura, M.; Ohkura, M.; Tsuchiya, F.(2006). The analysis of medical near-miss cases applying text mining method, The 36th Annual Meeting of the Kanto-branch Japan Ergonomics Society.

Hayasaka, T.; Kimura, M.; Ohkura, M.; Tsuchiya, F.(2007). The analysis of medical near-miss cases applying text mining method, Proceedings of IPSJ Annual Convention, 3J-3.

Hripcsak, G.; Bakken, S.; Stetson, D. P.; Patel, L. V.(2003). Mining complex clinical data for patient safety research: a framework for event discovery, Journal of Biomedical Infomatics, 36, pp.120-130.

Kimura, M.; Furukawa, H.; Tsukamoto, H; Tasaki, H.; Kuga, M; Ohkura, M.; Tsuchiya, F.(2005). Analysis of Questionnaires Regarding Safety of Drug Use, Application of Text Mining to Free Description Questionnaires, The Japanese Journal of Ergonomics, Vol.41 No.5 pp.297-3051.

Kimura, M.; Tatsuno, K.; Hayasaka, T.; Takahashi, Y.; Aoto, T.; Ohkura, M.; Tsuchiya, F.(2007). The Analysis of Near-Miss Cases Using Data-Mining Approach, Proceedings of the 12th International Conference on Human-Computer Interaction, pp.474-483.

Tatsuno, K.; Kimura, M.; Ohkura, M.; Tsuchiya, F.(2005). Applying the data mining technique to near-miss cases of medicine (III), The 35th Annual Meeting of the Kanto-branch Japan Ergonomics Society.

Takahashi, Y.; Kimura, M.; Ohkura, M.; Aoto, T.; Tsuchiya, F. (2004). Study on analysis for near-miss cases with medicine (II), The 34th Annual Meeting of the Kanto-branch Japan Ergonomics Society.

Takahashi, Y.; Kimura, M.; Ohkura, M.;Aoto, T.; Tsuchiya, F. (2005). Study on analysis for near-miss cases of Medication, Proceedings of IPSJ Annual Convention, 6V-6.

Tsumoto, S.; Hirano, S.(2007). Data Mining as Complex Medical Engineering, Journal of Japanese Society for Artificial Intelligence, Vol.22, No.2, pp.201-207.

Watabe, S.; Kimura, M.; Ohkura, M.; Tsuchiya, F.(2007).The analysis of the near-miss cases of medical equipments using the text-mining technique, The 37th Annual Meeting of the Kanto-branch Japan Ergonomics Society.

Watabe, S.; Kimura, M.; Ohkura, M.; Tsuchiya, F.(2008). The analysis of the near-miss cases of medical equipments using the text-mining technique, Proceedings of the IEICE General Conference, A-18-3.

8

Interactive Knowledge Discovery for Temporal Lobe Epilepsy

Mostafa Ghannad-Rezaie[1] and Hamid Soltanian-Zadeh[2]
[1]*University of Michigan, Ann Arbor, MI*
[2]*Henry Ford Hospital, Detroit, MI*
USA

1. Introduction

Medical data mining and knowledge discovery can benefit from the experience and knowledge of clinicians, however, the implementation of this data mining system is challenging. Unlike traditional data mining methods, in this class of applications we process data with some posterior knowledge and the target function is more complex and even may include the opinion of user. Despite the success of the classical reasoning algorithms in many common data mining applications, they failed to address medical record processing where we need to extract information from incomplete, small samples along with an external rulebase to generate 'meaningful' interpretation of biological phenomenon. Swarm intelligence is an alternative class of flexible approaches that is promising in data mining. With full control over the rule extraction target function, particle swarm optimization (PSO) is a suitable approach for data mining subject to a rulebase which defines the quality of rules and constancy with previous observations. In this chapter we describe a complex clinical problem that has been addressed using PSO data mining. A large group of temporal lobe epilepsy patients are studied to find the best surgery candidates. Since there are many parameters involved in the decision process, the problem is not tractable from traditional data mining point of view, while the new approach that uses the field knowledge could extract valuable information.

The proposed method allows expert to interaction with data mining process by offering manual manipulation of generated rules. The algorithm adjusts the rule set with regard to manipulations. Each rule has a reasoning which is based on the provided rulebase and similar observed cases.

Support vector machine (SVM) classifier and swarm data miner are integrated to handle joint processing of raw data and rules. This approach is used to establish the limits of observations and build decision boundaries based on these critical observations.

2. Background

2.1 Data mining in medicine

The overall process of knowledge discovery from database (KDD) is a multistage process. The main step in KDD, Data Mining (DM), is the most commonly used name to describe the computational efforts meant to process feature space information, in order to obtain

valuable high level knowledge, which must conform to three main requisites: accuracy, comprehensibility and interest for the user (Apte et la. 1997). DM discovers patterns among database-stored information to support special user interest such as data classification. Computer-aided diagnosis (CAD) systems are one the primary areas of interest in data mining (Lavarac 1999, Toivonen et la 2000).
Designers of computer-based diagnosis systems often view the physician's primary decision-making task as a differential diagnosis. This term refers to a type of analytical task wherein the decision maker is confronted with a fixed set of diagnostic alternatives.
Over the past two decades, a large number of specialized procedures have been developed to assist physician in differential diagnosis of a variety of well defined clinical problems. These have been extensively reported in the medical and computing literature. In addition, algorithms to deal with a host of common medical problems, expressed by means of detailed flowcharts, have increasingly found their way into the clinical application.
Many different techniques have been used in structuring these clinical algorithms. In some cases, special programs have been formulated to capture the logic involved in the workup of particular classes of clinical problems. In other cases, generalized procedures have been adopted that are tailored to a particular application by specification of certain parameters; for example, many diagnostic programs have been developed to use the normative models of statistical decision theory. In some complex diagnosis tasks too many parameters such as cancer staging and neurological disease, medical diagnosis systems evolve rapidly. Evaluation studies frequently show that these programs, whatever their basis, generally perform as well as experienced clinicians in their respective domains, and somewhat better than the non-specialist. It is interesting, therefore, to speculate on the reason that such programs have not had greater impact on the practice of medicine.
Resistance in the medical community is sometimes attributed to the natural conservatism of physicians or to their sense of being threatened by the prospect of replacement by machines. Some have argued that this can be resolved only on the basis of education and training, and that the next generation will be more comfortable with computer-based decision aids as these become routinely introduced into the medical community. Some clinicians argue rather forcefully that the real reason that they have not adopted computer-based decision aids is that these systems have often been based on unrealistic models, which fail to deal with the physicians' real problems.
Unlike most of data mining approaches, we propose to optimize the rule-discovery process by giving clinician flexibility of incorporating domain knowledge, in the form of desire rule formats, into the rule search.
There are many reasons why a physician might experience difficulty in formulating an appropriate differential diagnosis. It may be that the case involves a rare disease or unusual presentation. Often, such difficulties arise in clinical problems where two or more disease processes are at work, generating a complex sequence of abnormal findings that can be interpreted in a variety of ways. Supporting the results with human understandable evidences, rule based CAD systems may be able to eventually convince clinician to accept their proposed results.

2.2 Interactive data mining

Mining medical information is to discover useful and interesting information from raw patient's clinical and non-clinical data (Apte et la. 1997, Kim 1997, Chen 2007). Nowadays, huge amount of features are collected, thanks to recent progresses in medical information systems and novel medical instrument (Lavarac 1999). This wide range of knowledge is confusing. Traditional manual analysis methods can not discover complex relationships and knowledge potentially may embed inside raw data. Also, the more complexity is added to expertise's diagnosis process, the more time is required to make a reliable judgment. Therefore, automated data mining applications in medical domain has become a very active field during recent years.

In this section, we discuss on knowledge discovery from raw data in medical diagnosis systems. The primary application of our interest is surgery candidate selection in temporal lobe epilepsy. In some aspects, this problem is a prototype of many complex medical diagnosis problems. Low number of samples, large number of features, and missing data are common problems we are facing. Thus, the method can be extended to similar medical diagnosis problems. Medical knowledge extraction process is divided into five steps: data collection, data pre-processing, modelling, rule extraction and evaluation. Some primary processing is required to extract feature vector presentation of the data. Data mining block is the main part of the system that generates rules. Finally, comprehensibility and completeness of the generated rules are evaluated. The main contribution of most of knowledge discovery works is to find appropriate data classification and rule extraction algorithms. The result is a more intelligent and more robust system providing a human-interpretable, low cost, approximate solution, compared to the conventional techniques. This article focuses on advantages of association support vector machine (SVM) and partial swarm optimization (PSO) approaches in medical data mining (Botee et la1998).

In Medical information mining, comprehensibility has a special value. In a nutshell, data mining comprehends the actions of automatically seeking out, identifying, validating and is used for prediction, structural patterns in data that might be grouped into five categories: decision trees, classification rules, association rules, clusters and numeric prediction.

This article proposes a data discovery algorithm for a small data set with high dimensionality. Vector fusion algorithm is used to construct a single feature vector of non-commensurate data sources. Support vector machine is applied to classify the feature vectors. Finally, particle swarm agents are used to discover the SVM classification rules (Barakat et la 2005). It has been shown that this algorithm can manage the rule extraction task efficiently. Fig 1 shows the general structure of proposed algorithm. Raw data and external rules both can contribute in the final rule generation.

2.3 Terminology

A rule-base is a finite set of rules. There is no agreed on definition of rules for medical information, however, to have a consistence terminology we use a simple rule language based on rules used by the well known Jena framework. The rules are in the form of:

$$(?A,b,c) \leftarrow (?A,x,y)\ (?A,v,w)\ \ldots\ (?B,p,q)$$

The left hand side of (←) is the goal of the rule and the right hand side is the body of the rule. In this language, each triples represents a relationship, for example (?A,b,c) represent relationship b between variable A and value c.

Each rule has an active region in the feature space where the rule is valid. This area is defined by another rule, called primitive rule.

In data mining subject to a rulebase a set of rules derive from database where derived rules should be consistent with the given rulebase. Each rule and its primitive in the rulebase have a degree of preciseness is a positive value. An established fact has a large degree of

preciseness, while a weak rule may have a degree of preciseness around 0. The cost function of a data mining algorithm increases when invalidating a rule proportional to the preciseness of the rule.
Prooftree represent the interaction between rules and data that lead to the result. The prooftree is a tool to indentify the reason for unexpected results.

3. Method

In recent years, various soft computing methodologies have been applied to address data mining (Lan et la. 2002; et la. Susa 2004, Xu et la 2007). Generally, there is no universal best data mining algorithm. Choosing appropriate data mining algorithm utterly depends on individual applications. Social algorithms and Swarm intelligence (SI) algorithms are well-known alternatives of soft computing tools that can be used for retrieving information from raw data (Galea 2002). Distributed Genetic Algorithm, Ant Colony Optimizer (ACO) and Particle Swarm Optimizer (PSO) are the most commonly used evolutionary algorithms in this domain. The most interesting contribution of these methods is in flexible rule extraction where we are facing to Incomplete and Inaccurate Measured dataset (Galea 2002).

3.1 Rule extraction

According to previous discussions, finding a rule-based classifier and reasons behind the decision making process are essential parts of medical computer aided diagnosis systems. Also they are key parts of knowledge discovery from databases (KDD). This section discusses the mathematical modeling of rule extraction process and application of particle swarm optimization to find the rule set describing a support vector machine classifier.
Assume S is the search space and θi is a data point inside S and yi = V(θi) is the data point class. A classifier is define by $yi^1 = U(\theta_i)$. The target of rule extraction is to find a rule set $R^U_{1..n}$ that describes the *U* classifier.
Each rule is a "IF-THEN" statement with two clauses. In the simplest case, the former clause is a condition on the search space and the latter clause is the target class. This rule may express as (?A,x,c) ← (?A,x,y).
The structure of these two clauses is called rule set grammar limiting phrases in the rule clauses. The simpler the grammar, the more comprehensive statements can be retrieved. Rectangular grammar limits the IF-clause to intervals of each individual feature. Fig.2 shows an example of the rectangular rules. Decision tree is another alternative of rule set topology which is quite common in medical applications because of better interpretability and higher searching speed. In this structure the IF-part may also include another rule in addition to intervals but number of intervals is limited.

3.2 Rule-set evaluation

The value of a rule is evaluated using different parameters:

- *Accuracy*: this term stands for the percentage of data points correctly classified by the rule.

$$A_R = \frac{\#\theta : V(\theta) = R(\theta)}{\#\theta} = \frac{TP + TN}{TP + TN + FP + FN} \tag{1}$$

- *Quality*: this term is the popular classification quality measure for the rule set and can be obtained from the ROC curve:

$$Q_R = \text{sensitivity} \cdot \text{specificity} = \frac{TP \cdot TN}{(TP + FN) \cdot (TP + FN)} \tag{2}$$

- *Coverage*: this term describes the percentage of specific class data points that are covered by the rule set from total available data points. This percentage is represented by C_R.
- *Simplicity*: the number of terms in rule the clauses and the number of intervals on each term condition representation (S_R). Generally, a very complex rule can describe any classifier and achieve very high Coverage and Accuracy spontaneously. Comprehensibility as a critical parameter in medical data mining is measured by this term. The number of rules in a rule set, and the number of terms in a rule represent the complexity phenomena. Simplicity is defined as *1/Complexity*.
- *Rule interference*: Adding to the individual rule evaluating parameters, the final rule set is admirable when it can cover the entire search space while the conflict among rules is kept as low as possible. Interference parameter (I_R) is particularly considered for reasoning process and reliable decision making.

Finally, the rule set evaluation is $\text{Eval}(R) = \alpha A_R + \beta C_R + \gamma S_R - \delta I_R$. The accuracy measure can be replaced by the quality when the trade-off between sensitivity and specificity is highly interested. Finding the best rule set is a complex multi-objective process.

3.3 Swarm intelligence rule extraction

Previous work in the literature shows power of PSO in solving rule extraction problems in medical diagnosis systems. Many recommended modifications of PSO for providing a flexible approach to address common difficulties of medical information retrieval from databases (Jaganathan 2007). Here, we present hybrid approaches to overcome problems presented in earlier sections.

Ant Colony Optimizer (ACO) and ant miners is the first swarm intelligent data mining algorithm presented by Parpinelli (Parpinelli et al. 2002, Omkara 2008). The purpose of their algorithm, Ant-Miner is to use ants to create rules describing an underlying data set. The overall approach of Ant-Miner is a separate-and-conquer one as same as C4.5 (Quinlan 1993). It starts with a full training set, creates a best rule that covers a subset of the training data, adds the best rule to its discovered rule list, removes the instances covered by the rule from the training data, and starts again with a reduced training set. This goes on until only a few instances are left in the training data (fewer than max number allowed) or the fitness function meets the target, at which point a default rule is created to cover remaining instances. Once an ant has stopped building a rule antecedent a rule consequent is chosen. This is done by assigning to the rule consequent the class label of the majority class among the instances covered by the built rule antecedent. The rule is then pruned in order to improve its quality and comprehensibility. The basic idea is to iteratively remove one term at a time from the rule while this process improves the rule quality as defined by a fitness function. In the iteration, each term in turn is temporarily removed from the rule antecedent, a new rule consequent is assigned, and the rule quality is evaluated. At the end of the iteration, the term that has actually been removed is the one that improves the rule quality the most.

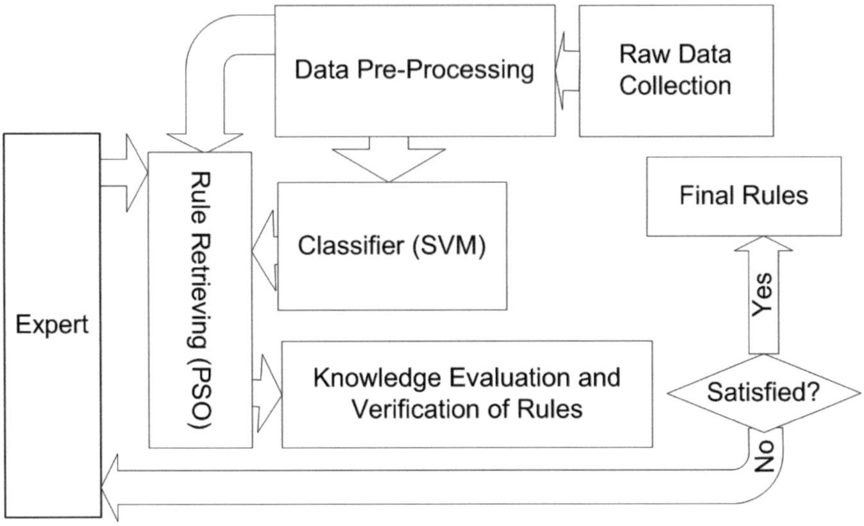

Fig. 1. General schematic of proposed rule extraction system.

4. Particle swarm intelligence

Rule discovery process can be done using a Particle Swarm Intelligence Algorithm. PSO imitates the intelligent behaviour of beings as part of a group to experience sharing in a society. In contrast to conventional learning algorithms with individual reaction to environment or searching space, PSO is based on adaptive social behaviours. The basic idea of the PSO model is constructed on three ideas: evaluation, comparison and imitation. Evaluation is the kernel part of any intelligent algorithm measuring quality of the result in the environment and usefulness inside the community. Some metrics are defined to represent the particle superiority. This evaluation is pointless without well-defined comparison process which is a sequential relationship in the particle space. The improvement of particles is made by imitating best solution up to now. Looking to best solution in the neighbourhood, a particle decides where to move in the next step. There are many alternatives for implementation of neighbourhood and distance between particle concepts.

4.1 PSO Algorithm

PSO is a set of individual agents simply searching for an optimal point in their neighbourhood. The movement of agents depends on behaviour of other agents in the vicinity and the best visited nodes. During PSO training particle's best met position (BPi) and the best solution met by neighbours (BPNi) is updated. A position vector and a velocity vector in the feature space are assigned to each particle. The standard PSO parameters update formulation is:

$$\begin{cases} v_i(t) = v_i(t-1) + \varphi_{1i}[BP_i - x_i(t-1)] + \varphi_{2i}[BP_{Ni} - x_i(t-1)] \\ x_i(t) = x_i(t-1) + v_i(t) \end{cases} \quad (3)$$

In the new version of PSO, a weight term is applied to prevent divergence of the velocity vector:

$$v_i(t) = \alpha(v_i(t-1) + \varphi_{1i}[BP_i - x_i(t-1)] + \varphi_{2i}[BP_{Ni} - x_i(t-1)]) \quad (4)$$

For a more general definition of the distance aspect, a more general form of position update equation is:

$$v_i(t) = \alpha(v_i(t-1) + \varphi_{1i}[Dis(BP_i, x_i(t-1))] + \varphi_{2i}[Dis(BP_{Ni}, x_i(t-1))]) \quad (5)$$

General optimization algorithm is summarized in Table 1.

```
Assume K particles
Distribute particles in the searching area

While (Fitness < TARGET_FITNESS && Epoch < MAX_EPOCH)
{
        evaluateTotalFitness();
        For any particle p
        {
          Evaluate(p);
          UpdateBestPosition(p);
          UpdateNeighborhoodList(p);
          UpdateBestPositionInNeighborhood(p);

          UpdatePositionInAllDimensions(p);

        }
}
```

Table 1. PSO pseudo-code.

4.2 PSO for database rule extraction

Rule extraction process usually contains two stages: rule set generation and pruning. Rule generation is a forward selection algorithm adding new rules to current rule-set. In contract, pruning or cleaning process is a backward elimination algorithm omitting extra rules form rule-set. PSO could efficiently apply in the rule generation process. While PSO is a strong optimization algorithm in the large search space, it could obtain rule-set with maximum fitness function, no mater how complex it is. Sousa (Sousa et al. 1999) proposed a particle swarm based data mining algorithm. Between different rule representation approaches, they followed Michigan rule where each particle encodes a single rule. Comparing different PSO implementations with C4.5 and other evolutionary algorithms, Sousa concluded PSO can obtain competitive results against other alternative data mining algorithms, although it need a bit more computational effort.

4.3 Neighbourhood structure effect on rule set

Neighbourhood and social networks phenomena are a new issues proposed in swarm intelligence by PSO. In (Clerc et al. 2002) Kennedy studies how different social network structures can influence the performance of the PSO algorithm, arguing that a manipulation affecting the topological distance among particles might affect the rate and degree to which individuals are attracted towards a particular solution. Four different types of neighbourhood topologies have been proposed in the previous works. In circles structure each individual is connected to number of its immediate neighbours. In wheels structure one individual is connected to all others, and these are connected only to that one. In star neighbourhood every individual is connected to every other individual. Finally random topology for some individuals, random symmetrical connections are assigned between pairs of individuals.

Structure of neighbourhood could affect data mining process. Rule-set fitness and convergence depend on neighbourhood structure. Experimental results have shown that the neighbourhood topology of the particle swarm has a significant effect on its ability in finding optima. Best pattern of connectivity among particles depends on fitness function. In single rule extraction such as Sousa (Sousa et al. 1999) wheel structure shows improvements in data mining convergence speed. However, random start neighbourhood is the better choice in multi-rule extraction approaches.

4.4 Decision tree rule indication using structured PSO

Decision trees are powerful classification structures. Standard techniques such as C4.5 can produce structured rules for decision tree. These techniques follow divide and conquer strategy on the data set to obtain two subsets. The algorithm is applied to subsets recursively. Each intermediate node tests a feature. Following path between leafs and root could take as a simple rectangular rule. PSO neighbourhood concept could design to extract tree based rules directly. In this structure each agent has a single decision node. Neighbourhood definition could force tree rule indication. Adjacent agents are defining as similar limitations on all features but one. The best point in the vicinity is the solution that satisfies neighbourhood condition while having lowest limitation. From decision tree point of view, best node in the neighbourhood is the root of its sub-tree and of course the best solution is decision tree root. The final solution presents by all agents together. Also the fitness function in this application is different from original target function and depends on the size of rule-set as well as accuracy parameters as described in the previous chapter.

4.5 Rule injection and rejection

Clinician involves in the rule-set instruction with rejecting an existed rule inside database or injection of new fact into the dataset. After injection or rejection process, other rules inside database may be affected. In the PSO algorithm there are two absorption points, local best solution and global best solution. New injection rule could model as a new absorption point. Injected rule could affect other solutions in the vicinity; however, training process is not applying to this rule. On the other hand, rejected rules are modelling as penalty term in the fitness function of the neighbourhood solutions. By adjusting mandatory conditions on the rules the target function changes to produce more realistic rule-set.

5. Extreme decision points and support vector machines

Classification is a valuable tool in data mining. Reasoning rules could extract from a classifier where we have more control on data analysis. Many successful decision support algorithm use well know pattern recognition algorithm. In this part we present the idea of extreme point from functional analysis. Through this part, we seem how its concept could be used as a valuable tool to make decision support structure. Also we propose support vector machine as a practical way to find critical points.

5.1 Extreme observation points for decision making

A point in a set is extreme if it could not express as an affine combination of other points. On the other hand, it is easy to show each member of a set could express as an affine combination of extreme points. Formally, the extreme points p of a decision boundary of R1 is defined as:

$$\exists w \mid wp + b > 0 \Rightarrow p \in R1 \tag{6}$$

Separation theory, which is the key theory in convex optimization, could express in term of extreme points: if two sets are linearly separable, their extreme points are separable or extreme points are sufficient to check linear separation of two set. In convex set case, this condition is sufficient for non-linear separation too. In other word, the nearest points of two decision boundary are always extreme points.

In practice the extreme theory is not very useful because of inaccuracy of data and limited observations. Since real-world data is quite noisy, identifying real extreme points are difficult. Also with limited observations of a set, there is not guarantee to have all extreme points in the observation set. Support vector machine is a powerful statistical learning tool that could use to find approximation of extreme points in the noisy observation.

5.2 Support vector machines and finding extreme points

Support vector machines (SVMs) have been successfully applied to a wide range of pattern recognition problems, including handwriting recognition, object recognition, speaker identification, face detection and text categorization (Zheng 1999; Majumder et la. , 2005, Valentini et la. 2005, Smach 2008). SVMs are attractive because they are based on an extremely well developed theory based on statistical learning. A support vector machine finds an optimal separating hyper-plane between members and non-members of a given class in the feature space. One can build a classifier capable of discriminating between members and non-members of a given class, such as feature vectors for a particular disease. Such a classifier would be useful in recognizing new members of the class. Furthermore, the classifier can be applied to the original set of training data to identify outliers that may have not been previously recognized.

In this section, we briefly introduce SVM. For detailed information, see (Cortes et la. 1995, Smach 2008).

For pattern recognition, we estimate a function using training data, where N is the feature space dimension (Webb et la. 2007).

To design learning algorithms, we need a class of functions. SV classifiers are based on the class of hyper-planes

$$(\vec{w} \cdot \vec{\theta}) - b = 0 \quad \vec{w} \in R^N, \, b \in R \tag{7}$$

They are corresponding to the decision functions

$$V(\vec{\theta}) = sign(\vec{w} \cdot \vec{\theta} - b). \tag{8}$$

Rescaling and such that the point(s) close to the hyper-plane satisfy implies:

$$y_i(\vec{w} \cdot \vec{\theta}_i - b) \geq 1, \; i = 1,2,\ldots N \tag{9}$$

The margin, measured perpendicularly to the hyper-plane, equals. To maximize the margin, we thus have to minimize subject to Equation 9. We then minimize the function:

$$\Phi\ (\vec{w}) = \frac{1}{2}\|\vec{w}\|^2 = \frac{1}{2}(\vec{w},\vec{w}) \tag{10}$$

The optimal hyper-plane can be uniquely constructed by solving a constrained quadratic programming problem whose solution is in terms of a subset of training patterns that lies in the margin. These training patterns are called support vectors.
To construct the optimal hyper-plane in the case when the data are linearly non-separable, we introduce nonnegative variables and the function

$$\Phi(\xi) = (\vec{w},\vec{w}) + C\sum_i \xi_i \tag{11}$$

Here is a regularization parameter used to allow a trade-off between the training error and the margin. We will minimize the above function subject to the constraints

$$y_i((\vec{w}\cdot\vec{\theta}_i) - b) \geq 1 - \xi_i \tag{12}$$

It can also be solved by quadratic optimization.

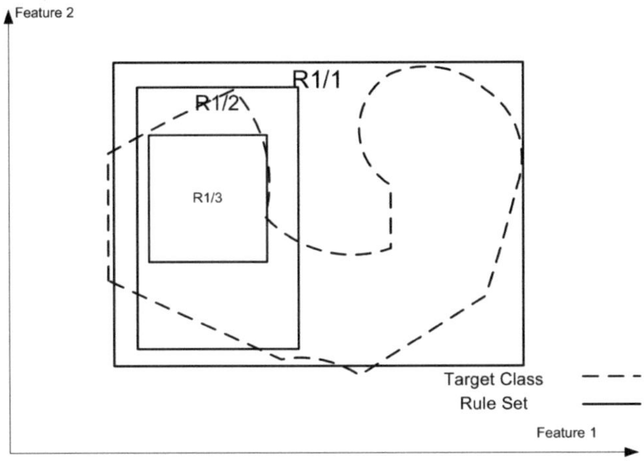

Fig 2. Hiercial rectangular rules to cover a non-covex rule-set.

6. Data mining for temporal lobe epilepsy

This section describes the main target problem of this article, epilepsy surgery candidate selection. In the following, we will describe the importance of the problem and the challenges we faces to find a solution. The problem is new in the area of soft computing but still can be considered as a prototype of common medical diagnosis problems such as breast cancer staging or leukaemia genome expression.

6.1 Problem statement

Epilepsy is recognized as an organic process of the brain. More formally, epilepsy is an occasional, excessive, and disorderly discharge of nerve tissue, seizure, which sometimes can be detected by electroencephalographic (EEG) recording. It is a complex symptom caused by a variety of pathological processes that result in treatment selection difficulties. Pharmacotherapy or surgical treatments are the neurologist alternatives. Optimal treatment selection in the first step may change the patient's life. Temporal lobe epilepsy is one of the most common types of known epilepsy. The main origin of seizures in this type is located in the hippocampus.

Despite optimal pharmacotherapy, about 20–30% of the patients do not become seizure-free (Sisodiya 1995). For some of these patients, surgery is a therapeutic option. Success of resective epilepsy surgery increased from 43% to 85% during the period 1986–1999 (Nei Et la 2000). Data from multiple sources suggest that 55–70% of patients undergoing temporal resection and 30–50% of patient undergoing extra-temporal resection become completely seizure-free (Tonini et la 2004). A recent prospective randomized controlled trial of surgery for temporal lobe epilepsy showed that 58% of patients randomized to surgery became seizure-free compared to 8% of the medical group (Wiebe 2001).

Surgery is considered a valuable option for medically intractable epilepsy even in the absence of a proven drug resistance; in addition, surgical outcome may be greatly influenced by the presence of selected prognostic indicators (Jeha et la. 2007). However, there are still uncertainties on who are the best surgical candidates, i.e., those who most likely will present good surgical outcome.

In a recent narrative literature review of temporal resections, good surgical outcome was associated with a number of factors (hippocampal sclerosis, anterior temporal localization of interictal epileptiform activity, absence of preoperative generalized seizures, and absence of seizures in the first post-operative week) (Sisodiya 1995). However, the published results were frequently confusing and contradictory, thus preventing inferences for clinical practice. Methodological issues (e.g., sample size, selection criteria, and methods of analysis) were indicated by the authors as the most likely explanation of the conflicting literature reports (Jeha et la. 2007).

For this reason, a quantitative review of the available literature has been undertaken in (Jeha et la. 2007) to assess the overall outcome of the epilepsy surgery and to identify the factors better correlating to seizure outcome. The aim of the study was to perform a meta-analysis of the results of published observational studies and assess the prognostic significance of the selected variables outlining the characteristics of the clinical condition, the correlations between the epileptogenic and functional lesion, and the type of surgical procedure.

6.2 Database for epilepsy patients

Human brain image database system (HBIDS) is under development for epilepsy patients at Henry Ford Health System, Detroit, MI (Ghannad-Rezaie et la. 2005; 2006). The proposed HBIDS will examine surgical candidacy among temporal lobe epilepsy patients based on their brain images and other data modalities. Moreover, it can discover relatively weak correlations between symptoms, medical history, treatment planning, outcome of the epilepsy surgery, and brain images. The HBIDS data include modalities such as MRI and SPECT along with patient's personal and medical information and EEG study (Ghannad-Rezaie et la. 2005, Siadat et la. 2005, 2003). The data has been de-identified according to HIPPA regulations (Ghannad-Rezaie et la. 2006).

For the first phase of the EEG study, the non-visual feature extractor is an expert or specialist. The experts do this routinely in the clinic based on well-defined standards. For un-structured text information, the wrapper is the expert or trained nurse. The structured data such as patient's personal information do not need to be analyzed by the wrapper, so they are directly stored in the database (Ghannad-Rezaie et la. 2006).

6.3 Candidate selection problem

Most of data mining methods are designed to work on a huge amount of data; thus KDD problem with small sample size does not broadly browse in the data mining literature. The most successful approach is to add classification or modelling stage before the rule extraction. A smart classifier can recover the patterns inside dataset and minder can recover the classification rules. In this approach, thoughtful selection of both steps is critical.

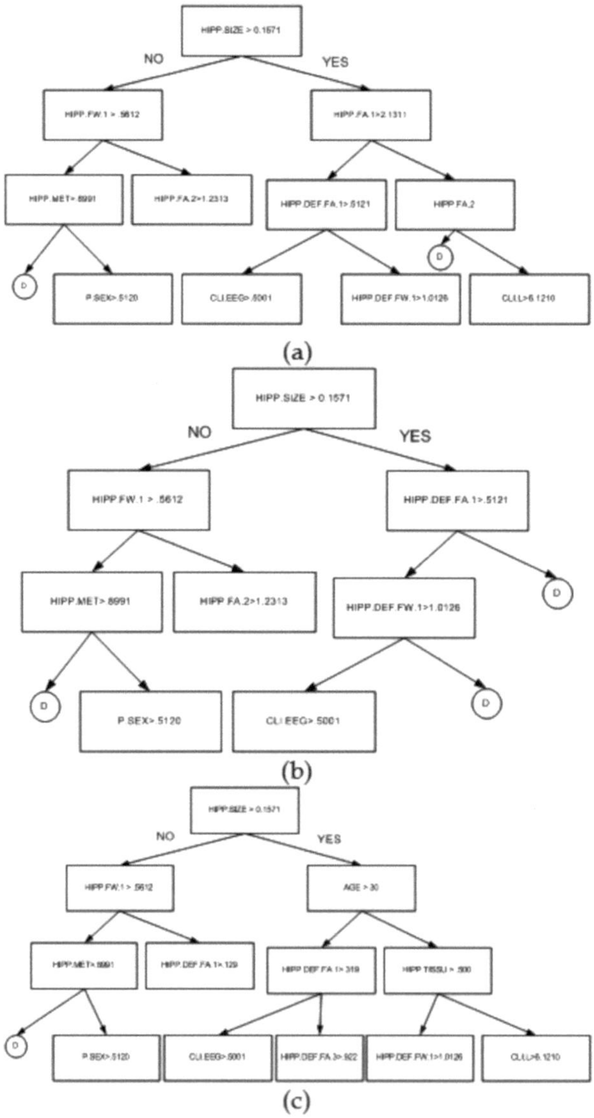

Fig. 3. a) Extracted rules in decision, b) rule injection, c) rule rejection.

Candidate selection in epilepsy, more generally in medical diagnosis, is a hard pattern recognition problem. As well as many current bioinformatics problems, the main challenge in candidate selection problem is to find an optimal point in a very large-dimensional data-space with few samples. As an example of other problems with the same challenge, functionally gene classification problem (Wallace 2006) has a reduced feature space with 200 dimensions while usually less than 50 samples are available in each case. Epilepsy problem has a 40-dimensions space and around 55 samples. Common soft computing tools such as neural networks are efficiently applicable only on large datasets. The longer feature vector, the larger database is required. Overtraining problem is always a threat for small samples machine learning. On the other hand, conventional feature space dimension reduction algorithms such as principle component analysis (PCA) are based on statistical computations that can not be applied to small number of samples. Other difficulties such as missing data, large variety of medical data types, feature disturbances, and prior knowledge make the problem more complicated. Furthermore, knowledge recovery in this problem is not straightforward.

7. Experimental results

7.1 Classifier evaluation

Medical classification accuracy studies often yield continuous data based on predictive models for treatment outcomes. Evaluation of the classifier efficiency is computed with regard to true or false classification results. True positive (TP), true negative (TN), false positive (FP) and false negative (FN) values are the basic evaluation measures for a classifier. The sensitivity and specificity of a diagnostic test depends on more than just the "quality" of the test---they also depend on the definition of what constitutes an abnormal test. A popular method for evaluating the performance of a diagnostic test is the receiver operating characteristic (ROC) curve analysis (Zhou 2005). ROC is a plot of the true positive rate against the false positive rate for the different possible cut-points of the classifier. Each point of the ROC curve is obtained by finding the true positive rate when the decision threshold is selected based on a specific false alarm rate.
The area under ROC curve represents accuracy of a classifier. In medical problems, false alarm rate as well as false rejection rate should be lower than pre-specified limits. The trade off between false alarm rate and false rejection rate is problem specific. In surgery decision-making problem, both rates must be considered; however, false alarm rate (doing surgery for a patient who does not need it) is more likely to be of concern.

7.2 Cross validation training

Because of a very low number of samples, complete separation of the test and train sets is not economical. Cross-validation is used to reuse train information in test process to measure the generalization error [20]. Assume is a set with cardinality of l and an algorithm maps F to VF in the results space. We would like to measure the generalization error. Cross-validation uses l-p samples to find the function of Vl-p where the generalization error is measured by:

$$e_1 = \sum_{x_i \in F_p} Eval(V_{l-p}(\vec{\theta}_i), y_i) \tag{13}$$

This process repeats M times and the final error expectation is

$$\hat{e} = \frac{1}{M}\sum_{i=1}^{M} e_i \tag{14}$$

which is expected to be the generalization error of Vl. When p is 1, it can be shown that the generalization error estimation is un-biased. Although this validation is time consuming, significantly increases the power of the training process. For most efficient use of the data, training and test sets are not separated. In each training epoch, 4/5 of the patients are randomly selected to train the classifier. The rest of the patients (1/5) are used to test. The final classifier is the average of many training processes. This training strategy provides maximum database usage efficiency at the cost of higher computational complexity. In this experiment, more than 50 train-test sets are used. The training process terminates when the classifier's mean squared error of the test-set increases in the last two epochs. The train and test vectors are the normalized classifications.

7.3 Performance

Here we present experimental result of comparison of four proposed algorithms: Structured decision tree training as the representative of classic mining algorithms, Ant colony miner as an evolutionary algorithm pioneer in medical data mining, previously proposed PSO database miner, hybrid approach. Common train and test dataset has been used for all data miners. Table 2 and 3 compare performance of different algorithms.

The performance of data mining algorithms is compared from different points of view. Performance of the generated rule sets has been compared using evaluation functions proposed in the previous parts. Relatively, C4.5 generates the most accurate solution. Actually it misses very few test cases but the overall score of this approach is quit low. Having a close look on simplicity metric and number of rules, it is obvious that the high accuracy of C4.5 is the result of a more complex rule set and the loss of generalization.

C4.5 is very fast algorithms compared with SI algorithm due to its iterative and divide/conquer strategy, thus can not be fairly compared with evolutionary data miners (Figure 4). It is especially designed to handle huge amount of data so obviously we expect very fast convergence. Among evolutionary algorithms, PSO shows a very good convergence speed. Simulation shows that even with an additional classification learning process, PSO is faster that conventional ACO miner while having the same performance.

Altogether, C4.5 shows to be a powerful method but the resulting rule is too complex to use. Fast convergence of C4.5 is impressive but for small databases it is not recommended. PSO after classification process obviously outperforms PSO direct knowledge recovery from database but it is comparable with ACO in some aspects. Generally, simulation results show that the proposed hybrid process has the best overall evaluation while is still somewhat faster than the previous evolutionary algorithms. Also a bit more memory usage can count as a drawback of the new approach compared to ACO and simple PSO. The effect of rule injection and rejection process has been shown Figure 6.

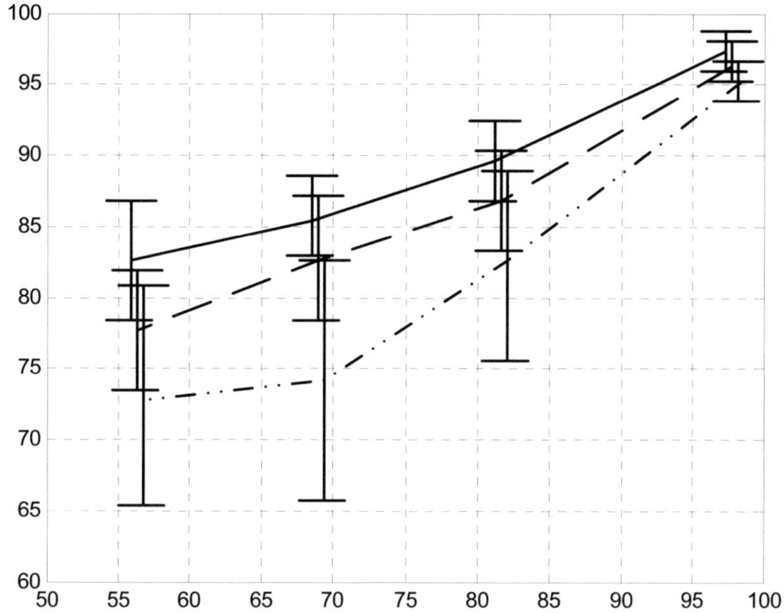

Fig. 4. New approach for different rule fitness factors.

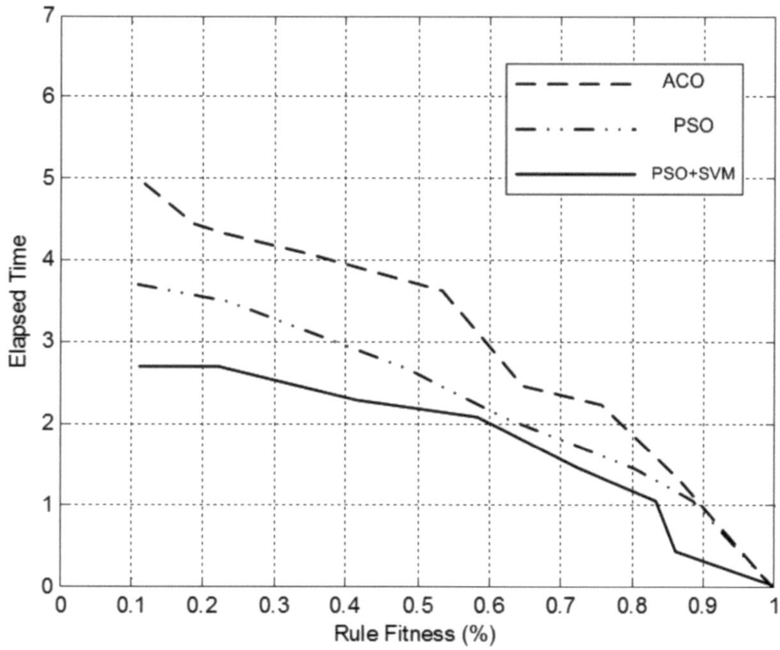

Fig. 5. Compare ACO and PSO rule extaction to new approach.

	Number of Total Terms in Rules	Accuracy (%)	Overall Evaluation (%)
C4.5 (J48)	9	92.9	81.7
ACO	8	76.5	88.3
PSO on Database	10	87.7	84.2
PSO on SVM Classifier	6	89.1	91.7

	Sensitivity (%)	Specificity (%)	Simplicity (%)
C4.5 (J48)	0.8421	0.9911	64.7
ACO	0.9521	0.9821	74.2
PSO on Database	0.8192	0.9541	53.8
PSO on SVM Classifier	0.9821	0.9781	87.5

Table 2. Acuracy paramenters for different apparoaches. The new approach gives the simplest rule expression while keeping good specificity.

Database	Percentage of dataset	Percentage of rule set	Accuracy on train set	Accuracy on test set	Traditional Method Performance
Breast Cancer	100%	0%	94.50	92.18	92.18
	50%	10%	90.31	89.51	89.52
	30%	15%	89.21	84.64	82.91
	25%	20%	86.69	84.88	80.94
Pima Diabetes	100%	0%	76.31	75.11	75.11
	50%	10%	74.12	72,05	70.82
	30%	15%	71.81	69.86	68.21
	25%	20%	72.92	70.45	62.94
Sonar	100%	0%	99.12	97.91	97.91
	50%	10%	93.21	91.96	91.21
	30%	15%	94.12	89.76	87.91
	25%	20%	91.49	88.29	85.63
Votes	100%	0%	88.21	85.41	85.41
	50%	10%	77.62	76.91	75.42
	30%	15%	79.21	78.81	76.65
	25%	20%	76.83	74.21	73.12

Table 3. UCI database (Hettich et la.1999) used to verified the approach.

	Accuracy (A %)	Quality (Q %)	Coverage (C %)	Simplicity (S %)	Interference (I %)	Overall (using A)	Overall (using Q)
C4.5	89	81	94	74	11	81	79
ACO	84	73	90	86	25	78	74
PSO	88	76	85	81	35	72	68
Hybrid	91	82	89	89	16	83	81

Table 4. Overall performance of different data miners on Wisconsin Breast Cancer data (*a*, *b*, *c*, *d* are set to 0.33).

8. Conclusion

We will develop and evaluate a new approach for interactive data mining based on swarm intelligence. The proposed method will process external rules along with the raw data to do reasoning. The proposed method is designed to work in low sample and high dimensional feature space conditions where statistical power of the raw data is not sufficient for a reliable decision. The proposed method will have both of the injection and rejection of rules to allow interactive and effective contributions provided by an expert user. The well-known support vector machine (SVM) classifier and swarm data miner will be integrated to handle joint processing of the raw data and the rules. The primary idea will be used to establish limits of observations and build decision boundaries based on these critical observations.

9. References

Apte C.; Weiss S. (1997) Data mining with decision trees and decision rules, *Future Generation Computer Systems*, Vol. 13, No 2-3, pp 197-210

Barakat N; Diederich, J;Eclectic rule-extraction from support vector machines, International Journal of Computational Intelligence

Botee, H. M.; Bonabeau, E.(1998) Evolving Ant Colony Optimization, ADVANCES IN COMPLEX SYSTEMS, Vol 1; No 2/3, pp 149-160

Clerc M.; Kennedy J. (2002) The particle swarm-explosion, stability and convergence in a multidimensional complex space, *IEEE Transactions on Evolutionary Computation*, Vol. 6, No 1, pp 58-73

Cortes C., Vapnik V. (1995) Support-vector networks, *Machine learning*, Vol. 20, Issue 3, 273–297

Chien C; Wanga W; Chenga J (2007) Data mining for yield enhancement in semiconductor manufacturing and an empirical study, Expert Systems with Applications, Vol 33, No 1,pp 192-198

Hettich S.; Bay S. D. (1999) The UCI KDD Archive [http://kdd.ics.uci.edu]. Irvine, CA: University of California, Department of Information and Computer Science

Galea M. (2002) Applying swarm intelligence to rule induction, MS Thesis, University of Edinburgh, Scotland

Ghannad-Rezaie M.; Soltanian-Zadeh H.; Siada M.; Elisevich K. V.(2005) Soft computing approaches to computer aided decision making for temporal lobe epilepsy, *Proc. of IEEE International Conf. on Fuzzy Systems (NAFIPS)*, Ann Arbor, Michigan, USA

Ghannad-Rezaie M.; Soltanian-Zadeh H.; Siadat M.-R.; K.V. Elisevich (2006) Medical Data Mining using Particle Swarm Optimization for Temporal Lobe Epilepsy, *Proceedings of the IEEE World Congress on Computational Intelligence*, Vancouver, Canada, July 15-21

Jaganathan P.; Thangavel K., Pethalakshmi A.; Karnan M. (2007) Classification rule discovery with ant colony optimization and improved quick reduce algorithm, *IAENG International Journal of Computer Science*, Vol. 33, No. 1 pp 50-55

Jeha, L. E. ;Najm, I.; Bingaman, W. ;Dinner, D. ;Widdess-Walsh, P. Luders, H.(2007) Surgical outcome and prognostic factors of frontal lobe epilepsy surgery, BRAIN, Vol 130; No 2, pp 574-584

Kim, S. H.; Hyun Ju Noh (1997) Predictability of Interest Rates Using Data Mining Tools, EXPERT SYSTEMS WITH APPLICATIONS, Vol 13; No 2, pp 85-96

Lan Y.; Zhang L.; Liu L. (2002) A method for extracting rules from incomplete information system, *Notes in Theoretical Computer Science*, Vol. 82, No. 4, pp. 312-315

Lavrac M. (1999) Selected techniques for data mining in medicine, Artificial Intelligence in medicine, Vol 6, No.1, pp 3-23.

Majumder S. K. ; Ghosh N.; Gupta P.K.(2005) Support vector machine for optical diagnosis of cancer, Journal of Biomedical Optics

Nei, M.; Ho, R. T. ;Sperling, M. R. (2000) EKG Abnormalities During Partial Seizures in Refractory Epilepsy, EPILEPSIA, VOL 41, No 5, pp 542-548

Omkara, S.N.;Karanth R (2008) Rule extraction for classification of acoustic emission signals using Ant Colony Optimisation, Engineering Applications of Artificial Intelligence, Vol 4, No 1, 320-324

Parpinelli R.S.; Lopes H. S.; Freitas A. A. (2002) Data mining with an ant colony optimization algorithm,IEEE Transactions on Evolutionary Computation,

Quinlan J. R. (1993) C4.5: Programs for Machine Learning, Morgan Kaufmann Inc.

Siadat M;Soltanian-Zadeh H; Fotouhi F;Elisevich K (2003) Multimodality medical image database for temporal lobe epilepsy, Proceedings of SPIE Vol. 5033, pp 487-491.

Siadat M;Soltanian-Zadeh H; Fotouhi F;Elisevich K (2005) Content-based image database system for epilepsy .Computer Methods and Programs in Biomedicine , Vol 79 , No 3 , pp 209 - 226

Sisodiya, S. M.; Free, S. L. ;Stevens, J. M. ;Fish, D. R. (1995) Widespread cerebral structural changes in patients with cortical dysgenesis and epilepsy, Brain, Vol 118, No4, pp 1039

Sousa T.; Silva A., Neves A. (2004) Particle Swarm based data mining algorithms for classification tasks, *Parallel Computing J.*, Vol. 30, pp. 767-783

Smach, F. (2008) Generalized Fourier Descriptors with Applications to Objects Recognition inÂ SVM Context, JOURNAL OF MATHEMATICAL IMAGING AND VISION, Vol 30, No 1, pp 43-71

Tonini C; Beghi E;Berg A.;Bogliun G;Giordano L;Newton R; Tetto A;Vitelli E;Vitezic D;Wiebe S(2004)Predictors of epilepsy surgery outcome: a meta-analysis, Epilepsy Research , Vol. 62 , No 1 , pp 75 - 87

Toivonen, H. T. T. Onkamo, P. Vasko, K. Ollikainen, V. Sevon, P. Mannila, H. Herr, M. Kere, J. (2000) Data Mining Applied to Linkage Disequilibrium Mapping,AMERICAN JOURNAL OF HUMAN GENETICS,Vol 67; No 1, pp 133-145

Wallace M.; Ioannou S., Karpouzis K.; Kollias S. (2006) Possibility rule evaluation: a case study in facial expression analysis, *International Journal of Fuzzy Systems*, Vol. 8, No 4,pp 219-23

Webb-Robertson B. J. M. ; Oehmen C. S. ; Cannon R.W.(2007) Support Vector Machine Classification of Probability Models and Peptide Features for Improved Peptide Identification from Shotgun Proteomics, Machine Learning and Applications,Vol 1,No 1, pp 500-505

Wiebe, S.; Blume, W. T.; Girvin, J. P.; Eliasziw, M.(2001)A Randomized, Controlled Trial of Surgery for Temporal-Lobe Epilepsy, NEW ENGLAND JOURNAL OF MEDICINE, Vol 345; No 5, pp 311-318

Valentini G. (2005) An experimental bias-variance analysis of SVM ensembles based on resampling techniques, IEEE Transactions on Systems, Man and Cybernetics, Part B,

Xu, J. Huang, Y. (2007) Using SVM to Extract Acronyms from Text, SOFT COMPUTING, Vol 11; No 4, pp 369-373

Zheng Z., Low BT, (1999) Classifying unseen cases with many missing values," *Proc. of Methodologies for Knowledge Discovery and Data Mining Conf.*, Vol. 2, pp. 370-372

Zou K. H.; Resnic F. S.; Talos I. (2005) A global goodness-of-fit test for receiver operating characteristic curve analysis via the bootstrap method, *J. of Biomedical Informatics*, Vol. 38, Issue 5, pp 395-403

9

Monitoring Human Resources of a Public Health-Care System through Intelligent Data Analysis and Visualization

Aleksander Pur[1], Marko Bohanec[2], Bojan Cestnik[4,2], and Nada Lavrač[2,3]
[1] *Ministry of Interior Affairs, Ljubljana,*
[2] *Jožef Stefan Institute, Ljubljana,*
[3] *University of Nova Gorica, Nova Gorica,*
[4] *Temida, d.o.o., Ljubljana,*
Slovenia

1. Introduction

According to the World Health Report (World Health Organization, 2000), a health-care system (HCS) is a system composed of organizations, institutions and resources that are devoted to producing a health action. Human resources are one of the main parts of this system.

This paper is focused on the model for monitoring and planning of human resources in the Slovenian public HCS. The HCS of Slovenia is divided into the primary, secondary and tertiary health-care levels. The primary health-care (PHC) is the patients' first entry point into the HCS. It is composed of four sub-systems: general practice, gynaecology paediatrics and dentistry.

We have developed a model for monitoring the network of physicians at the PHC level, taking into the account the physicians' specializations, their geographic and work-time dispersion, time capacity constraints and their availability for patients. The motivation for this development came from the Ministry of Health of the Republic of Slovenia, who need a holistic overview of the PHC network in order to make short- and long-term management decisions and apply appropriate management actions, as well as evaluate PHC target achievements.

The first step was to form a data warehouse; a corresponding Entity Relationship Diagram data model was composed of unique database entries from the following existing sources:

- Slovenian Social Security databases: the data about health-care providers together with assigned patients per individual general practitioner, assigned patients with social security, and the data about health-care centres,
- the database of Slovenian physicians and dentists (Slovenian Medical Chamber),
- the database of the National Institute of Public Health containing data about Slovenian health centres, and
- the database of the Slovenian Statistics Bureau concerning the demographic and geographic distribution of citizens and communities in Slovenia.

The next steps involved the development of the model for monitoring the network of primary-care professionals based on the established data warehouse. The model was used on real HCS data for the year 2006, which forms a part of a larger model for monitoring the responsiveness of the HCS for population, developed for the Ministry of Health of the Republic of Slovenia.

2. Methodology

Despite many frameworks related to performance and activity monitoring (Data-driven Decision Support System (DSS) (Power, 2002), Performance Monitoring, Business Performance Management (BPM), Business Activity Monitoring (BAM) (Dresner, 2003) etc.), there is a lack of methodologies for representing the concept of monitoring based on different data analysis methods. A similar methodology is addressing Performance Monitoring Protocols presented by the Working Party on Performance Monitoring in the Public Services (Bird, 2005). In this section, we present our approach to performance monitoring in modelling the PHC network in Slovenia.

2.1 Approach to human resources monitoring

Our model for monitoring the network of primary-care professionals in the Slovenian HCS consists of hierarchically connected modules. Each *module* is aimed at monitoring some aspect of the PHC network, which is of interest for decision-makers and managers of the network. Typical aspects about physicians are, for example: age and qualification of physicians, their workload and geographical distribution.

Each module involves a number of monitoring processes, which are gathered according to a given monitoring goal. Each *monitoring process* is characterised by: monitoring objectives, input data, data collecting methods, constraints on data, data dimensions, data analysis methods, output data, target criteria or target values of outputs, output data representation and visualisation methods, security requirements and the users of the monitoring system. Among these components, the *data analysis methods* transform the *input data* to *output data* represented using some *data representation formalism* according to the given *monitoring objectives*. The *target* is a level of performance that the organization aims to achieve for a particular activity. Information about *data collection* shows how and how often the data has been collected or needs to be collected (e.g., data can be collected by representative surveys or by standard procedures in organizations according to some refreshment rate). The *constraints* define the valid input and output data. *Security requirements* define the use and management of the monitoring processes and of the data.

This approach is not limited to any particular *data analysis method*. In principle, any methods can be used, such as Structured Query Language (SQL) procedures, On Line Analytical Process (OLAP) techniques for interactive knowledge discovering, as well as knowledge discovery in data (KDD) and data mining methods (Han, 2001) for discovering important but previously unknown knowledge. The same holds for *data representation* methods, which can include pivot tables, charts, network graphs and maps.

With respect to monitoring goals, *output variables* can be classified in different categories like *lead* and *lag* (Niven, 2003). The *lead* ones measure the performances that have influence on achieving the goals, whereas the *lag* are only related to the degree of achieving the goals.

In order to improve the comprehensibility of the model, its modules are hierarchically structured. The modules at the top level represent the main objectives. Usually all the main objectives can be incorporated in a single top-level module. The modules at a lower level are connected to the one at a higher level. Each connection represents a data channel that connects outputs of the lower level module with the inputs of a higher-level module. In principle, the hierarchy is constructed so that the results of lower-level processes could help to explain the results of monitoring processes at a higher level. For example, the module for the assessment of HCS responsiveness could be composed of the physical accessibility of Health Services, availability of resources of Health Services and the rate of visits of population to health-care provider.

2.2 The model of monitoring human resources in a HCS

The model of monitoring the network of physicians at the PHC level is made in accordance with the above described methodology. The real challenge was to improve the monitoring of human resources in the HCS by different KDD methods..

The main concept is described by the hierarchically connected modules, shown in Fig. 1. The module *human resources* represents the main aspect of monitoring. The included monitoring processes are aimed at the monitoring of anomalies, outliers and other interesting events related to the network of physicians. The lower-level modules intend to provide detailed explanations of these events.

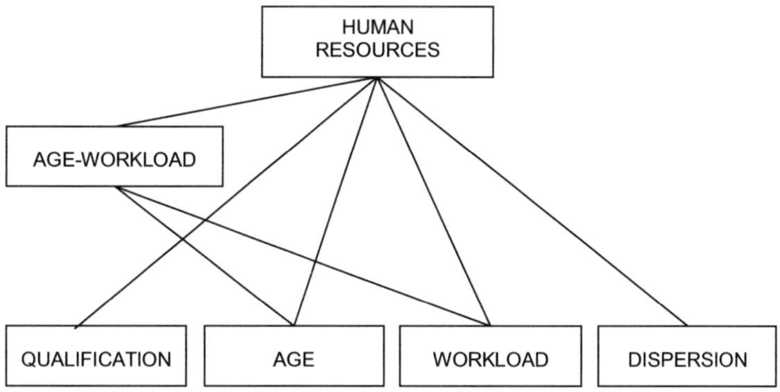

Fig. 1. The structure of the model for monitoring the network of physicians at a primary health-care level, represented by hierarchically connected modules.

3. Description of individual HCS modules

3.1 Monitoring of human resources

The main module *human resources* is aimed at a holistic monitoring of physicians' performance. In principle, the monitoring processes in this module must be able to process several input parameters. Therefore, different methods of KDD and multi-criteria decision models can be used for data analysis. The module includes a monitoring process that intends to represent the main aspects of physicians characterised by their *qualification, age, gender, workload* and *dispersion* (the number of locations where the physician works). The monitoring process is based on the OLAP model, which uses the dimensions: *time, location* where physicians work, *specialisation* and *gender*. The results based on a prototype application are presented by pivot tables and multidimensional charts, as shown in Fig. 2.

The scatterplot on the right side of Fig. 2 shows the average age, average workload, and average dispersion of physicians in communities for different specializations. The x-axis shows the average age of physicians, while the average workload is shown along the y-axis.

The communities are shown by shapes and colours of data points as explained in the legend. The size of these points is proportional to the average dispersion of physicians in the community. The specialization and gender of physicians could be selected using combo boxes in the top left corner. Thus, the scatterplot shows these average values for a gynaecologist working in some Slovenian community. For example, the workload and age of physicians shown on the top right corner are above the average. This presentation clearly shows outliers and anomalies in the HCS. Detailed information about these interesting aspects could be found in lower level modules. On the left side of Fig. 2, the same data is represented by the pivot table.

This module also includes a monitoring process aimed at discovering relations between the main aspects of physicians using the methods of association rules discovery (Srikant, 1996). The monitoring process tries to find the outliers overlooked by previous OLAP analyses. Table 1, for example, includes some rules focused on the relations between communities and physicians working in general practice. For example, for the community Škofja Loka it is characteristic that physicians younger than 40 years are underloaded (see the rules 2, 3). This module could also include the monitoring processes based on multi-criteria decision models (Bohanec, 2006).

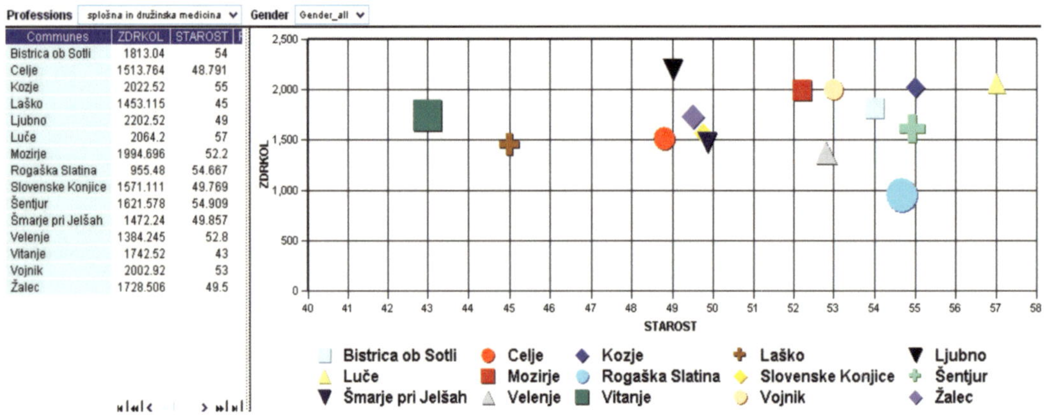

Fig. 2. The holistic aspect of physicians presented by OLAP techniques.

Rule	Supp.	Conf.	Lift
[age:60+]+[workload: middle] ==>Ptuj	0.51%	14.63%	5.99
[dispersion:1]+[age:to40]+[workload: small] ==>Škofja Loka	0.34%	5.97%	4.42
[age:to40]+[workload: small] ==> Škofja Loka]	0.34%	5.19%	3.85
[workload: large]+[age:40-60]+[gender] ==>Domžale	0.42%	7.04%	3.63
[age:to40]+[workload: middle] ==> Novo mesto	0.42%	9.62%	3.46
[gender:z]+[age:to40]+[workload: small]==> Domžale	0.34%	6.35%	3.27
[gender:z]+[age:to40]+[workload: middle]==> Novo mesto]	0.34%	8.89%	3.19
[workload: large]+[gender:m] ==>Domžale	0.51%	6.00%	3.09
[age:60+]+[workload: large] ==> Maribor	0.67%	25.81%	3.00
[age:60+]+[workload: large]+[gender:m]==> Maribor	0.59%	25.00%	2.90

Table 1. Association rules showing relations between communities and general practice physicians.

3.2 Qualification of physicians

The aim of this module is to enable monitoring of physicians' and dentists' qualification for the job they actually perform. The main performance indicator is the physician's specialization degree, granted by the Slovenian Medical Chamber, which must be verified every 7 years. The specialization degree is a prerequisite for getting a license for employment in a certain area of medicine.

To monitor the suitability of physicians for the job they are performing we have used social network visualization technique available in the social network analysis program named Pajek ("Spider" (Batagelj, 2006)). The monitoring of physicians' suitability is achieved by the monitoring of three variables: SPEC (specialization), LIC (luicence), and OPR (the type of patients that the physician is in charge of, categorized by patient type). The motivation for this analysis is based on the observation that physicians with a certain specialization may get different luicenses, and while a certain licence assumes that the physician will only deal with patients of a certain patient category, in reality she may be in charge of different types of patients (e.g., a paediatrician may provide health services to grown up patients, although she has a specialization in paediatrics and a licence in paediatrics).

It has also been observed that an individual physician may have several specializations, and several licences, and hence patients of different types. The Pajek diagram (Fig. 3) shows well the typical (thick lines - a high number of physicians) and atypical (thin lines - a low number of physicians) cases, which enable abnormality detection and further analysis of individual discovered anomalies.

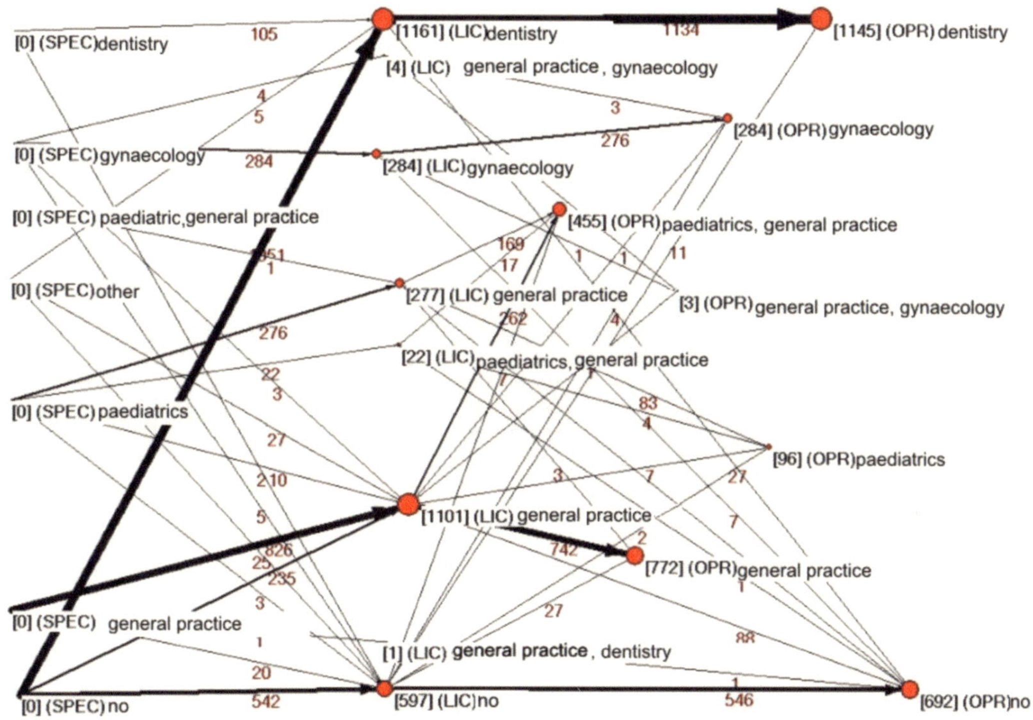

Fig. 3. The qualifications of physicians for the job they are performing.

3.3 Age of physicians

The monitoring processes in this module are aimed at age and gender analyses of physicians. The module includes a process based on the OLAP model. The dimensions of this model are *age*, *gender*, *specializations* and *locations* where they work. The main monitored quantity in the facts table is the number of physicians. The results are presented by pivot tables and different charts. For example, the number of gynaecologists by age and gender is presented in the chart in Fig. 4. The x-axis shows the age variable, while the number of doctors is shown along the y-axis. The gender is shown in the legend. Although relatively simple, this chart clearly shows a decline of the number of young male gynaecologists that have accomplished the studies in the last twenty years. Generally, the number of physicians is related to the number of students that have accomplished the studies at the Faculty of Medicine in Ljubljana that is the main source of doctors in Slovenia. Thus, this presentation can help planning the education system. The other process in this module provides a list of gynaecologists that are near retiring age. The list can be used to help planning missing human resources in the near future.

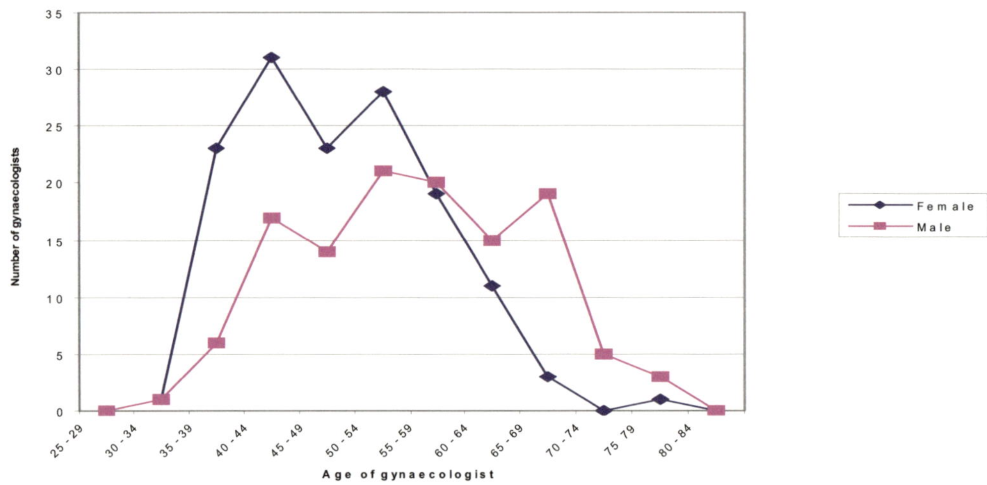

Fig. 4. The numbers of gynaecologists by age and gender.

3.4 Workload analysis

This module is aimed at monitoring the physicians' workload. Considering the available data, the assessment of workload is based on age-adjusted listed patients per physician. Each age group of listed patients is weighted according to use of health-care resources, e.g. the number of visits per physician. The physicians without registered patients are excluded from this analysis.

The monitoring process is based on the OLAP model. The dimensions of this model are: *time*, *specializations*, *locations* where the physicians work, the ratio between the number of listed patients and physicians, and the ratio between the age-adjusted number of listed patients and physicians. The measure in the fact table is the sum of physicians. Again, results are presented in pivot tables and different charts.

3.5 Age-workload analyses

The monitoring processes in this module are aimed at the combined analyses of physicians' age and their workload (number of patients per physician). The considered dimensions are: *time*, *locations* and *professions*. The monitoring process provides the state of each physician regarding their age and the number of patients. For example, Fig. 5 shows the age and workload of general practitioners. The x-axis shows the physicians' age, while the y-axis shows the number of their patients. Physicians aged between 40 and 50 have the most patients, but some of them have a large number of patients also after 50. The retirement of physicians having a large number of patients has an important impact on the PHC network. This impact is more precisely described by the next monitoring process, which is based on GIS.

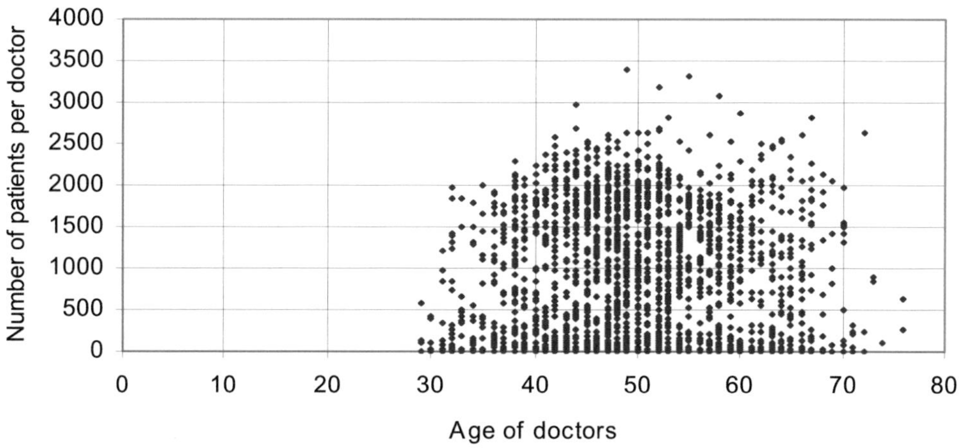

Fig. 5. The physicians in GP by age and listed patients.

The map in Fig. 6 shows the number and share of patients affected by the retirement of physicians in the next five years (until 2011). The assumption is that physicians will retire at the age of 65. In this map, each polygon represents a community. Their shade is proportional to the number of patients whose doctors will retire. The pie charts represent the ratio between the patients unaffected and affected by the retirement until 2011. Thus, this analysis provides information on the number of physicians and regions where they have to be replaced in the next five years.

From the implementation viewpoint, the latter module is composed of data about physicians' age, their registered patients and geographic data. The detailed information about physicians' age and patients is provided by subordinate modules *age* and *workload* (Fig. 1).

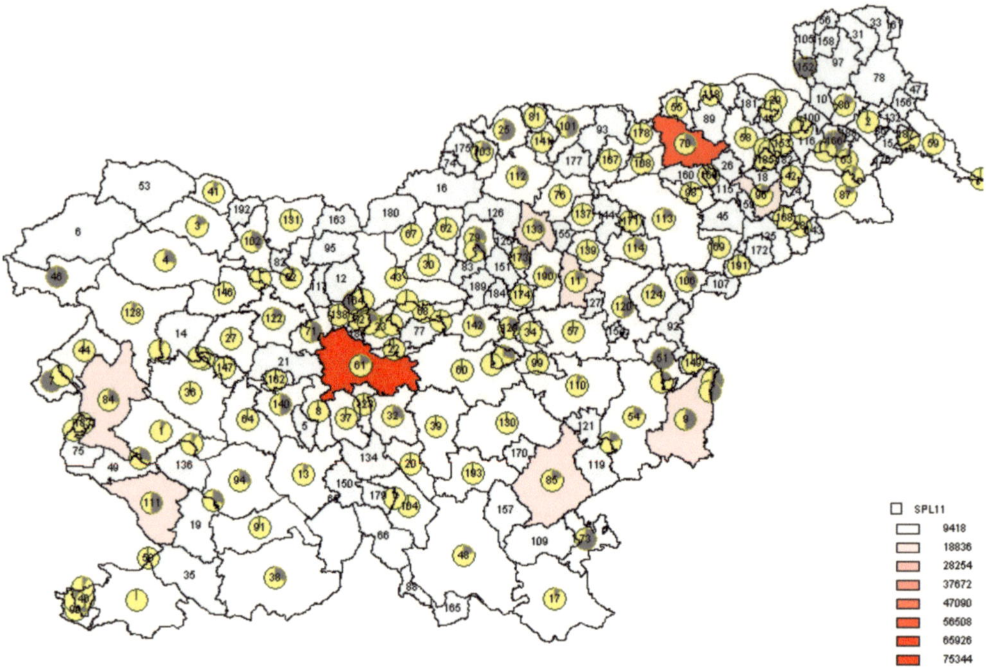

Fig. 6. The impact of physicians retiring until 2011.

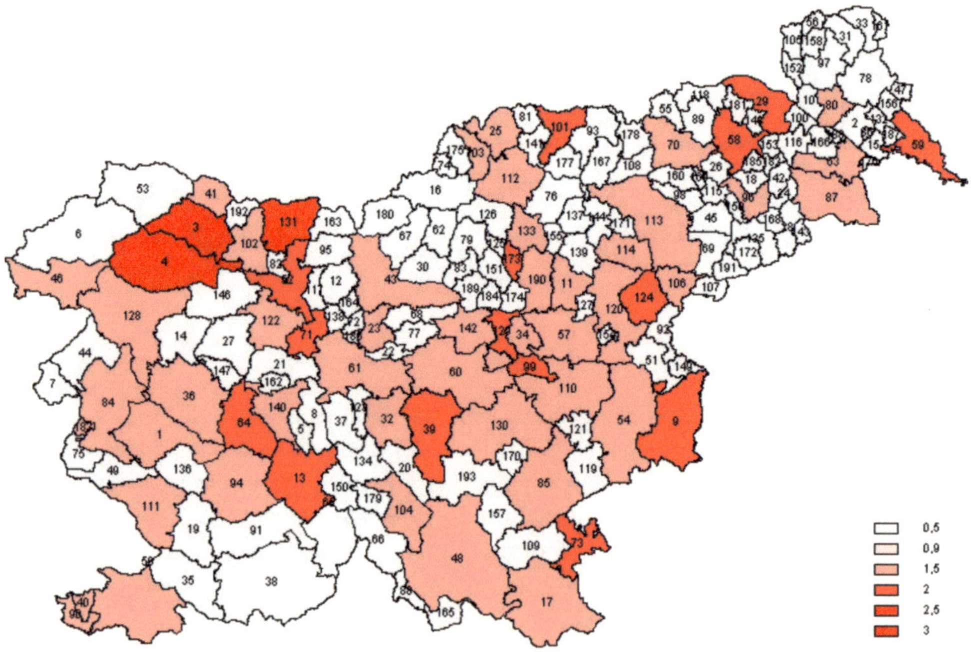

Fig. 7. Average dispersion of working locations.

3.6 Dispersion of working location

This module is aimed at monitoring the dispersion of locations where physicians work. Depending on the requirements, a physician may work on more than one location, but this dispersion usually means additional workload for physicians and their lower availability for patients at some location. The monitoring process provides the number of locations where physicians work, which are shown using the GIS techniques. Fig. 7, for example, shows the dispersion in 2005 for gynaecology. The darker the community are, the larger the average number of locations where physicians from this community work.

4. Conclusion

The aim of the presented human resource monitoring system is to assess performance and provide information necessary for the planning and management of primary health-care network in Slovenia. At the general level, the approach is based on a carefuly designed hierarchy of modules, each monitoring a specific aspect of the network - in particular physicians' age, qualifications, workload and dispersion. At the implementation level, the system uses a number of different techniques, including OLAP, KDD and data analysis (such as association rule mining). In most cases, the results are presented visually by charts, network graphs and maps. In this way, the monitoring system provides an information-rich picture of the network and its performance, and also helps detecting its critical aspects that require short- or long-term management actions. In principle, the higher levels of the model provide holistic information, while the lower levels provide more details that are useful for the explanation of observed phenomena.

The monitoring system has been developed in collaboration with the Ministry of Health of the Republic of Slovenia. Currently, it is implemented as a prototype and has been tested with real data for the year 2006. For the future, we wish that it becomes a regular tool for monitoring the health-care network in Slovenia. We also envision the application of the same methodology in other public networks, such as education and police.

5. References

World Health Organization: World Health Report 2000: Health Systems. Improving Performance, http://www.who.int/whr/2000/en/whr00_en.pdf, Accessed January 26, 2007 (2000)

Niven, R., P.: Balanced Scorecard for Government and Nonprofit Agencies, John Wiley and Sons, Inc (2003), ISBN 0-471-42328-9

Bird, M., S. (ed.): Performance indicators good, bad, and ugly, Working Party on Performance Monitoring in the Public Services, J. R. Statist. Soc. A (2005) 1-26

Bohanec, M.: DEXi, A Program for Multi-Attribute Decision Making. http://www-ai.ijs.si/MarkoBohanec/dexi.html, Accessed January 26, 2007 (2006)

Batagelj, V., Mrvar, A.: Program for Analysis and Visualization of Large Networks. Reference Manual, University of Ljubljana, Ljubljana (2006)

Dresner, H.: Business Activity Monitoring, BAN Architecture, Gartner Symposium ITXPO, Cannes, France (2003)

Power, J., D.: Decision Support Systems. Concepts and Resources for Managers, Quorum Books division Greenwood Publishing, ISBN: 156720497X (2002)

Han, J., Kamber, M.: Data Mining: Concepts and Techniques, Morgan Kaufmann Publishers (2001)
Srikant, R., Agrawal, R.: Mining Quantitative Association Rules in Large Relation Tables, IBM Almaden Research Center, San Jose (1996)

10

Data and Mined-Knowledge Interoperability in eHealth Systems

Kamran Sartipi, Mehran Najafi and Reza S. Kazemzadeh
McMaster University
Canada

1. Introduction

The advancement of software development through component technology and system integration techniques has resulted in a new generation of very large software systems. This new paradigm has intensified challenges including interoperability of heterogeneous systems, sharing and reusing services, management of complexity, and security and privacy aspects. Examples of such globalized systems include: communication systems, banking systems, air traffic systems, transportation systems, and healthcare systems. These challenges require new development and management technologies and processes that fulfill the emerging demands in the networked systems.

Modern healthcare is experiencing major changes and as a result traditional conceptions are evolving: from health provider-centric to patient and family-centric; from solitary decision making to collaborative and evidence-based decision making; from decentralized and generalized care to centralized and specialized care. The need for better quality of service, unique identification of health records, and efficient monitoring and administration requires a uniform and nation-wide organization for service and data access.

Among other requirements, these changes require extensive assistance from modern software and information technology domains. Until recently there has been little attention to the IT infrastructure of healthcare systems. However, global trends are shifting healthcare towards computerization by developing electronic health record systems, IT-standardization through HL7 (Health Level 7) initiatives and nation-wide infrastructure specifications (Canada Health Infoway) and utilization of current evidences in decision-making processes. Most current systems are monolithic, isolated, paper-based, error-prone legacy systems which cause huge costs for the governments and healthcare organizations. The new systems need to take advantage of modern information and distributed systems to meet the emerging demands in healthcare environments.

As a result governments and private sectors are investing on healthcare information technology infrastructures to reduce huge costs of the existing systems and improve the quality of public care.

Health informatics (eHealth) is a new field which embodies a variety of techniques in information and knowledge management, data mining, decision support systems, web services, and security and privacy. Therefore, researchers with multi-disciplinary research interests from these fields need to collaborate in order to advance the state of the art in eHealth. In this chapter, we attempt to cover the core technologies that need to work seamlessly to allow healthcare professionals and administration to use the available services effectively and efficiently. Also, we pay particular attention to the current research activities and issues regarding to the interoperbility of information and knowledge extracted from data mining operations. We propose a new architecture for interoperability of data and mined-knowledge (knowledge extracted from data mining algorithms). Finally, we propose new research avenues on the combination of data mining, eHealth, and service oriented architecture and discuss their characteristics.

The structure of this chapter is as follows: Section 2 presents the application of data mining in healthcare. Section 3 introduces different forms of knowledge representations in medical domain. Section 4, describes messaging standards in this domain. After these introductions to knowledge and messaging standards, we propose our framework in Section 5. In Section 6 an architecture for the framework is discussed and finally in Section 7, some research avenues are elaborated for applying our framework on the architecture that is explained in Section 6. We conclude the discussion of the chapter in Section 8.

2. Application of data mining in healthcare

Data mining or Knowledge Discovery from Databases (KDD) refers to extracting interesting and non-trivial relations and patterns from data in large databases. The results would be used for different purposes and domains stretching from marketing, administration, research, diagnosis, security, and decision making that are characterized by large amount of data with various relations. Healthcare is an important source for generating large and dynamic data repositories that can not be analyzed by professionals without help from computers. Typical healthcare databases containing information about patients, hospitals, bed costs, claims, clinical trials, electronic patient records, and computer supported disease management, are ideal sources to apply data mining operations for discovery purposes.

Data mining solutions have been used in healthcare to overcome a wide range of business issues and problems. Some of these problems include:

- Segmenting patients accurately into groups with similar health patterns.
- Evidence based medicine, where the information extracted from the medical literature and the corresponding medical decisions are key information to leverage the decision made by the professional. Therefore, the system acts as an assistant for the healthcare professionals and provides recommendations to the healthcare professionals.
- Planning for effective information systems management.
- Predicting medical diagnosis, treatment costs, and length of stay in a hospital.

After identifying an appropriate problem in a domain for applying data mining, we need a methodology. Different steps for applying data mining on a large database are as follows.

Data Selection: extract the data fields of interest. The selection is a subset of the data attributes that were collected in the data collection activity. For instance, in data collection the research team might choose to monitor or collect data from all of the patient's physical examinations, while in this step, particular fields, e.g., weight or height measurements are selected to be used for the data mining operation.

Data preprocessing: this step involves checking data records for erroneous values, e.g., invalid values for categorical data items, and out of range values for numerical attributes. In the real world practice, many records may have missing values. The researchers may decide to exclude these records from the data set, or substitute missing attributes with default or calculated values, e.g., the average of the values in other records for a missing numerical attribute.

Data transformations: several different types of transformations may be applied to the data items to make them more appropriate for the particular purpose of mining. The transformations can be considered as changing the basis of the space in which data records reside as points in this space. For example the patient's height in millimeter has probably too much precision; hence a conversion to centimeter or meter may be considered. Additionally, the data mining expert may choose to transform the weight value into discretized bins to further simplify things for the mining process. Also, there might be some fields that are derived from other data attributes, e.g., the duration of an infection can be derived by subtracting the initial diagnosis date from the date that the treatment was completed.

Data modeling: in this step, a data mining algorithm is applied to the data. The choice of the algorithm is decided by the researchers and depends on the particular type of analysis that is being carried out. There are wide ranges of algorithms available, but we can group them into two categories: those that describe the data and those that predict on future cases (Prudsys, 2006). The algorithms can also be grouped based on the type of mining they perform, e.g., clustering, classification, and association rules mining.

Evaluation and interpretation of results: it is essential that the results be evaluated in terms of meaningfulness, correctness, and usefulness. Based on the evaluation of results, the researchers may choose to go some steps back and perform them again differently. This makes the knowledge discovery process an iterative process. After completion of the discovery process, we refer to the extracted results as mined knowledge. These results are eventually stored in some application (data miner tool) specific format for future access and use.

Data mining models

Data mining models are data structures that represent the results of data mining analysis. There are many types of data mining models. In this section we briefly describe some major types: classification, clustering, and association-rules models. There are numerous algorithms in each category that typically differ in terms of their data or application specific fine tunings, their performance and approach in building the models, or the case or domain-specific heuristics they apply to increase the efficiency and performance of the mining process.

Classification models:

A classification algorithm (e.g., neural network or decision tree) assigns a class to a group of data records having specific attributes and attribute-values. The classification techniques in healthcare can be applied for diagnostic purposes. Suppose that certain symptoms or laboratory measurements are known to have a relation with a specific disease. A classification model is built that receives a set of relevant attribute-values, such as clinical observations or measurements, and outputs the class to which the data record belongs. As an example, the classes can identify "whether a patient has been diagnosed with a particular cancer or not", and the classifier model assigns each patient's case to one of these classes. Some classification techniques that are applied on healthcare include: i) Neural network which is modeled as a large number of inter-connected data processors (known as neurons) that possess a small amount of local memory. These neurons learn based on algorithms that are inspired by biological neurons. A neural network (Haykin, 1998) can be used as a tool in the data mining modeling step; and ii) Bayesian (statistical) modeling (Jensen, 1998) is another modeling alternative that uses conditional probability to form a model.

Association rules models:

Association rule $X \Rightarrow Y$ is defined over a set of transactions T where X and Y are sets of items. In a healthcare setting, the set T can be the patients' clinical records and items can be symptoms, measurements, observations, or diagnosis. Given S as a set of items, support(S) is defined as the number of transactions in T that contain all members of the set S. The confidence of a rule is defined as support($X \cup Y$)/support(X) and the support of the rule itself, is support($X \cup Y$). The discovered association rules can show hidden patterns in the mined data set. For example, the rule:

$$\{\text{People with a smoking habit}\} \Rightarrow \{\text{People having heart disease}\}$$

with a high confidence; might signify a cause-effect relationship between smoking and the diagnosis of heart disease. Although, this specific rule is a known fact that is expected to be valid, there are potentially many more rules that are not known or documented.

Clustering models:

Clustering is originated from mathematics, statistics, and numerical analysis (Berkhin, 2006). In this technique the data set is divided into groups of similar objects. The algorithms usually try to group elements in clusters in a way to minimize the overall distance measure (e.g., the Cartesian distance) among the cluster's elements. Data items are then assigned to the clusters based on a specific similarity measure, and the researchers study the other properties of the generated clusters.

Applications of the above data mining techniques in healthcare that have been reported in literature are as following:

- By applying the k-NN classifier (i.e., an instance based method (AhaD, 1989)), Burroni et al. developed a decision support system to assist clinicians with distinguishing early melanoma from benign skin lesions, based on the analysis of digitized images obtained by epiluminescence microscopy (Burroni et al., 2004).
- Neural networks have been used in the computer-aided diagnosis of solid breast nodules. In one study, ultrasonographic features were extracted from 300 benign and 284 malignant biopsy-confirmed breast nodules (Joo et al., 2004).
- Another application of neural networks is detection of the disposition in children presenting to the emergency room with bronchiolitis (inflammation of small airways) (Walsh et al., 2004).
- In (Perou et al., 2000), k-means clustering is used to explore breast cancer classification using genomic data.
- The usefulness of Bayesian networks in capturing the knowledge involved in the management of a medical emergency service have been studied by Acid et al. (Acid et al., 2004).
- Segal et al. have shown that by learning Bayesian networks from data it is possible to obtain insight into the way genes are regulated (Segal et al., 2003).

As far as we are concerned in our framework, we don't differentiate between different implementations and algorithms of any of the data mining categories, if their results can be represented by the general constructs of the corresponding data mining type. For instance, different association rules mining algorithms take different approaches in extracting the *frequent-itemsets* and opt to choose different measures to exclude intermediary sets and hence prevent explosion in the results set. Based on standard constraints of support and confidence, others may apply additional constraints on the size of the rules' antecedent and consequent.

As we discussed, data mining has been used widely in healthcare for extracting knowledge in medical data. Finally this knowledge helps physicians to make a better decision. In the following sections, we will introduce a framework for transferring the generated mined-knowledge along with the electronic health records (EHR) of patients from a source organization to the point of use in another organization.

3. Knowledge representations in medical domain

In this section, major international methodologies and standards for representing medical and healthcare body of knowledge will be discussed. Best practice clinical workflows known as "clinical guidelines" are developed by medical researchers and represent human-based medical knowledge through rule-based or flow-based guideline techniques. On the other hand mined-knowledge can be automatically extracted through data mining techniques to be incorporated into human-generated knowledge in order to enhance their decision-making processes. We will elaborate on different computer based knowledge representations (i.e., GLIF3 and PMML) that are used to represent and transfer extracted knowledge. Finally, at the point of care the medical experts need clinical decision support systems to use these knowledge.

Clinical Guidelines

In the healthcare domain, a medical guideline (Grimshaw & Russell, 1993) (or a clinical guideline) is a document that assists healthcare personnel in making decision with respect to diagnosis, management or treatment of disease. There are two major types of medical guidelines as rule based and flow based guidelines. Rule based guidelines (Quaglini et al., 2003) are built with decision tree or association rules mining. There is one corresponding decision tree for each rule based guideline. In other words, we can convert each decision tree to its corresponding rule based guideline and vice versa. Figure 1 (left) illustrates a decision tree representation of a rule-based guideline.

A flow-based guideline (Panzarasa & Stefanelli, 2006) consists of different steps that form a treatment or diagnostic process for a patient. In every implementation of a flow-based guideline, there is an engine that runs the workflow. At each step, the workflow either changes the state of the system or transfers the control to the next step based on the condition and constraints on the working information.

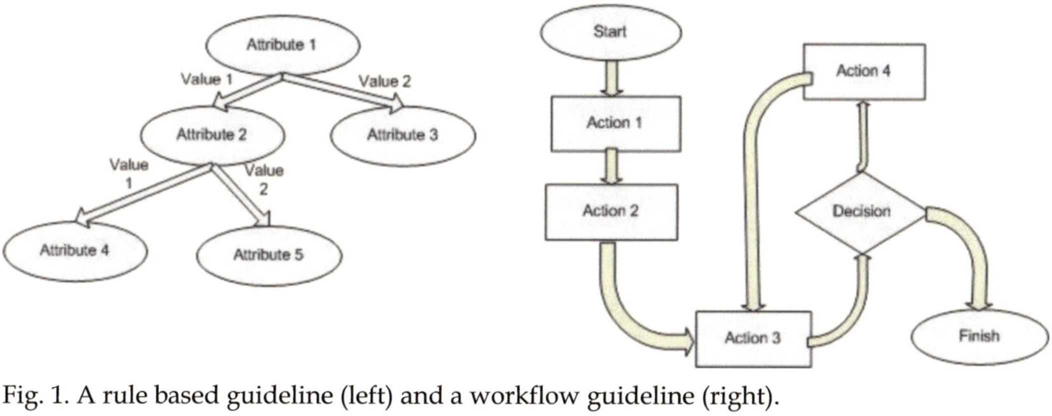

Fig. 1. A rule based guideline (left) and a workflow guideline (right).

GLIF (Guide Line Interchange Format)

Guideline Interchange Format 3 (GLIF3) (*Guideline Interchange Format)*, is a guideline modeling language that represents the clinical best practices as flowcharts. Expert medical researchers execute medical guidelines in GLIF3 format and in their Clinical Decision Support Systems to provide decision making support and clinical best practice. GLIF3 guidelines have been developed for a variety of purposes, including but not limited to heart failure, hypertension, thyroid screening, and many more. GLIF3 guidelines are defined in three levels of abstraction:

- **Conceptual level**: the first level is a flow chart that represents different states and actions in a structured graph. This level provides an easy to comprehend conceptualization of the guideline. At this level, the details of decision making are not provided and hence the guideline models are not computable. Different types of nodes in GLIF3 are as follows:
  - *Decision step* determines the direction of the flow based on a decision criterion specified in an expression language. For example, the age of the patient might be compared to a specific age as a decision criterion to direct the flow.
  - *Activity step* is a node that performs an action, e.g., prompts to prescribe medications; order tests; retrieve patient's medical records; or recommends treatments.
  - *Patient state step* is a node in the flow graph that designates a specific patient's condition, e.g., presence of a symptom, previous treatments, or diagnoses. Also, guideline models start with a patient state step.
  - *Branch step* is used to fork and generate two or more concurrent decision making guideline-flows, such as ordering a lab test and prescribing medication both at the same time.
  - *Synchronization step* is used to merge two or more concurrent decision flows into a single decision flow, such as receiving the lab test report, and observing the effectiveness of the prescribed medication, before continuing to proceed to the next step.
- **Computable level**: to allow a guideline flow to be computed, the author has to specify the control flow, decision criteria, medical concepts, and relevant patient data. These are specified in the computable level.
- **Implementation level**: for GLIF3 guidelines to be actually deployed at an institution site, the patient data and actions should be mapped to institution specific information systems. The required mappings are specified in this level.

Predictive Model Markup Language

Predictive Model Markup Language (PMML) (Data Management Group) is an XML-based language to describe data mining models (clustering, associations, etc.). Also it represents the required constructs to precisely describe different elements, input parameters, model specific parameters, transformations, and results of a variety of types of data mining models. PMML is meant to support the exchange of data mining models between different applications and visualization tools. PMML provides independence from application, platform, and operating system, and simplifies the use of data mining models by other applications (consumers of data mining models).

Clinical Decision Support System

Clinical (or diagnostic) Decision Support Systems (CDSS) (Spiegelhalter & Knill-Jones, 1984) are interactive computer programs which are designed to assist physicians and other health professionals with decision-making tasks. The basic components of a CDSS include a *dynamic* (medical) knowledge base and an *inference mechanism* (usually a set of rules derived from the experts and evidence-based medicine) and implemented through medical logic modules based on a language such as Arden syntax (Hripcsak, 1991). It could also be based on expert systems or neural network.

Some of the most common forms of decision support systems include: *drug-dosing calculators* which are computer-based programs that calculate appropriate doses of medications based on clinician's input key data (e.g., patient weight, indication for drug, serum creatinine). These calculators are especially useful in managing the administration of medications with a narrow therapeutic index. More complex systems include computerized diagnostic tools that, although labor intensive and requiring extensive patient-specific data entry, may be useful as an adjunctive measure when a patient presents with a combination of symptoms and an unclear diagnosis.

Both simple and complex systems may be integrated into the point-of-care and provide accessible reminders to clinicians based on previously entered data. These systems may be most practical when coupled with computerized physician order entry and electronic medical records. Finally, through their integration with practice guidelines and critical pathways, decision support systems may provide clinicians with suggestions for appropriate care, thus decreasing the likelihood of medical errors. For example, a guideline for the management of community-acquired pneumonia may include a clinical tool that, after the input of patient-specific data, would provide a recommendation regarding the appropriateness of inpatient or outpatient therapy.

An example of a clinical decision support system using decision trees can be found in a study by Gerald et al (Gerald et al., 2002). The authors developed a decision tree that assisted health workers in predicting which contacts of tuberculosis patients were most likely to have positive tuberculin skin tests. Also, a clinical decision support system for predicting inpatient length of stay is proposed in (Zheng et al., 2005).

In our proposed framework in Section 5, we use PMML to encode the result of data mining of the healthcare data and transfer this information to the point of care to be used by a clinical decision support system.

4. Communication standards for electronic health records

Standard-based interoperability between heterogeneous legacy systems is one of the main concerns in healthcare domain. Health Level 7 (HL7) is the most important standard messaging model that is widely adopted by the new healthcare systems. In addition to messaging standards, mapping clinical concepts and terms among different healthcare systems is an essential requirement for interorability provision. SNOMED CT is a comprehensive clinical terminology system that will be introduced in this section. Electronic Health Record (EHR) is a major component of the health informatics domain that is defined as: *digitally stored healthcare information about an individual lifetime with the purpose of supporting continuity of care, education and research.* It allows an information system engineer to represent data about observations, laboratory tests, diagnostic imaging reports, treatments, therapies, administrated drug, patient identifying information, legal permissions, etc. There are three main organizations that create standards related to EHR, including: HL7 (Dolin et al., 2005) in United States which is widely adopted, CEN TC 215 (De Moor et al., 2004) operates in most European countries, and ASTM E31 (Hripcsak et al., 1993) is specialized for commercial laboratory vendors in United States.

Health Level 7 (HL7)

HL7 is an international community of healthcare experts and information scientists collaborating to create standards for the exchange, management and integration of electronic healthcare information. HL7 version 3 (V3) has defined Reference Information Model (RIM) which is a large class diagram representation of the clinical data and identifies the life cycle of events that a message will carry. The HL7 messaging process applies object-oriented development methodology on RIM and its extensions to create messages. Then these standard messages are used to transfer EHR data between different healthcare systems.

HL7 message refinement process

HL7 methodology uses RIM, HL7-specified vocabulary domains, and HL7 v3 data type specification and establishes the rules for refining these base standards to specify Message Types and equivalent structures in v3. The strategy for development of these message types and their information structures is based upon the consistent application of constraints on HL7 RIM and HL7 Vocabulary Domains, to create representations that address a specific healthcare requirement. Figure 2 illustrates the refinement process specified in HL7 methodology, where the different parts are discussed below.

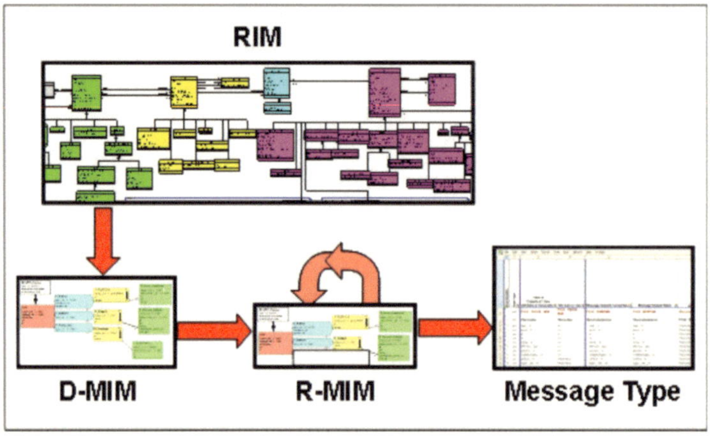

Fig. 2. Refinement process specified in HL7 methodology (Dolin R., Alschuler L., Beebe C., et al. The HL7 clinical document architecture.)

- *Domain Message Information Model* (D-MIM) is a subset of the RIM that includes a fully expanded set of class clones, attributes and relationships that are used to create messages for any particular domain (e.g., accounting and billing, claims, and patient administration)
- *Refined Message Information Model* (R-MIM) is used to express the information content for one or more messages within a domain. Each R-MIM is a subset of the D-MIM and only contains the classes, attributes and associations that are required to compose those messages.
- *Hierarchical Message Description* (HMD) is a tabular representation of the sequence of elements (i.e., classes, attributes and associations) represented in an R-MIM. Each HMD produces a single base message template from which the specific message types are drawn.
- *Message Type* represents a unique set of constraints on message identification that are presented in different forms such as: grid, table, or spreadsheet.

Clinical Document Architecture (CDA)

CDA is an XML-based markup standard intended to specify the encoding, structure and semantics of clinical documents to be exchanged. The content of a CDA document consists of a mandatory textual part (which ensures human interpretation of the document contents) and optional structured parts (for software processing). The structured part relies on coding systems (e.g., from SNOMED (Andrews et al., 2007) and LOINC (McDonald et al., 2003)) to represent concepts. The CDA standard doesn't specify how the documents should be transported. CDA documents can be transported using both HL7 v2 and HL7 v3 messages. CDA contributes in simplifying the healthcare message composition and transportation between non HL7 standard legacy systems, as well as to communicate more complex information.

Clinical terminologies (SNOMED CT)

A clinical terminology system facilitates identifying and accessing information pertaining to the healthcare process and links together terms with identical clinical meanings; hence it leverages the provision of healthcare services by the care providers.

SNOMED CT (Systematized Nomenclature of Medicine - Clinical Terms), is a systematically organized computerized collection of medical terminology that covers most areas of clinical information such as diseases, findings, procedures, microorganisms and pharmaceuticals. The terminology is comprised of concepts, terms and relationships with the objective of precisely representing clinical information across the scope of healthcare. It allows a consistent way to index, store, retrieve, and aggregate clinical data across specialties and sites of care. It also helps organizing the content of medical records, reducing the variability in the way data is captured, encoded and used for clinical care of patients and research. Concepts are clinical meanings and identified by a unique and human-readable numeric identifier (ConceptID) that never changes (e.g., 25064002 for "Headache").

In a clinical terminology system, *concepts* represent various levels of clinical detail, from very general to very specific with finer granularity. Multiple levels of granularity improve the capability to code clinical data at the appropriate level of detail. (e.g., *Dental Headache* is a kind of *Headache* in general). Concept descriptions are the terms or names assigned to a SNOMED CT concept. Multiple descriptions might be associated with a concept identified by its ConceptID. Every description has a unique DescriptionID.

So far, we introduced: i) standards for representing healthcare information and extracted mined-knowledge, ii) technology for a standard-based messaging mechanism, and iii) required healthcare terminology systems to provide unique medical concepts and terms. These together will allow the healthcare professionals to access to medical information and communicate their medical knowledge and use the computerized services available at other healthcare organizations. In the next section, we elaborate on a framework that allows both data and knowledge to be communicated and used.

5. A conceptual framework for data and mined knowledge interoperability

We have proposed a framework for interoperability of data and mined knowledge in clinical decision support systems which is based on HL7 v3 messaging, web services for communication, and flow-based clinical guidelines.

Figure 3 illustrates the overall view of the proposed distributed knowledge management framework. The framework consists of three phases, as: preparation, interoperation, and interpretation. The description of each phase follows.

Knowledge preparation

In this phase, the data mining knowledge is extracted from healthcare data in an off-line operation. For this purpose data is mined and a data mining model is fit to the data. This model might describe the data or be used to carry out future predictions on new data. Examples of such applications are: classifying a disease based on its symptoms to help diagnosis; clustering the patients based on relevant risk factors; verifying known medical facts; and expressing useful hidden patterns in data as in association rules mining. Different data mining techniques have been presented in Section 2. This phase starts by removing the healthcare data attributes that can identify a patient or reveal their private data. Some studies (Mielikainen, 2003) have also shown that the privacy breaches can occur even when the data is anonymized. After anonymization the knowledge extraction process starts through: data selection, data cleaning, and data transformation, which are followed by the actual data mining operation. Finally, the results are assessed in terms of usefulness, validity, and understandability.

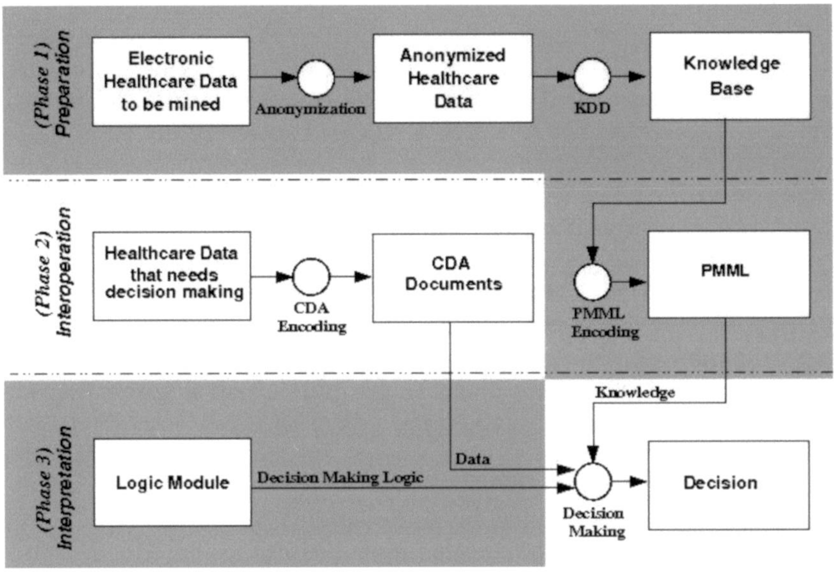

Fig. 3. Healthcare knowledge management framework. The shaded areas designate off-line parts.

Knowledge interoperation

In this phase, two separate flows of data and knowledge are properly encoded to be used at the point of care. This phase ensures the interoperability among the institutions with different data and knowledge representations. In an off-line operation, the extracted knowledge in phase 1 should be ported to the parties that will use it for decision making. This is performed by employing PMML specification to encode the mined results into XML based documents. The XML schema for each data mining result describes the input data items, data mining algorithm specific parameters, and the final mining results. In an on-line operation, the subject data (i.e., healthcare data that needs decision making) in a source institution's internal data representation (e.g., EMR systems) is encoded into HL7 v3 messages or a CDA document to be interpreted for decision making in a destination institution. The encoded PMML knowledge can also be stored and used locally by health care institutions. The PMML and CDA documents provide the interoperability of knowledge and data in our framework in the sense that the Decision Support System (DSS) will be independent of the proprietary data format of the involved institutions

Knowledge interpretation

In this phase, a final decision is made based on the results of applying the mined models to the subject data. The logic of decision making is programmed into the logic modules that access, query, and interpret the data and knowledge that flow from the previous phase. The final decision might be to issue an alert or to remind a fact. For the mined knowledge to be actually used at the point of care, the data mining models should be interpreted for the subject cases (patient data). Three different documents are involved in this phase. The first document is the CDA document from phase 2 that contains a case data for a patient (e.g., a particular laboratory report) and is accessed on-line; the second document is the PMML document, containing the knowledge extracted in an off-line data mining process in phase 1 that was made portable by proper encoding in phase 2; and the third document is a program (logic module) that contains the necessary logic to interpret the data and knowledge.

The logic modules are independent units, each responsible for making a single decision based on the facts extracted in phase 1. In principle, they are similar to the idea of Arden Syntax Medical Logic Modules (MLM) with the exception that they can access and query mined knowledge bases. Each logic module contains the core decision making operation for a specific application and is bound to a specified data mining model in a PMML file. The overall structure of a logic module is described below. The decision making is carried out in 3 main steps, retrieving the right data fields from the data source; applying the mined models to the data; and eventually taking an action or a set of actions. To do this, first the local variables in each logic module are populated by accessing the corresponding data fields in the CDA document. Before the model is applied to the data that was read, the required transformations are performed on the data. These transformations are specified in the transformation dictionary section of the PMML document. Based on the results of this application, the module takes an action. For example, if the module was invoked at a *Decision Step* in a guideline, it may branch to a specific path; or it may simply display the results in the form of a reminder or an alert.

The proposed framework is at the conceptual level and requires an infrastructure to be applied. In the next section, we discuss some of the existing architectures in this domain which allow our conceptual framework to be implemented.

6. Existing architectures for interoperability support

Healthcare systems are large and complex information systems that require huge investments from a government to provide a nation-wide infrastructure. Such an infrastructure implements an electronic health record (EHR) system that spans different jurisdictional regions and connect a large number of distributed healthcare systems. In this context, service oriented architecture (SOA) has been widely adopted to solve the interoperability of the involving heterogeneous distributed systems.

In the rest of this section, first we introduce SOA, then we describe web services as a implementation technology for SOA and finally, we elaborate on Canada Health Infoway as an example of a service based architecture that connects different healthcare systems.

Service Oriented Architecture

Service Oriented Architecture (SOA) (Krafzig et al., 2004) plays a key role in the integration of heterogeneous systems by the means of services that represent different system functionality independent from the underlying platforms or programming languages. SOA contributes in relaxing the complexity, leveraging the usability, and improving the agility of the business services. On the other hand, new services may need to be adopted by the SOA community. Service is a program that interacts with users or other programs via message exchanges. An (SOA) consists of the following concepts: *application frontend, service, service repository,* and *service bus;* each summarized as follows. Application frontends use the business processes and services within the system. A service consists of implementation, service contract, functionality and constraint specification, and service interface. A service repository stores service contracts. A service bus connects frontends to the services. A service-oriented architecture is a style of design that guides all aspects of creating and using business services throughout their lifecycle (from conception to retirement). An SOA is also a way to define and provide an IT infrastructure to allow different applications to exchange data and participate in business processes, regardless of the operating systems or programming languages underlying those applications.

Web Services

In more technical terms, a service is a program that interacts with users or other programs via message exchanges, and is defined by the messages not by the method signatures. Web services technology is defined as a systematic and extensible framework for application-to-application interaction built on top of existing web protocols. These protocols are based on XML and include: Web Services Description Language (WSDL) to describe the service interfaces, Simple Object Access Protocol (SOAP) for communication between web services and client applications, and Universal Description, Discovery, and Integration (UDDI) to facilitate locating and using web services on a network. These protocols are briefly defined below.

SOAP is an XML based protocol for messaging and remote procedure call using HTTP and SMTP. It defines how typed values can be transported between SOAP representation (XML) and application's representation by using XML schema definition. It also defines where various parts of Remote Procedure Call (RPC) are defined, including object identity, operation name, and parameters.

WSDL has an XML format that describes web services as a collection of communication end-points that can exchange certain messages. A complete WSDL service description has two parts: i) web service description (abstract interface), and ii) protocol-dependent details (concrete binding) that users must follow to access service at a service end- point.

UDDI is an XML based standard that provides a unified and systematic way to find service providers through centralized registry of services.

BPEL is a language for specifying business process behavior based on web services. These processes export and import functionality by using web service interfaces.

Web services are widely adopted as standard technology for implementation of service oriented architecture (SOA).

Infoway EHRi

Canada Health Infoway (EHRS Blueprint) is an organization that provides specifications for a standard and nationwide healthcare infrastructure. Infoway defines specifications and recommendations for development of an interoperable Electronic Health Record (EHR) system which is compatible with HL7 standards and communications technologies.

Infoway aims at integrating information systems from different health providers and administrations (e.g., hospitals, laboratories, pharmacies, physicians, and government agencies) within different provinces, and then connect them to form a nationwide healthcare network with standard data formats, communication protocols, and a unique health history file for each patient. In such a large infrastructure the individual's health information is accessible using common services according to different access privileges for patients and providers. Infoway provides EHRi (Electronic Health Record Infostructure) which is designed based on service oriented architecture technology and consists of several components, as illustrated in Figure 5. The SOA main components within Infoway are discussed below.

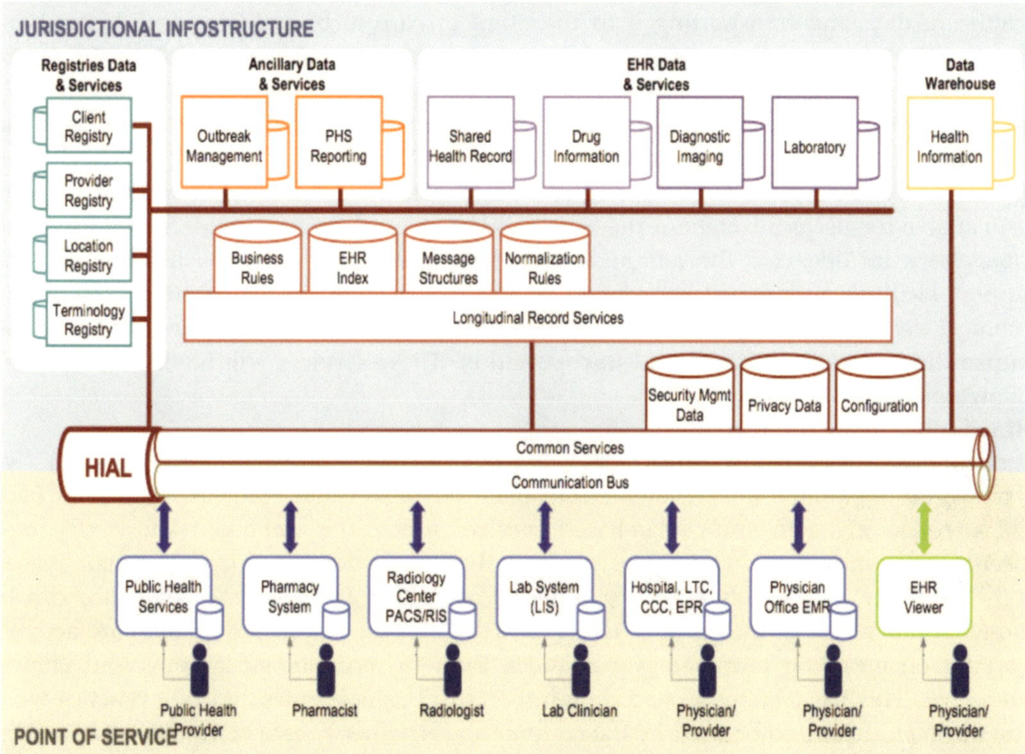

Fig. 5. Infoway EHRi (Source: Infoway (Canada Health Infoway))

As mentioned earlier, a typical SOA architecture consists of four main parts: frontend applications, service repository, services, and service bus. Application frontends are point-of-service components for physician, pharmacy, patient, and EHR viewer. Services are provided by different components; for an extended list of these services and their types, refer to (EHRS Blueprint). Service repositories consist of three groups "registries data & services", "ancillary data & services", and "EHR data & services". HIAL (Health Information Access Layer) is responsible for the functionality of the service bus. Considering the heterogeneity and age of the connected healthcare systems in a network, the integration process should be performed through a multi-technology facility, provided by "intermediary services" of SOA architecture. Infoway's Infostructure is mainly intended for transporting clinical documents through a communication framework. However, this architecture can also be used for other purposes such as tele-medicine, where performance guarantees are required. In such cases the performance of the service bus can be configured using technologies such as Message Oriented Middleware. Data warehouse represents a separate capability to compile, aggregate and consolidate EHR data for reporting and statistical or research analysis, as well as health prevention initiatives. After this introduction to Infoway Infostructure, in the next section we will discuss how to incorporate data mining services in such infrastructures.

7. Potential research avenues in electronic healthcare

In Section 5, we proposed a conceptual framework for data and mined-knowledge interoperabilty where the emphasize was put on the extraction of knowledge from healthcare data and transporting it to the point of care to be used by decision support systems. We discussed information and knowledge representation technologies (CDA and PMML) in an abstract manner.

In this section, we shift our focus towards research guidelines for defining new services for data and knowledge transportation based on SOA with emphasize on healthcare applications. We propose the enhancement of SOA services to allow domain knowledge to be available for users throughout the whole system as well as to provide monitoring and supervisory facilities for the administrative personnel. Other services include decision support facilities and mined-knowledge provisions that are crucial in administrative or technical decision making processes. The application domains include: financial analysis, tourism, insurance, healthcare, and transportation. These services will be discussed in the followings.

Mined-knowledge services

Current SOA services are either "data-centric", i.e., they transport data between two systems, or "logic-centric", i.e., they encapsulate business rules. However, there has been less attention given to knowledge-based services where the embodied knowledge in a specific application domain could be available through standard services. The main reason is the difficulty of precisely encoding different aspects of knowledge so that they can be correctly interpreted at the point of use. Researchers in the healthcare domain are actively working on encoding terminology semantics through terminology systems and clinical guidelines. This has resulted in encoding important business rules and best practice work flows into guidelines to be used by the community. Another source of valuable knowledge is the knowledge that is extracted from a large data set by applying data mining algorithms. This knowledge includes non-trivial patterns and trends among data that are not easily visible without computing assistance. We discussed different data mining algorithms and their applications in healthcare in Section 2. The application of the provided mined-knowledge at the point of use would boost the accuracy and convenience of decision making by the administrative personnel. In order to provide such mined-knowledge interoperability for large systems, enterprise service bus technology (Chappell, 2004) provides the required facilities.

Decision support system (DSS)

The proposed DSS component provides two types of services. I) Standard workflow services that reflect the best practices in a domain. In the healthcare domain, best clinical practices are developed by researchers and practitioners as clinical guidelines to help healthcare professionals and patients make decisions about screening, prevention, or treatment of a specific health condition. The DSS component offers these workflows to the users all over the system. COMPETE (COMPETE) is a pioneering Canadian healthcare project in electronic health research that is specialized in developing clinical guidelines based on different available resources. II) Customizable workflow generation services that allow users to define workflows for their enterprises. Such components may provide services for generating new guidelines by professionals as a part of standardization of workflows. This service for generating clinical guidelines would complement the service for accessing a predefined clinical guideline.

Supervisory and visualization services

We propose services that allow administrative personnel or government agencies to secure effective control and supervision over the quality of service of the networked systems through activity visualization and identification of distribution patterns of services and bottlenecks. The visualization of activities in a large network of systems is crucial for administrative personnel to obtain updated and comprehensive insight into the active or passive relationships among different systems within the network. Examples of such networks include: bus and train transportation systems, air traffic control systems, transactions between financial institutions, and healthcare systems. As an application, consider the integrated network of healthcare systems as a large graph with different types of nodes representing clinical and administrative institutions, and types of edges representing categories of interactions among these institutions. Specific software analysis techniques from software reverse engineering can be applied to visualize the static or dynamic architecture of a large region of healthcare infrastructure (e.g., a province) from different view points. In this approach, data mining techniques are used to discover complex patterns of interactions among the nodes of the network and to provide means for self-management of the network.

Case study for Healthcare Network Visualization

A domain model is required to specify the graph node-types (i.e., different kinds of healthcare institutions such as: hospitals, physicians, pharmacies, laboratories, and government agencies) and graph edge-types as abstractions of health related communications between any two nodes (e.g., lab referral, drug prescription, billing statements, and patient electronic record acquisition). In this context, each edge-type will have several sub-types; for example, an edge-type "drug prescription" can have sub-types that represent a specific category of drugs that can be prescribed. This service will be implemented as follows. A common service in each node of the network is needed so that it enables the "supervisory component" to inquire about the network transaction activities of every node in the network within a certain period of time. On a daily basis, the interactions among the healthcare institutions will be logged and at the end of the day these logs will be sent (through service invocation) to a supervisory component to be analyzed. Consequently, the supervisory component can provide different views of the graph of the healthcare network, where the nodes and edges are color-coded according to the type of institutions and the types of interactions. The application of association rules mining algorithms on the generated graph would identify groups of maximally associated graph nodes according to specific graph edge types. In this context, maximal association refers to a group of nodes that all share the same services from a maximal group of service providers (e.g., specific categories of medications in pharmacies; and blood tests, X-rays, and ultrasounds in laboratories). A variety of data mining applications can be used to explore nontrivial properties in this network such as: spread of epidemics; distribution patterns of patients in particular regions; or distribution patterns of specific health services. The discovery of such patterns would enable the healthcare administrations and government agencies to restructure the service locations in order to reduce the cost of services and to increase the accessibility of services to a larger population. The results would be available through a set of "monitoring and supervisory services" to the healthcare administrative personnel for analysis and policy decisions.

8. Conclusion

Current healthcare infrastructures in the advanced societies can not fulfil the demands for quality public health services which are characterized by patient-centric, seamless interoperation of heterogeneous healthcare systems, and nation-wide electronic health record services. Consequently, the governments and healthcare institutions are embracing new information and communication technologies to provide the necessary infrastructures for healthcare and medical services. In this chapter, we attempted to cover background preparation, advanced technology, architectural considerations, and research avenues within the new and critical domain of electronic health to address these emerging demands and presented the state-of-the-art solutions. The emphasize has been on the exploration power of data mining techniques to extract patterns and trends from large healthcare databases, and the means to deliver these knowledge along with the healthcare data to the point of use for enhanced decision making by professionals. Also, we discussed the trends towards raising the level of abstraction of services to the users which resulted in adopting service oriented architecture by the nation-wide healthcare infrastructures. Such high-level abstraction of healthcare services provides ease of use, vendor-independence, and seamless integration of the legacy systems with new systems. Healthcare domain is pioneer in systematically tackling the semantic interoperability by providing large and comprehensive terminology systems that allow common understanding of the medical terms and concepts. Furthermore, healthcare domain provides a well-defined process for representing and refining the whole body of medical information to develop standard HL7 messages for communication. As a result, the healthcare domain has acquired the necessary means to evolve towards a nation-wide and fully interoperated network of healthcare systems. Such a healthcare network is characterized by collaborating service providers and service users and enhanced techniques for more accurate clinical decision making.

9. References:

Prudsys A. *XELOPES,* library documentation - version 1.3.1. URL= http://www.prudsys.com/Service/Downloads/bin/1133983554/Xelopes1.3.1_Intro.pdf, 2006.

Haykin S., *Neural Networks: A Comprehensive Foundation*, book, Prentice Hall PTR, 1998.

Jensen F., *Introduction to Bayesian Networks*, book, Springer, 1998.

Berkhin P., *Survey of clustering data mining techniques.* URL = http://www.ee.ucr.edu/~barth/EE242/clustering_survey.pdf, 2006.

AhaD W. *,Incremental, instance-based learning of independent and graded concept descriptions.* International Workshop on Machine Learning, pp. 387–391, 1989.

Burroni M., Corona R., Dell'Eva G., et al., *Melanoma computer-aided diagnosis: reliability and feasibility study,* Clin Cancer Res, pp.1881–1886,2004.

Joo S.,Yang Y., Moon W., Kim H., *Computer-aided diagnosis of solid breast nodules: use of an artificial neural network based on multiple sonographic features.* IEEE Transact Med Imaging, pp 1292–1300, 2004.

Walsh P., Cunningham P., Rothenberg S., O'Doherty S., Hoey H., Healy R. *An artificial neural network ensemble to predict disposition and length of stay in children presenting with bronchiolitis*. Eur Journal Emerg Med. pp 259–564, 2004.

Perou C., Sorlie T., Eisen M., et al. *Molecular portraits of human breast tumours*, Nature, pp. 747–752, 2000.

Acid S., De Campos LM., Fernandez-Luna J., Rodrguise S., Rodrguise J., Salcedo J., *A comparison of learning algorithms for Bayesian networks: a case study based on data from an emergency medical service*. Artificial Intelligence in Medicine; pp 215-232, 2004.

Segal E., Shapira M., Regev A., Pe'er D., Botstein D., Koller D., Friedman N., *Module networks: identifying regulatory modules and their condition-specific regulators from gene expression data*., Nat Genet; pp 16-176, 2003.

Grimshaw J., Russell I., *Effect of clinical guidelines on medical practice: a systematic review of rigorous evaluations*. Lancet. pp. 1317–1322, 1993.

Quaglini S., Stefanelli M., Cavallini A., Micieli G., Fassino C., Mossa C., *Guideline-based careflow systems*, Artificial Intelligence in Medicine , pp. 5 - 22, 2003.

Panzarasa S., Stefanelli1 M., *Workflow management systems for guideline implementation*, Neurological Sciences, pp. 245-249, 2006.

Guideline Interchange Format (GLIF)3.5 - technical specification. URL = http://smi-web.stanford.edu/projects/intermed-web/guidelines/GLIF_TECH_SPEC_May_4_2004.pdf, 2004.

Data Management Group (DMG). *Predictive model markup language (pmml) version 3.0 specification*. URL =http://www.dmg.org/pmml-v3-0.html.

David J. Spiegelhalter and Robin P. Knill-Jones, *Statistical and Knowledge-Based Approaches to Clinical Decision-Support Systems, with an Application in Gastroenterology*, Journal of the Royal Statistical Society. Series A (General), pp. 35-77, 1984.

Hripcsak G., *Arden Syntax for Medical Logic Modules*, MD Compution, 1991

Gerald L.,Tang S., Bruce F., et al. *A decision tree for tuberculosis contact investigation*. Am J Respir Crit Care Med, pp. 1122–1127, 2002.

Zheng Y., Peng L., Lei J., *R-C4.5 decision tree model and its applications to health care dataset*, Services Systems and Services Management conference, pp. 1099- 1103, 2005

Dolin R., Alschuler L., Beebe C., et al. *The HL7 clinical document architecture*. J Am Med Inform Assoc, pp.552–569, 2005.

De Moor g., Claerhout B., van Maele G., Dupont D., *e-Health Standardization in Europe: Lessons Learned*, E-Health: Current Situation and Examples of Implemented and Beneficial E-Health Applications, book, Publisher: IOS Press, Pages233-237, 2004.

Hripcsak G., Wigertz O., Kahn M., Clayton P. , *ASTM E31.15 on health knowledge representation: the arden syntax* , book, progress on standardization in health care informatics, IOS press, 1993.

Andrews J., Richesson R., and Krischer J. ,*Variation of SNOMED CT Coding of Clinical Research Concepts among Coding Experts*, J. Am. Med. Inform. Assoc., pp. 497 - 506, 2007.

McDonald C., Huff S., Suico J., Hill G., Leavelle D., Aller R., Forrey A., Mercer K., DeMoor G., Hook J., Williams W., Case J., Maloney P. , *LOINC, a universal standard for identifying laboratory observations: a 5-year update*, MEDLINE, pp.624-33, 2003.

Mielikainen T., On inverse frequent set mining. *Workshop on Privacy Preserving Data Mining (PPDM)*, pp 18–23, 2003.

Krafzig D., Banke K., Slama D.,Enterprise *SOA: Service-Oriented Architecture Best Practices*, Book, Prentice Hall PTR, 2004.
Canada Health Infoway, http://www.infoway-inforoute.ca/.
EHRS Blueprint - Infoway Architecture Update. http://www.infoway-inforoute.ca/.
Chappell D., *Enterprise Service Bus: Theory in Practice*, book, O'Reilly, 2004.
COMPETE. Computerization of Medical Practice for the Enhancement of Therapeutic Effectiveness. http://www.compete-study.com/index.htm.

11

A Scalable Healthcare Integrated Platform (SHIP) and Key Technologies for Daily Application

Wenxi Chen, Xin Zhu, Tetsu Nemoto[1], Daming Wei and Tatsuo Togawa[2]
Biomedical Information Technology Lab., the University of Aizu
[1]*School of Health Sciences, Faculty of Medicine, Kanazawa University*
[2]*School of Human Sciences, Waseda University*
Japan

1. Introduction

A ubiquitous era has arisen based on achievements from the development of science and technology over the previous 1,000 years, and especially the past 150 years. Among the numerous accomplishments in human history, four fundamental technologies have laid the foundation for today's pervasive computing environment.
The electromagnetic wave theory, established by James Maxwell in 1864, predicted the existence of waves of oscillating electric and magnetic fields that travel through empty space at a velocity of 310,740,000 m/s. His quantitative connection between light and electromagnetism is considered one of the great triumphs of 19th century physics. Twenty years later, through experimentation, Heinrich Hertz proved that transverse free space electromagnetic waves can travel over some distance, and in 1888, he demonstrated that the velocity of radio waves was equal to the velocity of light. However, Hertz did not realize the practical importance of his experiments. He stated that, "It's of no use whatsoever … this is just an experiment that proves Maestro Maxwell was right - we just have these mysterious electromagnetic waves that we cannot see with the naked eye. But they are there." His discoveries were later utilized in wireless telegraphy by Guglielmo Marconi, and they formed a part of the new "radio communication age".
The second fundamental technology is spread-spectrum telecommunications, whose multiple access capability allows a large volume of users to communicate simultaneously on the same frequency band, as long as they use different spreading codes. This has been developed since the 1940s and used in military communication systems since the 1950s. Realization of spread-spectrum technology requires a large computational capacity and leads to a bulky size and weight. Since the initial commercial use of spread spectrum telecommunications began in the 1980s, it is now widely used in many familiar systems today, such as GPS, Wi-Fi, Bluetooth, and mobile phones. This was made possible by the invention of computing machines and integrated circuits, the third and fourth tremendous triumphs.
The first automatic computing machine, known as ENIAC, was built using 18,000 vacuum tubes, 1,500 relays, 70,000 resistors, and 10,000 condensers. It performed 35,000 additions per

second and cost US$487,000 (Nohzawa, 2003). The latest CPU, the Yorkfield XE, contains 820 million transistors on 2 × 107 mm^2 dies and features a 1333 MT/s FSB and a clock speed of 3 GHz (Intel Corp., 2007).

Since the first integrated circuit (IC), which contained a single transistor and several resistors on an 11 × 1.6 mm^2 germanium chip, was fabricated by Jack Kilby in 1958, advanced 45 nm semiconductor technology makes it possible to condense an entire complicated spread-spectrum telecommunication system into a magic box as small as a mobile phone.

Today, we are interconnected through wired and wireless networks, and surrounded by an invisible pervasive computing environment. This makes "information at your fingertips" and "commerce at light speed" possible. We are already acclimatized to enjoy everything worldwide conveniently, wherever we are. We enjoy online shopping and share information with friends from the other side of the Earth in an instant.

However, this is a double-edged sword. Our daily lifestyle has changed dramatically. While we may benefit from the advantages of today's society, at the same time, we face many unprecedented problems in the health domain, which have emerged with all of these changes.

One of the greatest concerns is the ascent of chronic illness that has occurred concurrently with the accompanying lifestyle changes. Figure 1 shows the change in mortality among different diseases from acute to chronic over the past 100 years in Japan. There has not been a large change in conventional causes of death, such as contingency, caducity, and pneumonia. Acute infectious diseases, such as tuberculosis, have disappeared completely since the 1980s. However, death due to chronic conditions is increasing. The leading causes of death are the three "C" top killer diseases: cerebral, cardiovascular, and cancer (malignant neoplasm), which account for 60 per cent of total deaths.

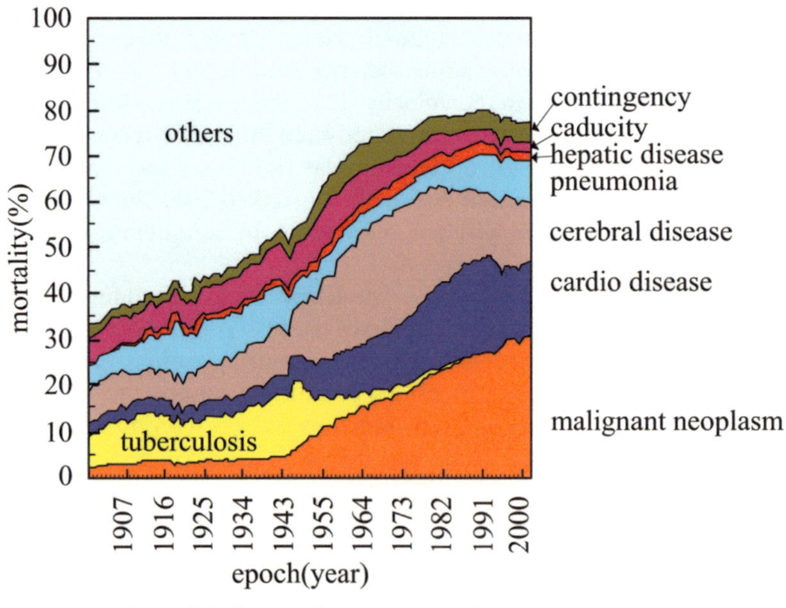

Fig. 1. Change in mortality of different diseases over the previous century in Japan. (Adapted from the Japanese Ministry of Health, Labour, and Welfare).

Rapid changes in both societal environment and daily lifestyle are responsible for most of these chronic illnesses. Treatment of chronic conditions is now recognized as a problem of all society and no longer just a private issue. To elevate all citizens' awareness of the importance of health promotion and disease prevention in response to the steep increase in long-term healthcare requirements, it is indispensable to be involved in every aspect and to take creative action. A variety of innovative strategies and activities are now being explored nationwide in Japan at three levels: macro (administration), meso (community, organization, and company), and micro (personal) levels.

At the macro level, a 12-year health promotion campaign, known as "Healthy Japan 21" (Japan Health Promotion and Fitness Foundation, 2000), has been advocated nationwide since 2000 and is financially supported by the Japanese Ministry of Health, Labour, and Welfare. Furthermore, a "health promotion law" (Japanese Ministry of Health, Labour and Welfare, 2002) was issued by the Japanese parliament. This reconfirmed that the national goal of medical insurance reconstruction was health promotion and disease prevention, and it defined individual responsibility and coordination among citizens, community, and government organizations.

At the meso level, industrial organizations and research institutions have developed many Internet-based systems and related devices for daily healthcare. Professional organizations and academic associations have established a series of educational programs and accreditation systems for professional healthcare promoters. Citizen communities have boosted health promotion campaigns through various service options.

At the micro level, more and more people are aware of the importance of health promotion and chronic prevention, and are becoming more active in participating in daily personal healthcare practices. They spend a lot of time and money on exercise, diet, and regular medical examinations to keep their biochemical indices as good as possible.

This trend turns out that in the US only, the healthcare domain is now growing up into a giant industrial territory worthy of about US$2 trillion annually (MarketResearch.com. 2008). In terms of building a better healthcare environment, and as one of the initiatives in the arena of human welfare in long-term chronic treatment, we are confronting the challenges of providing effective means for vital sign monitoring technologies suitable for daily use, and large-scale data mining and a comprehensive interpretation of their physiological interconnection. These solutions are being developed across the world. Many companies are already engaged in and placing priority on, providing a total solution to these ever-increasing demands.

The "Health Data Bank" ASP service platform was released as a multifaceted aid for the health management of corporate employee medical exam results (NTT Data Corp., 2002). The service supplies healthcare personnel with a set of tools for effective employee health guidance and counselling, and takes into account factors such as an employee's current physical condition, as well as living habits and environment, and age-related changes in longitudinal management in accumulated individual data. Individual corporate employees can browse their personal data through Internet channels, and view records of their check-ups, as well as graphs detailing historical changes in their health condition, thus facilitating improved personal health management.

Companies and research institutes in the European Union have launched several multinational projects to develop wearable and portable healthcare systems for personalized care. The "MyHeart" project is a framework for personal healthcare applications led by Philips, which aims to develop on-body sensors/electronics and appropriate services to help fight cardiovascular disease through prevention and early diagnosis. It can monitor vital signs and physical movement via wearable textile technology, process the measured data, and provide the user with recommendations (Philips Electronics, 2004). After the completion of the "MyHeart" program, a continuation "HeartCycle" project began in March 2008. Many new sensors and key technologies, such as a cuff-less blood pressure sensor, a wearable SpO2 sensor, an inductive impedance sensor, an electronic acupuncture system, a contactless ECG, arrays of electret foils, a motion-compensation system for ECG, and a cardiac performance monitor (from bioimpedance) will be developed and built into the system. A patient's condition will be monitored using a combination of unobtrusive sensors built into the patient's clothing or bed sheets and home appliances, such as weighing scales and blood pressure meters. Data mining and decision support approaches will be developed to analyse the acquired data, to predict the short-term and long-term effects of lifestyle and medication, and to obtain an objective indicator of patient compliance (Philips Electronics, 2008).

"MobiHealth" was a mobile healthcare project funded by the European Commission from 2002 to 2004. Fourteen partners from hospitals and medical service providers, universities, mobile network operators, mobile application service providers, mobile infrastructure, and hardware suppliers across five European countries participated in the project. It allowed patients to be fully mobile while undergoing health monitoring without much discomfort in daily activities. The patients wore a lightweight unit with multiple sensors connected via a Body Area Network (BAN) for monitoring ECG, respiration, activity/movement/position, and a plethysmogram over short or long periods with no need to stay in hospital (European Commission, 2002).

The "AMON" system was designed to monitor and evaluate human vital signs, such as heart rate, two-lead ECG, blood pressure, oxygen blood saturation, skin perspiration, and body temperature using a wrist-mounted wearable device. The device gathers the data and transmits it to a remote telemedicine centre for further analysis and emergency care, using a GSM/UMTS cellular infrastructure (Anliker et al., 2004; European Commission, 2001).

"HealthVault" aims to build a universal hub of a network to connect personal health devices and other services that can be used to help store, and manage personal medical information in a single central site on the Web (Microsoft Corp., 2008). It will provide a seamless connection interface scheme for various home health and wellness monitoring devices, such as sport watches, blood glucose monitors, and blood pressure monitors marketed by medical equipment manufacturers worldwide.

On the other hand, many explorative studies on fundamental technology for vital signs monitoring have been conducted in the academic world and in research institutes. Much innovative instrumentation suitable in daily life has emerged and is gradually being commercialized.

Since the first accurate recording of an ECG reported by Willem Einthoven in 1895, and its development as a clinical tool, variants, such as Holter ECG, event ECG, and ECG mapping are now well known and have found a variety of applications in clinical practice. Measurement of ECG is now available from various scenarios. Whenever a person sits on a chair (Lim et al., 2006) or on a toilet (Togawa et al., 1989), sleeps in a bed (Kawarada et al., 2000; Ishijima, 1993), sits in a bathtub (Mizukami et al., 1989; Tamura et al., 1997), or even takes a shower (Fujii et al., 2002), his/her heart beat can be monitored, with the person unaware.

The smart dress, "Wealthy outfit", weaves electronics and fabrics together to detect the wearer's vital signs, and transmits the data wirelessly to a computer. The built-in sensors

gather information on the wearer's posture and movement, ECG, and body temperature. Despite having nine electrodes and conductive leads woven into it, the suit looks and feels completely normal (Rossi et al., 2008; Marculescu et al., 2003).
The wellness mobile phone, "SH706iw", manufactured by the Sharp Corp. (Japan), has been released by NTT DoCoMo Corp. (Japan) in September 2008. It will have all the standard features of a mobile phone but will also act as a pedometer, a body fat meter, a pulse rate, and a breath gas monitor. Moreover, a built-in game-like application will support daily health management for fun and amusement (Sharp Corp., 2008; DoCoMo Corp., 2008).
According to an investigation report from the World Health Organization (WHO, 2002), most current healthcare systems still have some common issues that need to be addressed. (a) The difference between acute and chronic care is not sufficiently emphasized. The overall concept in system development has not shifted enough towards chronic conditions, and has not evolved to meet this changing demand. (b) Despite the importance of patients' health behaviour and adherence to improvement for chronic conditions, patients are not provided with a simple way to involve themselves in self-management and to have essential information to handle their condition to the best extent possible. (c) Patients are often followed up sporadically, and are seldom provided with a long-term management plan for chronic conditions to ensure the best outcomes.
Indeed, they are large obstacles in front of us that need to be cleared. We consider these issues a long-term difficult challenge to governments, communities, and individuals alike. We deem two main aspects should be paid primary attention. The first aspect is that vital-sign monitoring for chronic conditions requiring different philosophy and strategy tends to be ignored. Long-term chronic care is mostly oriented to untrained users in the home environment. However, many devices are far from being "plug and play", and require tedious involvement in daily operation. The second aspect is the lack of interconnection between multifarious physiological data within existing medical systems, as medication is usually decided by interpretation based on fragmented data and standards based on acute and emergent symptoms, and is often provided without the benefit of complete long-term physiological data.
To meet current needs, and to tackle the two problems above, our studies focus on developing a series of wearable/invisible vital-sign measurement technologies to facilitate data collection in the daily environment in perpetuity, and on applying data mining algorithms to conduct comprehensive interpretation of multifarious long-term data fusion, and ultimately to build a scalable healthcare integrated platform, SHIP, for various applicable domains, wherever vital signs are conducive.

2. Methods and results

Our studies included developing a series of instrumental technologies and data mining mathematical algorithms to construct finally a versatile platform, SHIP, integrated with wired and wireless network technologies. The following paragraphs describe an overall vision of SHIP and introduce three related constitutional technologies that we have been developing since 2002 (Chen et al., 2004).

2.1 SHIP

SHIP was conceived to provide three functions: (a) detection (monitoring multifarious vital signs by wearable/invisible means, (b) analysis (comprehensive interpretation of long-term

physiological data using data mining mathematics), and (c) service (providing customizable services to various human activity fields by a combination of multiple key technologies).
As shown in Fig. 2, SHIP was constructed in a three-layer model which was supported by five pillars and many bricks.

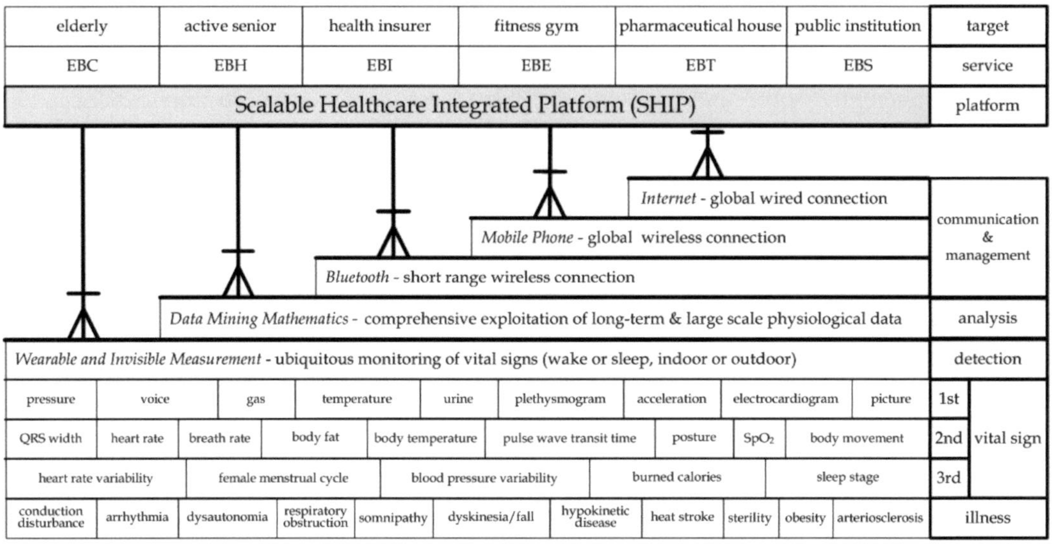

Fig. 2. Systemic architecture of the scalable healthcare integrated platform is founded on bricks, and supported by five pillars in a three layers structure. A variety of application domains can be created using the SHIP.

The first layer consists of a series of bricks for physiological data detection in three orders. Each brick in the first order can be considered as being a wearable/invisible measurement method, which can be used either indoors or outdoors, either awake or asleep. While each brick in the second and third orders indicates a data mining approach to derive information from the other bricks. The direct measurement signals are denoted as first-order vital signs. Second-order vital signs, such as heart rate, are derived from the first-order parameters. Third-order signs originate from the first- and second-order parameters.
Some of direct measurement objects are: pressure, voice, gas, temperature, ECG, acceleration, plethysmogram, and urine. The second-order vital signs are derived from the first-order vital signs, such as the QRS width and heart rate from ECG, the pulse rate and breathing rate from the pressure (Chen et al., 2005), posture and body movement from acceleration (Zhang et al., 2007), and pulse wave transit time from the ECG and plethysmogram. The third-order vital signs are derived from both the second-order and the first-order vital signs. For example, the variability in heart rate is derived from the heart rate profile. The female menstrual cycle is estimated from the body temperature (Chen et al., 2008a), and the variation in blood pressure is estimated from the pulse wave transit time (Chen et al., 2000). Changes in these parameters are indicators of specific ailments, such as arrhythmia from the variability in heart rate, somnipathy from body movements and sleep stage, and respiration obstruction from SpO2. We combined the directly measured and derived parameters to treat related illnesses such as cardiovascular disease, obesity, and respiratory obstruction.

Data mining mathematics for data analysis resides in the second layer. Most of statistical approaches and data warehouse technologies are applicable to conduct a comprehensive exploitation of the large volume of long-term accumulated physiological data. Innovative findings and understanding from this layer will be one of five pillars to support various application domains.

The third layer consists of three pillars and is responsible for data communication and management through wireless and wired networking technology. Bluetooth telemetry technology is adopted as one pillar to support short-range wireless communication of data between sensor devices and home units or mobile phones. Mobile telephony and the Internet are two other pillars and used for wide-range data telecommunication and management.

SHIP has four characteristic features. (a) Its ubiquity makes it possible to detect and collect vital signs either asleep (unconscious status) or awake (conscious status), and either outdoors or indoors through wearable/invisible measurements and wired or wireless networks. (b) Its scalability allows users to customize their special package to meet individual needs, and also service providers to match different requests from medical/clinical use, industries, government agencies, and academic organizations through a variety of partnership options. (c) Its hot-line connectivity is realized by either mobile telephony or Internet (indoors or outdoors) and guarantees that any emergent event can be captured and responded to in real time. (d) Its interoperability is provided through a data warehouse that is configured in two formats. An exclusive format maintains security and enables high-speed data transmission within SHIP, and an externally accessible format ensures that SHIP is open to other allied systems through the HL7 standard (Health Level Seven Inc., 1997) to provide a seamless interface that is compatible with other existing medical information systems.

SHIP is intended to create a flexible platform for the exchange, management, and integration of long-term data collected from a wide spectrum of users, and to provide various evidence-based services to diverse domains. Subjects in target services are not only elderly and active seniors in healthcare but also subjects such as pharmaceutical houses for therapeutic effect tracing, insurance companies involved in risk assessment and claim transactions, transportation system drivers, fire fighters, and policemen involved in public security.

The layer and brick model in the SHIP architecture makes it possible to integrate many elementary achievements from ourselves and co-workers. Three different types of fundamental instrumentation (invisible/wearable/ubiquitous) and the results of data mining from our studies are introduced in the following sections.

2.2 Invisible sleep monitor

Invisible measurement means that a sensor unit can be deployed in an unoccupied area and is unobtrusive and concealable. Monitoring of vital signs can be performed in an invisible way, such that a user is unaware of its existence and does not have to take care that the device is present at all.

A schematic illustration of invisible sleep monitoring is shown in Fig. 3. There is a sensor plate and a bedside unit in the system configuration. A sensor unit is placed beneath a pillow, which is stuffed with numerous fragments of soft comfortable materials formed from synthetic resins. Two incompressible polyvinyl tubes, 30 cm in length and 4 mm in diameter, are filled with air-free water preloaded to an internal pressure of 3 kPa and set in parallel at a distance of 11 cm from each other. A micro tactile switch (B3SN, Omron Co. Ltd) is fixed along the central line between the two parallel tubes. The two tubes above and the micro switch are sandwiched between two acrylic boards, both 3 mm thick. One end of each tube is hermetically sealed and the other end is connected to a liquid pressure sensor head (AP-12S, Keyence Co. Ltd). The inner pressure in each tube includes static and dynamic components, and changes in accordance with respiratory motion and cardiac beating. The static pressure component responds to the weight of the user's head, and acts as a load to turn on a micro tactile switch. The dynamic component reflects the weight fluctuation of the user's head due to breathing movements and pulsatile blood flow from the external carotid arteries around the head. Pressure signals beneath the near-neck and far-neck occiput regions are amplified and band-pass filtered (0.16–5 Hz), and the static component is removed from the signal. Only the dynamic component is digitized at a sampling rate of 100 Hz and transmitted to a remote database server through an Internet connection. The tactile switch is pressed to turn on a DC power supply via a delay switch (4387A-2BE, Artisan Controls Corp.) when the user lies down to sleep and places his/her head on the pillow.

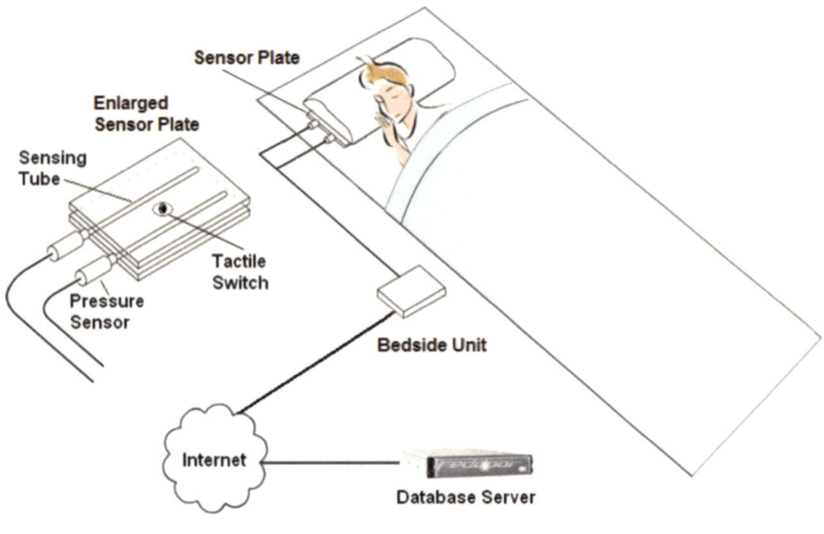

Fig. 3. Schematic illustration of the invisible monitoring of vital signs during sleep. A sensor plate is placed beneath a pillow. Signals reflecting pressure changes under the pillow are detected, digitized, and transmitted to a database server via the Internet by a bedside unit.

A 60 s fragment of raw signal measured under the near-neck occiput region during sleep is shown in Fig. 4(a). The breathing rate (BR), heart rate (HR), and body movements can be detected from the raw data measurements.

The BR and HR are detected by wavelet transformation on a dyadic grid plane using a multiresolution procedure, which is implemented by a recursive à trous algorithm. The Cohen–Daubechies–Fauraue (CDF) (9, 7) biorthogonal wavelet is the basis function used to design the decomposition and reconstruction filters (Daubechies, 1992). The raw measured signal is decomposed into an approximation and multiple detailed components through a cascade of filter banks (Mallat & Zhong, 1992; Shensa, 1992). Further mathematical theories can be found in Daubechies, 1992 and Akay, 1998. Implementation details are given in Chen et al., 2005, and Zhu et al., 2006.

The wavelet transformation (WT) of a signal, $x(t)$, is defined as follows:

$$W_s x(t) = \frac{1}{s}\int_{-\infty}^{+\infty} x(\tau)\psi(\frac{t-\tau}{s})d\tau, \tag{2-2-1}$$

where s is the scale factor and $\psi(t)$ is the wavelet basis function. This is called a dyadic WT if $s = 2^j$ ($j \in Z$ and Z is the integral set). Two filter banks, the low-pass and high-pass decomposition filters $\mathbf{H}_0$ and $\mathbf{H}_1$, and associated reconstruction filters, $\mathbf{G}_0$ and $\mathbf{G}_1$, can be derived from the wavelet basis function and its scaling function, respectively. Using Mallat's algorithm, the dyadic WT of the digital signal, $x(n)$, can be calculated as follows:

$$A_{2^j} x(n) = \sum_{k\in Z} h_{0,2n-k} A_{2^{j-1}} x(k), \tag{2-2-2}$$

$$D_{2^j} x(n) = \sum_{k\in Z} h_{1,2n-k} A_{2^{j-1}} x(k), \tag{2-2-3}$$

where $A_{2^j}x(n)$ and $D_{2^j}x(n)$ are the approximation and detail components, respectively, in the 2^j scale, and $x(n)$ (or $A_{2^0}x(n)$) is the raw data signal. The terms h_0 and h_1 are the filter coefficients of $\mathbf{H}_0$ and $\mathbf{H}_1$, respectively. Therefore, $A_{2^j}x(n)$ and $D_{2^j}x(n)$ ($j \in Z$) can be extracted from $x(n)$ (or $A_{2^0}x(n)$) using equations (2-2-2) and (2-2-3) recursively. The 2^{j-1} scale approximation signal can also be reconstructed from the 2^j scale approximation and the detail component:

$$\hat{A}_{2^{j-1}} x(n) = \sum_{k\in Z} g_{0,n-2k} A_{2^j} x(k) + \sum_{k\in Z} g_{1,n-2k} D_{2^j} x(k), \tag{2-2-4}$$

where g_0 and g_1 are the filter coefficients of $\mathbf{G}_0$ and $\mathbf{G}_1$, respectively. The terms $\hat{x}(n)$ (or $\hat{A}_{2^0}x(n)$) can be finally reconstructed by repeatedly using equation (2-2-4). Any noise in $D_{2^j}x(n)$ can be removed using a soft or hard threshold method before $\hat{A}_{2^{j-1}}x(n)$ is reconstructed. It should be pointed out that the sampling rate of the 2^j scale approximation and detail is $f_s/2^j$, where f_s is the sampling rate of the raw signal.

Because the 2^6 scale approximation waveform is close to a human breathing rhythm, while the detail waveforms of both the 2^4 and 2^5 scales contain peaks similar to those of human heartbeats, the 2^6 scale approximation component, A6, is used to reconstruct the waveform for obtaining the BR, and the D4 and D5 detail components at the 2^4 and 2^5 scales are combined into a single synthesized waveform and then reconstructed to detect the HR. Figure 4(b) shows the reconstructed waveforms for HR detection, and Fig. 4(c) shows the reconstructed waveforms for BR detection.

During a night's sleep, over a period of 4–8 h, a regular pulsation due to either the heart beating or breathing is not always detectable. Body movements may greatly distort the pressure variation signal pattern. In such a time slot, either the BR or the HR, and sometimes even both, are barely detectable. Instead, body movements are detected using a statistical method in such time slots. If a very large change, whose absolute value is four times larger than the standard deviation of the preceding detected movement-free raw signal, is detected in the incoming signal, the preceding and succeeding 2.5 s periods from the movement detection point are treated as being body movement periods and not used to estimate the BR and HR. Detection of the BR is more sensitive to body movements than detection of the HR is.

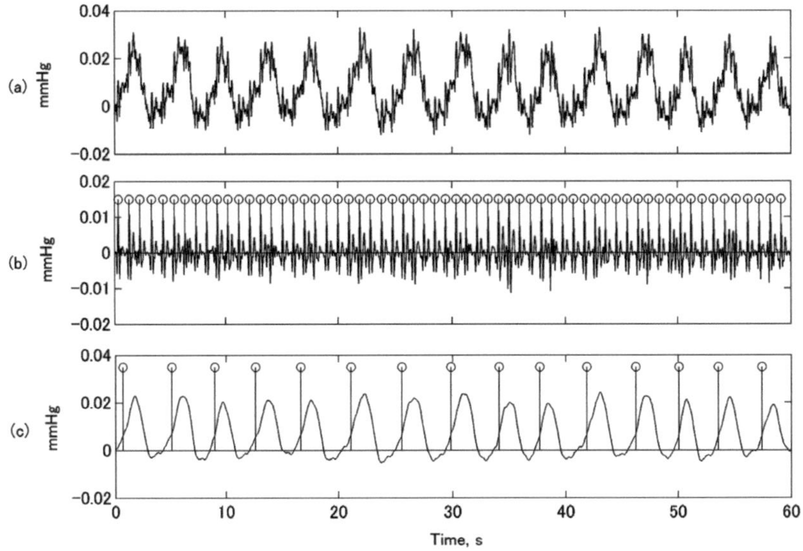

Fig. 4. A body movement-free sample and the detected BR and HR beat-by-beat. (a) The raw pressure signal data measured under the near-neck occiput region. (b) The pulse-related waveform reconstructed from the D4 and D5 components. (c) The breath-related waveform reconstructed from the A6 component. The open circles indicate the detected characteristic points for BR/HR determination.

Figure 5(a) shows a 60 s segment of a raw signal, which includes body movement during unstable sleep. When the pressure signal is distorted by a body movement, the periods detected that are from two reconstructed waveforms (HR-related and BR-related) are not always identical in both time and length. Because HR detection is usually more robust than BR detection, body movement detection from reconstructed BR-related waveforms is longer than that from HR-related waveforms. The final body movement outcome is an OR operation of both results. In the case shown in Fig. 5, the body movement period in terms of HR-related waveform detection is counted as 15.4 s, while that in terms of BR is 35.9 s. The final body movement outputs as 37.8 s from the OR operation of both results in the time domain.

Figure 6 shows a profile of the BR and the HR obtained from measurements over a single night. The vertical axis denotes the BR/HR in units of breaths per minute or beats per minute (bpm). The black dots and vertical bars, terminated at the upper and lower ends by short horizontal lines, show the mean values and standard deviation on a beat-by-beat basis for the HR and a breath-by-breath basis for the BR for each minute. Discontinuities in the estimation of the BR/HR are denoted by the vertical bars occurring sporadically over time, and their widths denote periods of body movement. The broader vertical bars correspond to longer body movement periods.

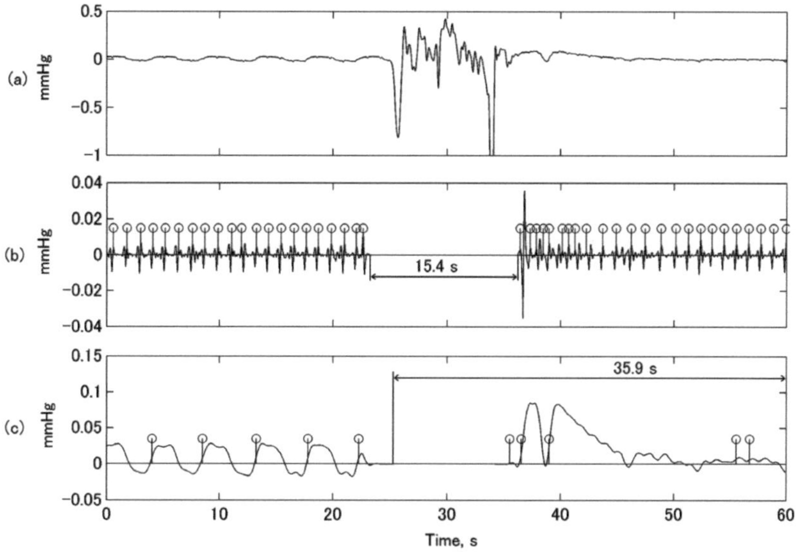

Fig. 5. An example of body movement in which both the BR and the HR are not fully detectable in a given period with different spans. The horizontal arrows indicate the body movement period in seconds. (a) Measured pressure signal distorted by body movements. (b) Reconstructed waveform and detected HR, as well as the detected body movement period. (c) Reconstructed waveform and detected BR as well as the detected body movement period.

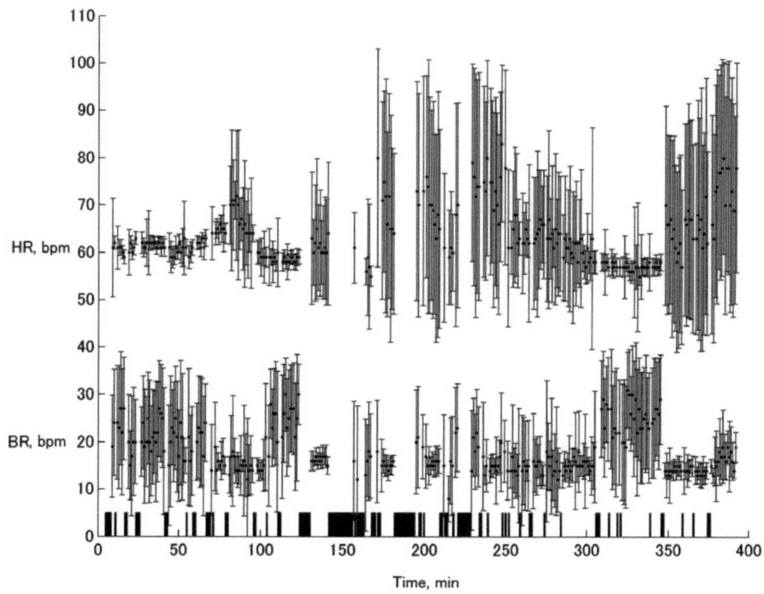

Fig. 6. Two profiles of the BR/HR obtained from measurements over a single night. The solid dots and vertical bars, terminated at the upper and lower ends by short horizontal lines, show the mean values and standard deviation within a period of one minute. The body movement periods are indicated by the variable-width vertical bars.

Figure 7 shows the complete profiles of the BR and HR during sleep over a period of 180 nights. The data were collected from a healthy female volunteer in her thirties at her own house over a period of seven months, under an informed agreement for the use of the data for research purposes. During this period, data over about 30 d were not measured. Therefore, data from a period of 180 d were recorded. The data are plotted on a day-by-day basis. The vertical axis represents the BR/HR in units of bpm. The symbols and vertical bars, terminated at the upper and lower ends by short horizontal lines, show the mean values and standard deviation of the detected HR (o) and the BR (*) in the corresponding night. The bold line is derived by filtering the mean values of the HR using a five-point Hanning window. The dashed line is an empirical estimate to indicate the possible trend of the average day base heart rate during those nights when data were not measured. Surprisingly, it is observed that the profile of the mean heart rate probably reveals a periodic property that corresponds to the female monthly menstrual cycle.

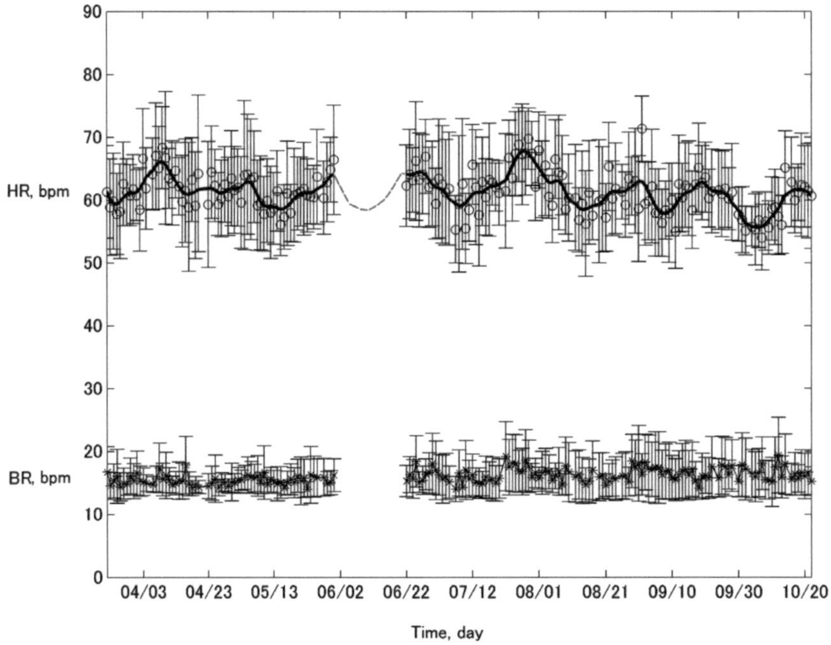

Fig. 7. Two complete profiles of the BR/HR over 180 nights. Data are plotted on a day-by-day basis. The symbols and vertical bars, terminated at the upper and lower ends by short horizontal lines, show the mean values and standard deviation of the detected HR (o) and the BR (*) in the corresponding night.

The devised system is completely invisible to the user during measurements. "Plug is all" is one of its significant characteristics in securing perpetuity in data collection. All a user has to do is just to plug in an AC power cable and a LAN cable. A user can even forget the existence of the device and perform no other operation once it is installed beneath a pillow on a bed. This property will substantially enhance its feasibility and usability in the home environment.
A subtle variation in pressure under the pillow is detected as a first-order signal. The BR/HR and body movements are derived as second-order parameters. Sleep stage estimation, assessment of sleep quality, and biphasic menstrual cycle properties are third-

order parameters. In the end, a comprehensive interpretation of the multiple parameters obtained and a fully automatic operation property would increase its applicability in sleep lab studies, and also for screening patients who do not need a full sleep diagnosis at an early stage.

2.3 Wearable monitor for body temperature

Body temperature is one of the most important barometers indicating human health status. Moreover, the basal body temperature (BBT) is usually used for women to help estimate ovulation and to manage menstruation. However, a reliable evaluation of the menstrual cycle based on the BBT requires measurement of a woman's temperature under constant conditions for long periods. It is indeed a tedious task for a woman to measure her oral or armpit temperature under similar conditions when she wakes up every morning over a long period, because it usually takes an average of 5 min to measure temperature orally, or 10 min under the armpit. Moreover, the traditional method for evaluating ovulation or menstrual cycle dynamics in clinical practice is often based on a physician's empirical observations on serial measurements of BBT. It has been pointed out that the BBT failed to demonstrate ovulation in approximately 20% of ovulation cycles among 30 normally menstruating women (Moghissi, 1980). To improve user accessibility and the accuracy of the application of the BBT, we have developed a tiny wearable device for cutaneous temperature measurements and a Hidden Markov Model (HMM) based a statistical approach to estimate the biphasic properties of body temperature during the menstrual cycle using a series of cutaneous temperature data measured during sleep.

The wearable monitor can be attached to a woman's underwear or brassiere when asleep to measure the cutaneous temperature around the abdominal area or between the breasts, as shown in Fig. 8.

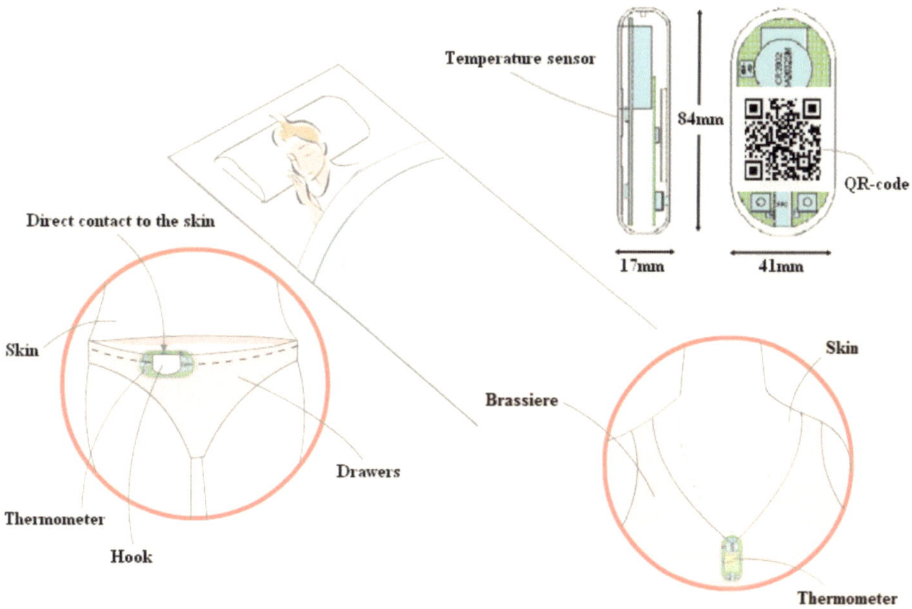

Fig. 8. A small, light wearable device (size = 41 × 84 × 17 mm^3, weight = 59 g) for cutaneous temperature measurements during sleep (QOL Co. Ltd., 2008).

The device is programmed to measure temperature over 10 min intervals from midnight to 6 am. At most, 37 data points can be collected during the six hours. Outliers above 40 °C or below 32 °C are ignored. The collected temperature data are encoded in a two-dimensional bar code, known as "Quick Response" code (QR code) (Denso Wave Inc., 2000) and depicted on an LCD display. As shown in Fig. 9, the user uses the camera built into a mobile phone to capture the QR code image (a) on the device display (shown in the circle on the left-hand side of Fig. 9). Once the QR code is captured into the mobile phone (b), the original temperature data (c) are recovered from the captured image and transmitted to a database server via the mobile network for data storage and physiological interpretation through data mining.

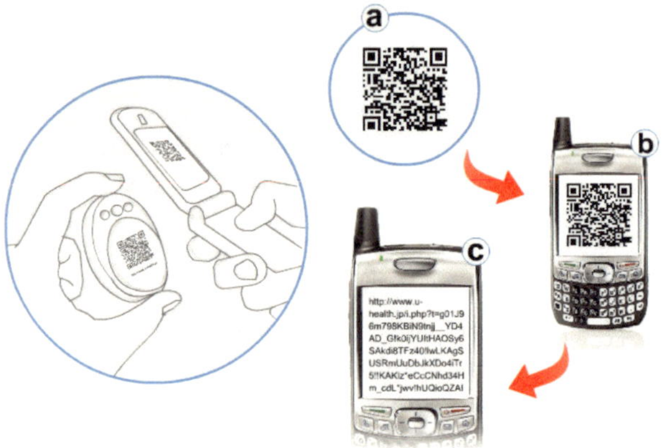

Fig. 9. A procedure for temperature data collection using a wearable sensor and a mobile phone. (a) A QR code image. (b) A QR code captured by a camera built into a mobile phone. (c) Original data recovered from the image captured by a mobile phone (QOL Co. Ltd., 2008).

The temperature data measured during sleep over a six-month period are shown in Fig. 10(a). The nightly data are plotted in the vertical direction and have a range of 32 to 40 °C. The purpose of data mining in this study was to estimate the biphasic properties in the temperature profile during the menstrual cycle from cutaneous temperature measurements.

As shown in Fig. 11, the biphasic properties of the menstrual cycle can be modelled as a discrete Hidden Markov Model (HMM) with two hidden phases. The measured temperature data are considered to be observations being generated by the Markov process from an unknown phase: either a low-temperature (LT) phase or a high-temperature (HT) phase, according to the probability distribution. The probability $b_L(k)$ is indicative that the value k is generated from the hidden LT phase. The probability $b_H(k)$ is indicative that the value k is generated from the hidden HT phase. The probability a_{ii} is indicative of a hidden phase transition between LT and HT phases.

Figure 10(b) shows the results after pre-processing to removing outliers from the raw data and eliminating any discontinuities from non-data-collection days. Figure 10(c) shows the HMM estimation output using the pre-processed data from Fig. 10(b) as the input. Figure 10(d) shows the estimation of the biphasic properties after post-processing. The superimposed black symbols "*" denote the menstrual periods recorded by the user. A transition from the HT phase to the LT phase denotes a menstrual period, while the reverse transition denotes ovulation.

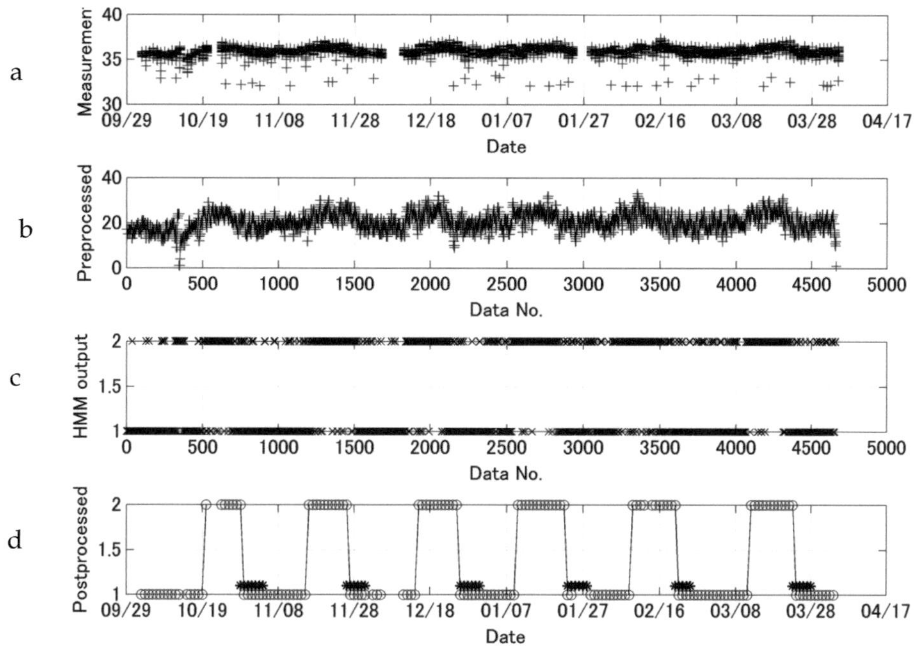

Fig. 10. Estimation procedure of a biphasic temperature profile. (a) Raw temperature data measured over a period of six months. (b) Pre-processed results. (c) Biphasic estimation based on an HMM approach. (d) Post-processed results. The symbol "*" denotes a menstrual period recorded by the user.

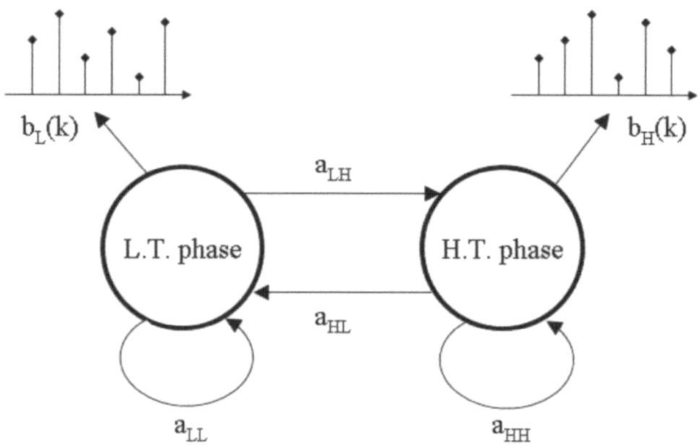

Fig. 11. A discrete hidden Markov model with two hidden phases for estimating biphasic property in a menstrual cycle from cutaneous temperature measurements.

The biphasic properties shown in Fig. 10(c) were estimated by finding an optimal HMM parameter set that determines the hidden phase from which each datum arises. This is based on a given series of measured temperature data, as shown in Fig. 10(b). The parameter set $\lambda(A,B,\pi)$ is assigned randomly in the initial condition and optimized through the forward-backward iterative procedure until $P(O|\lambda)$ converges to a stable maximum value or until the absolute logarithm of the previous and current difference in $P(O|\lambda)$ is not greater than δ.

The algorithm for calculating the forward variable, α, the backward variable, β, and the forward–backward variable, γ, are shown in equations (2-3-1) to (2-3-3).
The forward variable, $\alpha_t(i)$, denotes the probability of phase, q_i, at time, t, based on a partial observation sequence, $O_1, O_2, \ldots, O_t$, until time t, and can be calculated using the following steps for a given set of $\lambda(A,B,\pi)$.

$$\alpha_t(i) = P_r(O_1, O_2, \ldots, O_t, i_t = q_i \mid \lambda)$$

$$\alpha_1(i) = \pi_i b_i(O_1), \qquad 1 \le i \le N, t = 1$$

$$\alpha_{t+1}(j) = \left[\sum_{i=1}^{N} \alpha_t(i) a_{ij}\right] b_j(O_{t+1}), \qquad 1 \le j \le N, t = 1, 2, \ldots, T-1 \tag{2-3-1}$$

The backward variable, $\beta_t(i)$, denotes the probability of phase, q_i, at time, t, based on a partial observation sequence, $O_{t+1}, O_{t+2}, \ldots, O_T$, from time t+1 to T, and can be calculated using the following steps for a given set of $\lambda(A,B,\pi)$.

$$\beta_t(i) = P_r(O_{t+1}, O_{t+2}, \ldots, O_T \mid i_t = q_i, \lambda)$$

$$\beta_T(i) = 1, \qquad 1 \le i \le N, t = T$$

$$\beta_t(i) = \sum_{j=1}^{N} a_{ij} b_j(O_{t+1}) \beta_{t+1}(j), \qquad 1 \le i \le N, t = T-1, T-2, \ldots, 1 \tag{2-3-2}$$

To find the optimal sequence of hidden phases for a given observation sequence, O, and a given model, $\lambda(A,B,\pi)$, there are multiple possible optimality criteria.
Choosing the phases, q_t, that are individually most likely at each time, t, i.e., maximizing $P(q_t = i \mid O, \lambda)$, is equivalent to finding the single best phase sequence (path), i.e., maximizing $P(Q \mid O, \lambda)$ or $P(Q, O \mid \lambda)$. The forward–backward algorithm is applied to find the optimal sequence of phases, q_t, at each time, t, i.e., to maximize $\gamma_t(i) = P(q_t = i \mid O, \lambda)$ for a given observation sequence, O, and a given set of $\lambda(A,B,\pi)$.

$$\begin{aligned} \gamma_t(i) &= P(q_t = i \mid O, \lambda) \\ &= \frac{P(O, q_t = i \mid \lambda)}{P(O \mid \lambda)} = \frac{P(O, q_t = i \mid \lambda)}{\sum_{i=1}^{N} P(O, q_t = i \mid \lambda)} \\ &= \frac{P(o_1 o_2 \ldots o_t, q_t = i \mid \lambda) P(o_{t+1} o_{t+2} \ldots o_T \mid q_t = i, \lambda)}{\sum_{i=1}^{N} P(o_1 o_2 \ldots o_t, q_t = i \mid \lambda) P(o_{t+1} o_{t+2} \ldots o_T \mid q_t = i, \lambda)} \\ &= \frac{\alpha_t(i) \beta_t(i)}{\sum_{i=1}^{N} \alpha_t(i) \beta_t(i)} \end{aligned} \tag{2-3-3}$$

The most likely phase, q_t^* at time t can be found as:

$$q_t^* = \arg\max_{1\le i\le N}\left[\gamma_t(i)\right], \qquad 1 \le t \le T. \tag{2-3-4}$$

As there are no existing analytical methods for optimizing λ(A,B,π), P(O|λ) or P(O,I|λ) is usually maximized (i.e., $\lambda^* = \arg\max_{\lambda}[P(O\mid\lambda)]$ or $\lambda^* = \arg\max_{\lambda}[P(O,Q\mid\lambda)]$) using gradient techniques and an expectation-maximization method. In this study, the Baum–Welch method was used because of its numerical stability and linear convergence (Rabiner, 1989). To update λ(A,B,π) using the Baum–Welch re-estimation algorithm, we defined a variable, $\xi_t(i,j)$, to express the probability of a datum being in phase *i* at time *t* and phase *j* at time *t*+1, given the model and the observation sequence:

$$\xi_t(i,j) = P(q_t = i, q_{t+1} = j \mid O, \lambda) = \frac{P(q_t = i, q_{t+1} = j, O \mid \lambda)}{P(O\mid\lambda)}. \tag{2-3-5}$$

From the definitions of the forward and backward variables, $\xi_t(i,j)$ and $\gamma_t(i)$, can be related as:

$$\xi_t(i,j) = \frac{\alpha_t(i)a_{ij}b_j(o_{t+1})\beta_{t+1}(j)}{P(O\mid\lambda)} = \frac{\alpha_t(i)a_{ij}b_j(o_{t+1})\beta_{t+1}(j)}{\sum_{i=1}^{N}\sum_{j=1}^{N}\alpha_t(i)a_{ij}b_j(o_{t+1})\beta_{t+1}(j)}, \tag{2-3-6}$$

$$\gamma_t(i) = P(q_t = i \mid O, \lambda) = \sum_{j=1}^{N} P(q_t = i, q_{t+1} = j \mid O, \lambda) = \sum_{j=1}^{N}\xi_t(i,j), \tag{2-3-7}$$

where $\sum_{t=1}^{T-1}\gamma_t(i)$ denotes the expected number of transitions from phase *i* in *O*. The term $\sum_{t=1}^{T-1}\xi_t(i,j)$ denotes the expected number of transitions from phase *i* to phase *j* in *O*.

Therefore, λ(A,B,π) can be updated using equations (2-3-8) to (2-3-10) as follows.
As π_i is the initial probability and denotes the expected frequency (number of times) in phase *i* at time *t* = 1 as $\pi_i = \gamma_1(i)$, it can be calculated using the forward and backward variables.

$$\pi_i = \frac{\alpha_1(i)\beta_1(i)}{\sum_{i=1}^{N}\alpha_1(i)\beta_1(i)} = \frac{\alpha_1(i)\beta_1(i)}{\sum_{i=1}^{N}\alpha_T(i)}, \tag{2-3-8}$$

The transition probability from phase *i* to phase *j*, a_{ij}, can be calculated from the expected number of transitions from phase *i* to phase *j* divided by the expected number of transitions from phase *i*.

$$a_{ij} = \frac{\sum_{t=1}^{T-1}\xi_t(i,j)}{\sum_{t=1}^{T-1}\gamma_t(i)} = \frac{\sum_{t=1}^{T-1}\alpha_t(i)a_{ij}b_j(o_{t+1})\beta_{t+1}(j)}{\sum_{t=1}^{T-1}\alpha_t(i)\beta_t(i)}, \tag{2-3-9}$$

The term $b_j(k)$ is the expected number of times in phase j and the observed symbol o_k divided by the expected number of times in phase j, and it can be calculated using:

$$b_j(k) = \frac{\sum_{\substack{t=1 \\ s.t. O_t = o_k}}^{T} \gamma_t(j)}{\sum_{t=1}^{T} \gamma_t(j)}. \qquad (2\text{-}3\text{-}10)$$

The initial input quantities are the known data N, M, T, and O and the randomly initialized $\lambda(A,B,\pi)$. Once α, β, and γ are calculated using equations (2-3-1) to (2-3-3), then $\lambda(A,B,\pi)$ is updated using equations (2-3-8) to (2-3-10), based on the newly obtained values of α, β, and γ. The search for the optimal parameter set, λ_{opt}, is terminated when $P(O\,|\,\lambda)$ converges to a stable maximum value or when the absolute logarithm of the previous and current difference in $P(O\,|\,\lambda)$ is equal to or smaller than δ. Thus, the most likely phase from which a datum is observed can be estimated using equation (2-3-4). A sample result estimated using the HMM algorithm is shown in Fig. 10(c).

The algorithmic performance is evaluated by comparing the user's own record of their menstrual periods with the algorithmically estimated result. When a transition line coincides with a self-declared menstrual period, then it is counted as a "true positive". If a transition line does not coincide with a self-declared menstrual period, then it is counted as either a "false negative" or a "false positive".

Figure 12 shows a poor sample with two different estimation errors. One is a false negative estimation occurring around November 14, where there was a menstrual period but it was not detected. Another is a false positive error, occurring around July 17, where an HT to LT transition was detected but there was no actual menstrual period.

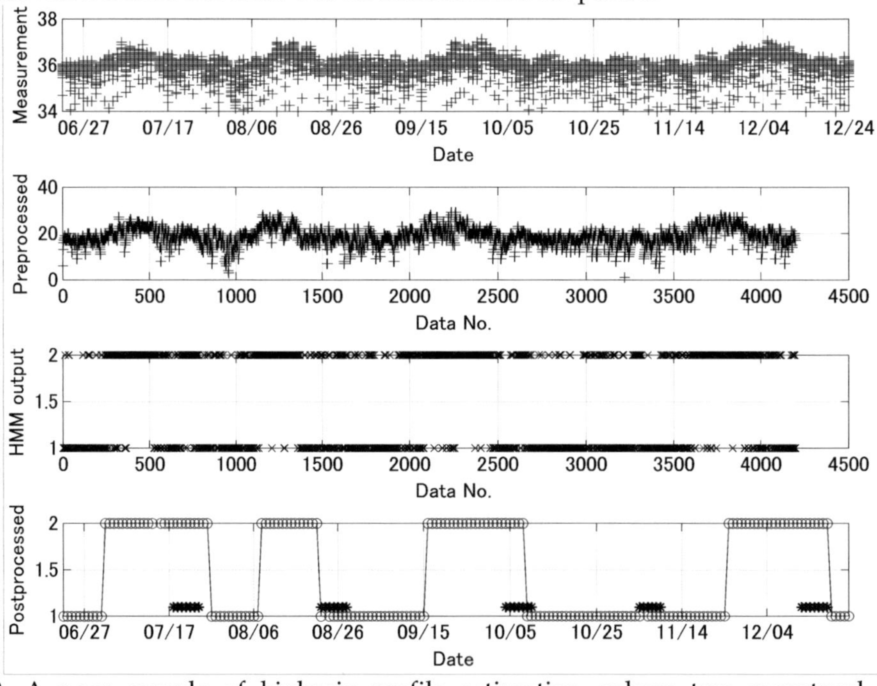

Fig. 12. A poor sample of biphasic profile estimation, where two menstrual periods occurring around July 17 and November 14 were not detected correctly by the algorithm.

To evaluate the algorithmic performance in finding the biphasic properties of the temperature data during menstrual cycles, both sensitivity and positive predictability are introduced. The sensitivity (Sens) denotes an algorithm's ability to estimate correctly the biphasic properties that coincide with the user's records of menstrual periods. This value is calculated using equation (2-3-11). When Sens has a value close to 1.0, then it means that there is less underestimation.

$$Sens = \frac{TP}{TP + FN}, \tag{2-3-11}$$

The positive predictability (PP) denotes the confidence of the positive estimation. This is calculated using equation (2-3-12), and when PP has a value that is close to 1.0, then it means that there is less overestimation:

$$PP = \frac{TP}{TP + FP}, \tag{2-3-12}$$

where *TP* denotes a true positive where the algorithmic estimation and the user's records coincide. *FN* is a false negative, and it counts the number of undetected menstrual periods. *FP* is a false positive, and it counts the number of detected HT to LT transitions where no actual menstrual period occurred.

In this study, a tiny wearable thermometer and an HMM-based data mining approach were developed and validated using data collected over a period of six months from 30 female volunteers. For a total of 190 self-declared menstrual cycles, the number of estimated cycles was TP = 169, the number of undetected cycles was FN = 15, and the number of falsely detected cycles was FP = 6. Therefore, by applying equations (2-3-11) and (2-3-12), the sensitivity was 91.8% and the positive predictability was 96.6%.

The device automatically collected the cutaneous temperature around the abdominal area or between the breasts without much discomfort during sleep. This met the requirement for perpetuity in body temperature measurements due to a low disturbance to daily life. The algorithm estimated the biphasic cyclic properties of the temperature profiles during menstrual cycles based on a series of long-term temperature data, with no need for any experimental or subjective involvement. This provides a promising approach for managing female premenstrual syndromes and birth control.

2.4 Ubiquitous monitoring based on a mobile phone

The voice is the sound made by the vibration of the vocal cords, caused by air passing through the larynx and bringing the cords closer together. Voice production is a complex process that starts with muscle movement and involves: phonation (voice), respiration (breathing process), and articulation (throat, palate, tongue, lips, and teeth). These muscle movements are initiated, coordinated, and controlled by the brain, and monitored through hearing and touch. A variety of changes in voice, such as pitch, intensity, and fundamental frequency, can take place when any of the above factors change, and will be one of the first and most important symptoms of mental depression, or some physical diseases, such as cancer, Parkinson's disease, epilepsy, stroke, and Alzheimer's disease, which means that early detection significantly increases the effectiveness of any treatment (France & Kramer, 2001; O'Shaughnessy, 1999; Mathieson, 2001).

Recently, many studies have been conducted to identify pathological voices by applying various classifiers to acoustic features, such as cepstral coefficients and pitch dynamics using Gaussian mixtures in a Hidden Markov Model (HMM) classifier. These have obtained a 99.44% correct classification rate for discrimination of normal and pathological speech using the sustained phoneme "a" from over 700 subjects (Dibazar et al., 2002). In contrast to sustained vowel research, the effectiveness of acoustic features extracted from continuous speech has also been evaluated. A joint time-frequency approach for classifying pathological voices using continuous speech signals was proposed to obviate the need for segmentation of voiced, unvoiced, and silence periods. The speech signals were decomposed using an adaptive time-frequency transform algorithm, and several features, such as the octave max, octave mean, energy ratio, length ratio, and frequency ratio were extracted from the decomposition parameters and analysed using statistical pattern classification techniques. Experiments with a database consisting of continuous speech samples from 51 normal and 161 pathological talkers yielded a classification accuracy of 93.4% (Umapathy et al., 2005).

On the other hand, mobile phones are a pervasive tool, and not only are they able to be used in voice communication but also they are an effective voice collector in daily conversation. This study aims to develop a ubiquitous tool for identifying various pathological voices using mobile phones and support vector machine (SVM) mathematics through the classification of voice features.

A. Voice data and acoustic features

The voice data used in this study were excerpted from the Disordered Voice Database Model 4337 v2.7.0 (Key Elemetrics Corp., 2004). Because parts of the recordings and clinical information were incomplete, we only chose 214 subjects aged from 13 to 82 years (mean ± STD = 45 ± 16 years) whose records were fully contained. The selected dataset included 33 healthy subjects (14 males and 19 females) and 181 patients (86 males and 95 females) who suffered from various voice disorders, such as polypoid degeneration, adductor spasmodic dysphonia, vocal fold anomalies, hyperfunction, and erythema, totalling more than 40 types of abnormality. The 25 acoustic features are listed in Table 1. They were calculated using the voice data, which were sampled from the vowel "a" pronunciation by each subject. The calculation method for each feature can be found in detail in the CDROM (Key Elemetrics Corp., 2004).

B. SVM principle

As a related supervised learning method used for classification and regression, SVM is a generalized linear classifier, but it differs from other methods because of its largest margin and its simplest form among several others. The optimal separation hyperplane was determined to maximize the generalization ability of the SVM. However, because most real-world problems are not linearly separable, the SVM introduced kernel tricks to deal with the linearly inseparable problems. Therefore, in theory, a linearly inseparable problem in the original data space can be completely transformed into a linearly separable problem in high-dimensional feature space.

No	Feature	Meaning	No	Feature	Meaning
1	APQ	Amplitude perturbation quotient	14	PPQ	Pitch period perturbation quotient
2	ATRI	Amplitude tremor intensity index	15	RAP	Relative average perturbation
3	DSH	Degree of subharmonic components	16	sAPQ	Smoothed amplitude perturbation quotient
4	Fatr	Amplitude-tremor frequency	17	Shdb	Shimmer in dB
5	Fftr	Fo-tremor frequency	18	Shim	Shimmer per cent
6	Fhi	Highest fundamental frequency	19	SPI	Soft phonation index
7	Flo	Lowest fundamental frequency	20	sPPQ	Smoothed pitch period perturbation quotient
8	Fo	Average fundamental frequency	21	STD	STD of fundamental frequency
9	FTRI	Frequency tremor intensity index	22	To	Average pitch period
10	Jita	Absolute jitter	23	vAm	Coeff. of amplitude variation
11	Jitt	Jitter per cent	24	vFo	Coeff. of fundamental frequency variation
12	NHR	Noise-to-harmonic ratio	25	VTI	Voice turbulence index
13	PFR	Phonatory fundamental freq. range			

Table 1. Abbreviations of acoustic features and their physical meanings.

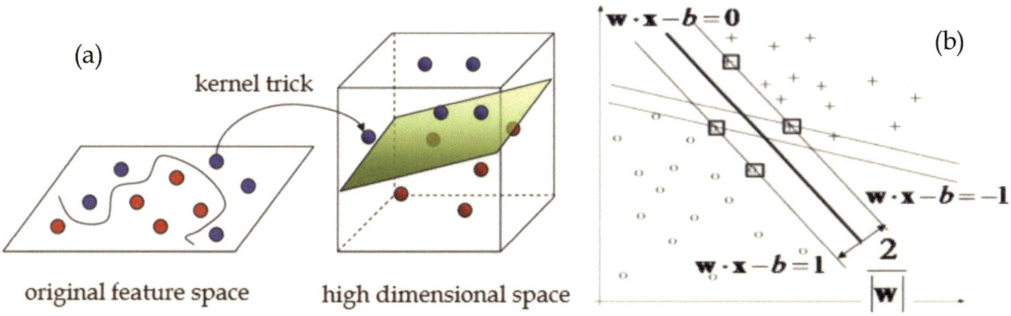

Fig. 13. Principle of the SVM. A separating hyperplane in high-dimensional feature space and a maximum margin boundary between two data sets. (a) A non-linear classification problem in an original lower-dimensional feature space is transformed into a linear classification problem in a higher-dimensional feature space through a non-linear vector function, or a kernel trick. (b) An optimal hyperplane to separate two classes of data in high-dimensional space with the largest geometric margin.

As shown in Fig. 13, suppose we have an original dataset, $\{x_i, y_i\}$, $x_i \in \mathbf{R}^d$, $y_i \in \{-1,1\}$, $i = 1,\ldots,M$. A separating hyperplane separates the positive from the negative subdataset. The points, x_i, which lie on the hyperplane satisfy $\mathbf{w}\cdot\mathbf{x}_i + b = 0$, where $\mathbf{w}$ is normal to the hyperplane,

$|b|/\|\mathbf{w}\|$ is the perpendicular distance from the origin to the hyperplane, and $\|\mathbf{w}\|$ is the Euclidean norm of **w**. Let d_+ and d_- be the shortest distances from the separating hyperplane to the closest positive data point and the closest negative data point, respectively. The margin of a separating hyperplane is defined as $d_+ + d_-$. In the linearly separable case, all the data points satisfy the following constraints.

$$\mathbf{x}_i \cdot \mathbf{w} + b \geq +1 \text{ for } y_i = +1 \tag{2-4-1}$$

$$\mathbf{x}_i \cdot \mathbf{w} + b \leq -1 \text{ for } y_i = -1 \tag{2-4-2}$$

These can be combined into one set of inequalities.

$$y_i(\mathbf{x}_i \cdot \mathbf{w} + b) - 1 \geq 0 \ \forall I \tag{2-4-3}$$

Clearly, the data points, which lie in the hyperplane H_1, $\mathbf{w} \cdot \mathbf{x}_i + b = 1$, lie at a perpendicular distance $|1 - b|/\|\mathbf{w}\|$ from the origin. Similarly, the data points that lie in the hyperplane H_2, $\mathbf{w} \cdot \mathbf{x}_i + b = -1$, lie at a perpendicular distance $|-1 - b|/\|\mathbf{w}\|$ from the origin. Hence, the margin is simply $2/\|\mathbf{w}\|$. Therefore, we can find an optimal separating hyperplane that has the largest margin by minimizing $\|\mathbf{w}\|^2$, subject to the constraints in equation (2-4-3).

The data points that lie on hyperplanes H_1 or H_2 are called support vectors. Their removal would change the solution found. This problem can now be solved through a Lagrangian formulation by introducing non-negative Lagrangian multipliers, α_i, $i = 1,\ldots,M$, for each of the inequality constraints (2-4-3). The Lagrangian takes the form:

$$L_P \equiv \frac{1}{2}\|\mathrm{w}\|^2 - \sum_{i=1}^{M} \alpha_i y_i (\mathrm{x}_i \cdot \mathrm{w} + b) + \sum_{i=1}^{M} \alpha_i . \tag{2-4-4}$$

By taking the gradient of L_P with respect to **w**, b vanishes, giving the outcome:

$$\mathrm{w} = \sum_{i=1}^{M} \alpha_i y_i \mathrm{x}_i , \tag{2-4-5}$$

$$\sum_{i=1}^{M} \alpha_i y_i = 0, \ \alpha_i \geq 0, \ i = 1,\ldots,M. \tag{2-4-6}$$

Substituting equations (2-4-5) and (2-4-6) into equation (2-4-4) gives:

$$L_P = \sum_{i=1}^{M} \alpha_i - \frac{1}{2} \sum_{i=1,j=1}^{M} \alpha_i \alpha_j y_i y_j \mathrm{x}_i \cdot \mathrm{x}_j . \tag{2-4-7}$$

Maximizing equation (2-4-7) under the constraints in equation (2-4-6) is a concave quadratic programming problem. If the dataset is linearly separable, then the global optimal solution, α_i, $i = 1,\ldots,M$, can be found. Then, the boundary decision function is given by:

$$D(\mathrm{x}) = \sum_{i \in i_S} \alpha_i y_i \mathrm{x}_i \cdot \mathrm{x} + b , \tag{2-4-8}$$

where, i_S is the set of support vector indexes, and b is given by:

$$b = y_i - \mathbf{w} \cdot \mathbf{x}_i,\ i \in i_S. \tag{2-4-9}$$

To tackle linearly inseparable problems, the SVM is extended by incorporating slack variables and kernel tricks. The non-negative slack variables determine the trade-off between maximization of the margin and minimization of the classification error. The kernel tricks use a non-linear vector function, $g(\mathbf{x})$, to map the original dataset into a higher-dimensional space. Therefore, the linear decision function in the new feature space can be given by:

$$\begin{aligned} D(\mathbf{x}) &= \mathbf{w} \cdot \mathbf{g}(\mathbf{x}) + b \\ &= \sum_{i \in i_S} \alpha_i y_i \mathbf{g}(\mathbf{x}_i) \cdot \mathbf{g}(\mathbf{x}) + b = \sum_{i \in i_S} \alpha_i y_i H(\mathbf{x}_i, \mathbf{x}) + b' \end{aligned} \tag{2-4-10}$$

where $H(\mathbf{x}_i, \mathbf{x})$ is the Mercer kernel. The advantage of using the kernel trick is that the high-dimensional feature space can be treated implicitly by calculating $H(\mathbf{x}_i, \mathbf{x})$ instead of $g(\mathbf{x}_i) \cdot g(\mathbf{x})$.

Twenty-five acoustic features were calculated from each subject's voice data, and 214 data segments from 214 individuals were labelled as "–1" for a healthy voice and "1" for a pathological voice. There are two major steps in voice classification. Firstly, a principal component analysis (PCA) was used to reduce the original feature dimensions as much as possible by ignoring correlated features while retaining the most significant information in the new dataset. Secondly, a transformed subdataset in the new coordinate system was applied to the SVM to elucidate the identification boundary for healthy and pathological voices. Two kernels, Gaussian and polynomial, with different parameter combinations, were evaluated, as shown in Figs 14 and 15. The black contours refer to the identification boundaries, the white contours to the margins, and the symbols on the white contours to the support vectors.

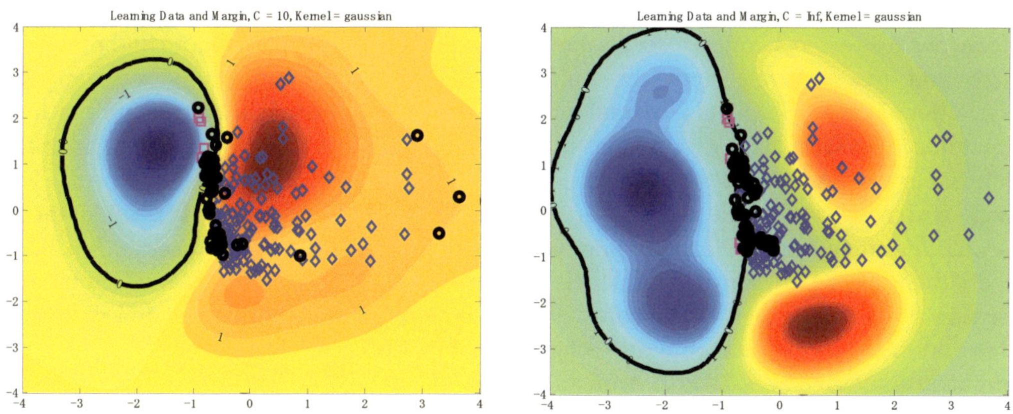

Fig. 14. Identification boundary, margin, and support vectors obtained using the Gaussian kernel with different slack variables ξ (left = 10 and right = +∞).

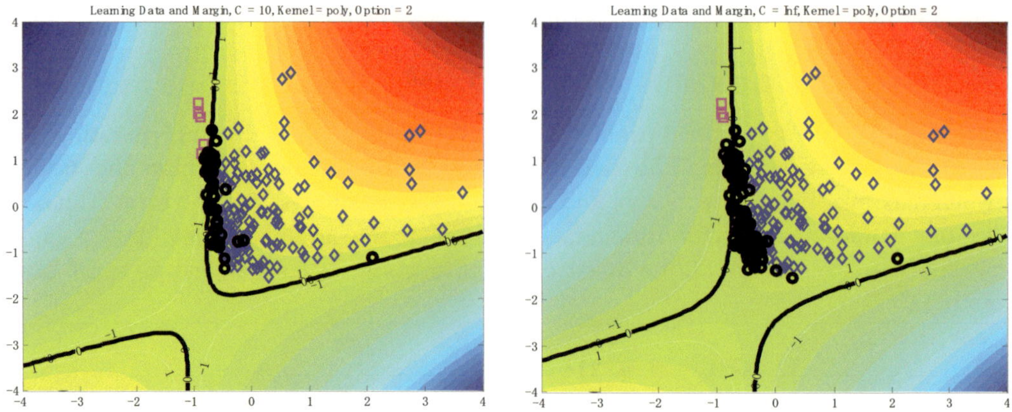

Fig. 15. Identification boundary, margin, and support vectors obtained using the polynomial kernel with d = 2 and different slack variables ξ (left = 10 and right = $+\infty$).

In this study, 25 acoustic features derived from a single vowel sound "a" were used to identify pathological and healthy voices. The accuracy under different combinations of features was tested using a fivefold cross-validation method. The results show that the STD, Fatr, and NHR were the most sensitive features in detecting pathological changes. Moreover, the length of the voice sample, the number of voice segments, and the total number of detected pitch periods affected the identification accuracy. The highest accuracy in detecting pathological voices from healthy voices was 97.0% (Peng et al., 2007a; Peng et al., 2007b).

Not only its mathematical elegance but also the practical advantage of simplicity means the SVM approach is promising for implementing in any portable device. A mobile phone's built-in microphone works perfectly as a "one-stone-kills-two-birds" solution for identifying subtle distinctions in voices ubiquitously without any inexpediency during daily conversation.

3. Discussion

Life is not just a biochemical process but rather is a symphony of many rhythms on the micro and macro levels from the milliseconds of single-neuron activity to monthly procreation, and yearly developmental aging. However, intrinsic biorhythms are gradually stupefying in modern lifestyles because of artificial lighting and controlled environments. A healthy life is considered a state or process of complete physical, mental, and social well-being, and not merely the absence of disease or infirmity (WHO, 1948). Even though research that may unravel the interplay between depression and other diseases has barely begun, there is a strong statistical link between the incidence of depression and several other diseases, including cancer, Parkinson's disease, epilepsy, stroke, and Alzheimer's disease. More and more doctors and patients recognize that mental state and physical well-being are intimately connected (Wisneski & Anderson 2005).

Because many currently used vital signs, such as blood pressure, ECG, and metabolized chemicals, are so important in life processes, the body must exert itself through the feedback regulatory mechanisms of the autonomic nervous system and the immune system to avoid disorders. In the case where these parameters are detected out of range, it is actually a sign that the body has become intolerant, and this is indicated by its exhaustion in maintaining proper biological functions. By then, it is already too late for us to take action. We should look for more sensitive symptoms that can reflect any small changes in the early stages of the development of ailments. Extrinsic extremities, such as capillary vessels and peripheral tissues, are less important in body functioning, and these areas are the first candidates to be deserted to guarantee that vital organs and tissues do not malfunction. Traditional Chinese Medicine (TCM) diagnoses by observing the colour of skin and the tones of sound by skilful means of inquiry, smell, and touch to acquire insight into pathological changes in a patient (Qu, 2007).

Much effort is being conducted towards chronic illness prevention and early warning. It has been found that the correlation between the blood sugar level and the acetone in a patient's breath is significant in the diagnosis of diabetes (Zhang et al., 2000). More barometers, such as the colour and texture of the skin, nails, palms, and tongue, are worthy of further investigation.

Application of these new approaches in treating chronic conditions requires advanced sensory technology feasible for daily monitoring, and a flexible platform for users, physicians, and allied health workers to manage the long-term data, as well as data mining mathematics suitable for the comprehensive interpretation of multiple data fusion.

Innovative sensory instrumentation technologies are indispensable for monitoring a wide range of physiological data in the environment of everyday living, because most users are not trained professionally, and as perpetual monitoring is preferable in chronic conditions, the sensory device should have some key advantages, such as zero administration, easy manipulation, automatic fault recovery, and the absence of unpleasantness or disturbance to everyday living. Fortunately, changes in long-term physiological data are much more important than the absolute values in long-term application, measurement resolution is prior to the accuracy, and this partly relieves the requirements to sensory instrumentation. Studies in this direction in several of our projects have been conducted using three main models of sensory technologies and real data validation in their field tests.

Invisible instrumentation - e.g., the sleep monitor - requires no user intervention at all during monitoring. This "plug is all" property makes it possible for a user to plug in several cables, such as a power supply and LAN, and the system then works automatically. Users do not have to remember how to use the machine and notice what it is doing behind them.

A wearable device - e.g., the women's temperature monitor - is worn as if a part of the underwear or brassiere with little discomfort. The feedback from the participants in our feasibility study indicated that taking a magic-like QR-code picture is much more enjoyable than taking an oral or armpit BBT measurement after morning arousal from sleep. Many of the participants found "play and fun" in this routine activity.

Ubiquitous monitoring technology based on a mobile phone has been developed for carry-on usage, at any time or place, without any need for attention. Indeed, a mobile phone is a marvellously powerful portable machine that has many built-in sensors, such as a microphone for sound, a camera for pictures, and a touch panel for pressure measurement, applicable for detecting vital signs. An additional built-in gas sensor would make it possible for a mobile phone to monitor breath gases.

As more and more innovative vital signs are detected in the environment of everyday living from a large number of the population and are accumulated over a longer period, a flexible data warehouse for facilitating the large volume of data is necessary. SHIP was devised as a scalable and customizable platform to make it possible to integrate a broad spectrum of physiological data, and also to perform multiple data fusion through comprehensive data mining to provide versatile services in diversified application domains.

By mining the long-term physiological data accumulated from the large-scale population, more physiological insights related to physical and mental ailments will be discovered from changes in the biorhythms in the long-term profiles, which are important for chronic conditions but is unable to be derived from fragmentary data collected over the short term.

Biological rhythms are found in a wide range of frequencies from seconds to years, and in different biological levels from the entire body to individual cells. Much research has been conducted on different scales, such as circadian, diurnal, monthly, and seasonal rhythms. Many rhythmic events are already well known. Sudden death due to cardiovascular disease happens mostly in the early morning. A high risk of stroke and silent cerebral infarct are related to the morning surge of blood pressure that occurs on waking. One of the most prominent biorhythms is the heartbeat, which is currently used to obtain insight into many cardiovascular-related diseases (Malik et al., 1996). There is growing evidence indicating that a marked diurnal variation exists in the onset of cardiovascular events, with a peak incidence of myocardial infarction, sudden cardiac death, and ischemic and hemorrhagic stroke occurring in the morning (from 6 am to noon), after a nadir in these events during the night (Kario et al., 2003).

On the other hand, the "Medical Classic of Emperor Huang" (Wikipedia, 2008), one of the TCM representative masterpieces published more than 2,000 years ago, divided a day into 12 time slots. Each time slot is two hours long and is responsible for alternating metabolic oscillations in different visceral organs. Each visceral organ has its optimal on-duty and off-duty time slot. During the period 5–7 am, the cardiovascular system is on duty and is most active. This leads to an increase in the burden on the heart and induces a morning surge in blood pressure. Even worse, patients suffering from cardiovascular disease are subject to sudden death. Such rhythmic concepts are close to current understanding (Qu, 2007).

In contrast, a dualism that considered mind and body to be separate prevailed until René Déscartes in the 17th century. Oriental medicine treats the body and mind as a whole and aims to enhance holistic balance and visceral organic harmony through enhancing self-healing functions by offering a series of therapies, such as herbal medicine, meditation, acupuncture, and osteopathy in the early stage of illness development, or "un-illness status".

The term "un-illness status" is used in the "Medical Classic of Emperor Huang". The proposed prescriptions, such as shadow boxing and rhythmic gymnastics, are still effective for the present management of most lifestyle-related chronic diseases, such as hypertension, hyperlipidaemia, diabetes, obesity, hyperuricaemia, arteriosclerosis, osteoporosis, hepatitis, asymptomatic stroke, potential heart attack, and fatty liver. The Japan Mibyou System Association (JMSA) was founded in 2005, and it defined "mibyou" (un-illness) as a situation between health and disease (JMSA, 2006). JMSA's mission is committed to the better control of un-illness situations and to improving human wellness. JMSA established an official accreditation system for health promoters that aim to provide wholesome and secure care to all citizens.

A "challenge to 100 years of age" project in the county community of Nishi-Aizu in central Japan has been mobilized since 1994 with governmental financial support of 2 billion Japanese yen (Nishi-Aizu, 2003). The fundamental goal is to increase healthy longevity by providing a total solution package to villagers. They built an ICT infrastructure, improved the soil, enhanced the nutritional balance, and initiated a health promotion campaign.

Homecare devices were distributed to 687 families among a total of 2,819 families. These devices can measure blood pressure, ECG, photoelectric plethysmograms, body temperature and weight, and can receive answers to queries. These endeavours increased the villagers' longevity from 73.1 years (80.0 years for females) in 1985 to 77.6 years (84.1 years for females) in 2000 and decreased the mortality from stomach cancer from 138.9% (125.4% for females) in 1988 to 91.7% (66.7% for females) in 2002.

In their "China study", Campbell et al. described a monumental survey of diet and death rates from cancer in more than 2,400 Chinese counties, and its significance and implications for nutrition and health. They showed that by changing their behaviour based on nutritional balance and lifestyle, patients can dramatically reduce their risk of cancer, diabetes, heart disease, and obesity (Campbell & Campbell, 2005).

Both oriental and occidental professional societies have now converged to a common understanding that many chronic problems can be avoided through practicing a total solution package, including nutritional balance, rhythmic lifestyle, duly exercise, and mental wellness.

With an increasing global penetration of mobile telephony and a mature ICT infrastructure, as illustrated in Fig. 16, a future SHIP must be built by integrating modern approaches, such as network technology, wearable/invisible sensory instrumentation, and data mining mathematics, with ancient wisdom from both oriental and occidental philosophy. An overall strategy and tactics for healthcare and allied applications can then be provided. Many new areas and industries, such as public transportation security, fire fighting and police, senior health insurance, professional athlete training, home-based care, and the tracking of the effects of pharmaceuticals will blossom.

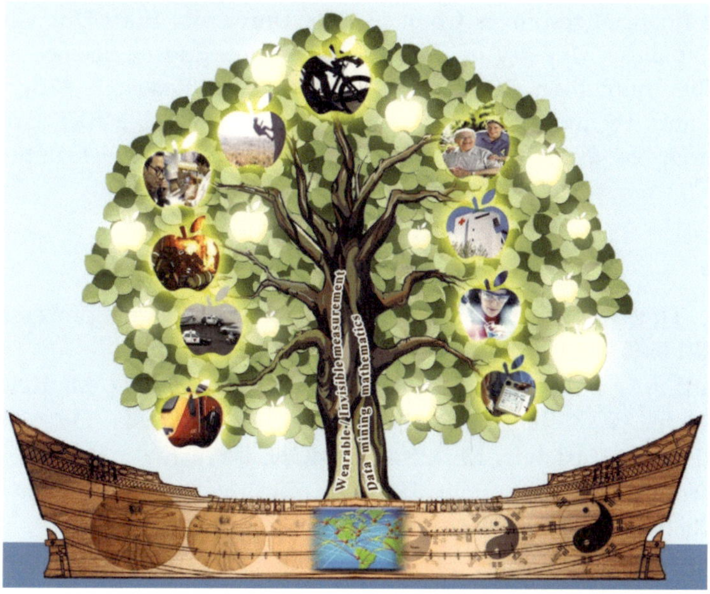

Fig. 16. Conceptual illustration of a future SHIP showing its constitutional fundamentals and application domains. This will be built by merging oriental holistic philosophy and occidental accurate treatment and the latest achievements in network technology, wearable/invisible measurements, and data mining mathematics. The SHIP will be applied in the chronic illness prevention domain, and also in a variety of applications, wherever vital signs are helpful.

4. Conclusions

In a series of R&D projects, our initiative endeavour was focused on SHIP architecture design and system integration. We have developed several sensory technologies for vital-sign monitoring in environments of everyday living, and data mining algorithms for the interpretation of comprehensive large-scale data. However, much new knowledge remains to be discovered from long-term data mining. The open architecture of SHIP makes it possible to integrate diversified vital signs and data mining algorithms, either from ours or from cooperative partners.

We also realize that radical societal change demands an active paradigm shift from acute disease treatment based in hospitals towards preventative care in lifelong activities, and in addition, individuals and also organizations and communities must be involved in daily efforts. We are optimistic in our belief that the global epidemic of chronic diseases can be relieved or controlled by using the latest research achievements, and by advocating healthy living behaviour, such as a positive attitude, sound nutritional balance, and regular physical exercise.

5. Acknowledgements

The authors thank all our colleagues and students from universities, academic institutions and companies for co-work in the above studies, and we thank participants for their enduring efforts in long-term data collection. The projects mentioned were supported in part by several financial resources from: (a) The University Start-Ups Creation Support System of the Japanese Ministry of Education, Culture, Sports, Science and Technology (MEXT); (b) The Innovation Technology Development Research Program under JST (Japan Science and Technology Agency) grant H17-0318; (c) MEXT Grants-In-Aid for Scientific Research No. 20500601; and (d) The University of Aizu Competitive Research Funding.

6. References

Akay, M. (1998). Time frequency and wavelets in biomedical signal processing. IEEE Press, 0-12-047145-0, New York.

Anliker, U.; Ward, J.A.; Lukowicz, P.; Troster, G.; Dolveck, F.; Baer, M.; Keita, F.; Schenker, E.B.; Catarsi, F.; Coluccini, L.; Belardinelli, A.; Shklarski, D.; Alon, M.; Hirt, E.; Schmid, R. & Vuskovic, M. (2004). AMON: a wearable multiparameter medical monitoring and alert system. IEEE Transactions on Information Technology in Biomedicine, Vol. 8, No. 4, pp. 415–427.

Campbell, T. C. & Campbell, T. M. (2005). The China Study, Benbella Books, 978–1932100389, Dallas, Texas, USA.

Chen, W.; Kitazawa, M. & Togawa, T. (2008a). HMM-based estimation of menstrual cycle from skin temperature during sleep. Proceedings of the 30th Annual International Conference of the IEEE Engineering in Medicine and Biology Society (EMBC'08), accepted, IEEE, Vancouver, Canada, August 20–24, 2008.

Chen, W.; Kobayashi, T.; Ichikawa, S.; Takeuchi, Y. & Togawa, T. (2000). Continuous estimation of systolic blood pressure using the pulse arrival time and intermittent calibration. Medical & Biological Engineering & Computing, Vol. 38, No. 5, pp. 569-574.

Chen, W.; Wei, D.; Cohen, M.; Ding, S.; Tokinoya, S. & Takeda, T. (2004). Development of a scalable healthcare monitoring platform. Proceedings of the Fourth International Conference on Computer and Information Technology (CIT'04), pp. 912-915, IEEE, 0-7695-2216-5, Wuhan, China, September 14 - 16, 2004.

Chen, W.; Zhu, X.; Nemoto, T.; Kanemitsu, Y.; Kitamura, K. & Yamakoshi, K. (2005). Unconstrained detection of respiration rhythm and pulse rate with one under-pillow sensor during sleep. Medical & Biological Engineering & Computing, Vol. 43, No. 2, pp. 306-312, 0140-0118.

Chen, W.; Zhu, X.; Nemoto, T.; Kitamura, K.; Sugitani K. & Wei, D. (2008b). Unconstrained monitoring of long-term heart and breath rates during sleep. Physiological Measurement, 29 N1-N10, 0967-3334.

Daubechies, I. (1992). Ten Lectures on Wavelets, SIAM, 0-89871-274-2, Philadelphia

Denso Wave Incorp. (2000). QR code, http://www.denso-wave.com/qrcode/aboutqr-e.html.

Dibazar, A.A.; Narayanan, S. & Berger, T.W. (2002). Feature Analysis for Automatic Detection of Pathological Speech. Proceedings of the Second Joint EMBS/BMES Conference, IEEE, Houston, TX, USA, pp. 182-183.

DoCoMo Corp., (2008). Wellness mobile phone. http://www.nttdocomo.co.jp/product/foma/706i/sh706iw/index.html

European Commission. MobiHealth project, http://www.mobihealth.org/

European Commission. AMON project, http://cordis.europa.eu/data/PROJ_FP5/ACTIONeqDndSESSIONeq112422005919ndDOCeq144ndTBLeqEN_PROJ.htm

France, J. & Kramer, S. (eds.) (2001). Communication and Mental Illness - Theoretical and Practical Approaches, Jessica Kingsley, 978-1853027321, London.

Fujii, M.; Dema, H. & Ueda, T. (2002). Liquid Jet Electrode and Surface Potential Detector, Japanese Patent No. JP2002-65625A, 5 March 2002.

Health Level Seven, Inc. (1997). Health Level Seven Standard, http://www.hl7.org/

Intel Corp., (2007). Yorkfield XE processor. http://en.wikipedia.org/wiki/Intel_Core_2#Yorkfield

Ishijima, M. (1993). Monitoring of electrocardiograms in bed without utilizing body surface electrodes. IEEE Trans. Biomed. Eng., Vol. 40, No. 6, pp. 593-594.

Japanese Ministry of Health, Labour and Welfare, Mortality change due to different disease over the past century in Japan. http://www.mhlw.go.jp/toukei/sippei/index.html

Japanese Ministry of Health, Labour and Welfare. (2002). Health promotion law. http://www.ron.gr.jp/law/law/kenko_zo.htm

Japan Health Promotion and Fitness Foundation. (2000). Healthy Japan 21. http://www.kenkounippon21.gr.jp

Japan Mibyou System Association. (2006). http://www.mibyou.gr.jp/

Kario, K.; Pickering, T.G.; Umeda, Y.; Hoshide, S.; Hoshide, Y.; Morinari, M.; Murata, M.; Kuroda, T.; Schwartz, J.E. & Shimada, K. (2003). Morning surge in blood pressure as a predictor of silent and clinical cerebrovascular disease in elderly hypertensives: a prospective study. Circulation, Vol. 18, pp. 1401-1406.

Kawarada, A.; Nambu, M.; Tamura, T.; Ishijima, M.; Yamakoshi, K. & Togawa, T. (2000). Fully automated monitoring system of health status in daily life, Proceedings of the 22nd Annual International Conference of the IEEE Engineering in Medicine and Biology Society, Vol. 1, pp. 531 - 533.

Kay Elemetrics Corp., (2004). Disordered Voice Database, Model 4337, Version 2.7.0 (CDROM). Lincoln Park, NJ.

Lim, Y.G.; Kim, K.K. & Park, K.S. (2006). ECG measurement on a chair without conductive contact, IEEE Trans. Biomed. Eng., Vol. 53, No. 5, pp. 956–959.

Malik, M. & Writing Committee of the Task Force of the European Society of Cardiology and the North American Society of Pacing and Electrophysiology. (1996). Guidelines, Heart rate variability, Standards of measurement, physiological interpretation, and clinical use. European Heart Journal, vol. 17, pp. 354–381.

Mallat, S. & Zhong, S. (1992). Characterization of signals from multi-scale edges. IEEE Trans. Pattern Anal. Mach. Intell., Vol. 14, No. 7, pp. 710–732.

Marculescu, D.; Marculescu, R.; Park, S. & Jayaraman, S. (2003). Ready to wear, Spectrum, IEEE, Vol. 40, No. 10, pp. 28–32.

MarketResearch.com. (2008). The Long-Term Care Market: Nursing Homes, Home Care, Hospice Care, and Assisted Living, Pub ID: KLI1729220, USA.

Mathieson, L. (2001). The Voice and Its Disorders, 6th edition. Wiley Blackwell, 978-1861561961, London and Philadelphia.

Microsoft Corp., (2008). HealthVault. http://www.healthvault.com/

Mizukami, H.; Togawa, T.; Toyoshima, T. & Ishijima, M. (1989). Management of pacemaker patients by bathtub ECG, Report of the Institute for Medical & Dental Engineering, Tokyo Medical and Dental University, 23, pp. 113–119.

Moghissi, K. S. (1980). Prediction and detection of ovulation. Fertility and Sterility, Vol. 32, pp. 89–98

Nishi-Aizu, (2003). Challenge to 100 Years of Age - The Making of a Healthy Village through a Total Care Solution, Zaikai21, 4-901554-07-7, Japan.

Nohzawa, T. (2003). Inventions of Computers - Engineering Trail, Techno Review Inc., 4-902403-00-5, Tokyo, Japan

NTT Data Corp., (2002). Health Data Bank. http://www.nttdata.co.jp/en/media/2002/080101.html

O'Shaughnessy, D. (1999). Speech Communications - Human and Machine, 2nd edition. Wiley-IEEE Press, 978-0780334496, New York.

Peng, C.; Xu, Q.; Wan, B. & Chen, W. (2007a). Pathological voice classification based on features dimension optimization, Transactions of Tianjin University, Vol. 13, No. 6, pp. 456–461.

Peng, C.; Yi, X.; Chen, W. & Wan, B. (2007b). Optimization and selection of feature parameters in dysphonia recognition. Chinese Journal of Biomedical Engineering, Vol. 26, No. 5, pp. 675–679, 1004–0552.

Philips Electronics. HeartCycle project. http://www.heartcycle.eu/

Philips Electronics. MyHeart project. http://www.research.philips.com /technologies/healthcare/homehc/heartcycle/myheart-gen.html

QOL Co. Ltd., (2008). Ran's Night. http://rans-night.jp/

Qu, L. (2007). Medical Classic of Emperor Huang - the Wisdom for Regimen, 1st edition. Lu Jiang Publisher, 978-7-80671-821-6, Xiamen, China.

Rabiner, L. R. (1989). A tutorial on hidden Markov models and selected applications in speech recognition. Proc. IEEE, Vol. 77, No. 2, pp. 257–286.

Rossi, D. D. (2008). Ready to wear: clothes that look hip and track your vital signs, too. http://www.wired.com/techbiz/startups/magazine/16-02/ps_smartclothes, Wired Magazine, Vol. 16, No. 2, p. 55.

Sharp Corp., (2008). Wellness mobile phone. http://plusd.itmedia.co.jp/mobile/articles/0805/27/news064.html

Shensa, M. (1992). The discrete wavelet transformation, wedding the à trous and the Mallat algorithm. IEEE Trans. Signal Processing, Vol. 40, No. 10, pp. 2464–2484.

Tamura, T.; Yoshimura, T.; Nakajima, K.; Miike, H. & Togawa, T. (1997). Unconstrained heart-rate monitoring during bathing. Biomedical Instrumentation & Technology, 31(4), pp. 391–396.

Togawa, T.; Tamura, T.; Zhou, J.; Mizukami, H. & Ishijima, M. (1989). Physiological monitoring systems attached to the bed and sanitary equipments. Proceedings of the Annual International Conference of the IEEE Engineering in Engineering in Medicine and Biology Society, Vol. 5, pp. 1461–1463

Umapathy, B.; Krishnan, S.; Parsa, V. & Jamieson, D.G. (2005). Discrimination of pathological voices using a time–frequency approach. IEEE Trans. Biomedical Engineering, Vol. 52, No. 3, pp. 421–430

WHO. (1948). Definition of Health, Official Records of the World Health Organization, No. 2, pp. 100.

WHO. (2002). A Long-Term Care Futures Tool-Kit, Pilot edition, 92–4–156233–1.

Wikipedia, (2008). Medical Classic of Emperor Huang. http://en.wikipedia.org/wiki/Huangdi_Neijing

Wisneski, L. A. & Anderson, L. (2005). The Scientific Basis of Integrative Medicine, CRC Press, 0-8493-2081-X, Florida, USA.

Zhang, B.; Kanno, T.; Chen, W.; Wu, G. & Wei, D. (2007). Walking stability by age - a feature analysis based on a fourteen-linkage model. Proc. of the 7th IEEE International Conference on Computer and Information Technology (CIT'07), 16-19 Oct. pp. 145-150

Zhang, Q.; Wang, P.; Li, J. & Gao, X. (2000). Diagnosis of diabetes by image detection of breath using gas-sensitive laps. Biosensors and Bioelectronics, Vol. 15, No. 5–6, pp. 249–256.

Zhu, X.; Chen, W.; Nemoto, T.; Kanemitsu, Y.; Kitamura, K.; Yamakoshi, K. & Wei, D. (2006). Real-time monitoring of respiration rhythm and pulse rate during sleep. IEEE Trans. Biomedical Engineering, Vol. 53, No. 12, pp. 2553–2563, 0018-9294.

12

A Mobile Device Based ECG Analysis System

Qiang Fang, Fahim Sufi and Irena Cosic
School of Electrical and Computer Engineering, RMIT University
Australia

1. Introduction

Coronary heart disease (CHD) such as ischemic heart disease is the most common cause of sudden death in many countries including USA and Australia (Roberts, 2006). Its main manifestations consist of Acute Myocardial Infarction (AMI, or heart attack) and angina. Stroke (or cerebrovascular disease) is Australia's second biggest killer after CHD as well as the leading cause of long term disability in adults (Access Economics Pty Limited, 2005). Heart failure and stroke cause a big burden on society due to their high costs of care, lower quality of life and premature death. Among Australians having a heart attack, about 25% die within an hour of their first-ever symptoms and over 40% will be dead within a year (Access Economics Pty Limited, 2005). So, for the 40% who would generally be dead in one year, prognostic telemonitoring can be a life saver.
More than half of the 8000 home care agencies in US are currently using some forms of telemonitoring (Roberts, 2006). Only in US, sales of services and devices associated with telemonitoring are projected to rise from $461 million in 2005 to over $2.5 billion in 2010 (Roberts, 2006). Comparing with monitoring at hospital premises, home based telemonitoring not only provides great financial advantage but also gives patients freedom of staying home and living a normal life with their family. Moreover, rural hospitals with limited healthcare resources also benefit from telemonitoring service if those hospitals are connected with major advanced hospitals in metropolitan areas. The Electrocardiograph (ECG) is the electric signal generated by the heart activities. ECG is of significant diagnostic value to various cardiovascular and cerebrovascular diseases. ECG signal is one vital physiological signal that telemonitoirng systems normally pay attention.
A typical telemonitoring system includes medical signal or image acquisition, data storing, data analysis, and data transmission subsystems. Some advanced systems even incorporate data mining and knowledge management techniques. Thus a telemonitoring system needs to have sufficient data processing power and processing speed to handle the required high computation overhead.
With the recent advance in IC design, the computing power and the memory size of mobile device have increased considerably. This development makes many mobile devices, even some low end mobile phone handsets, capable of carrying out complex computing tasks. Especially after the recent release of iPhone and the powerful mobile programming platforms such as J2ME from Sun Microsystems™, Android from Google™ (code.google.com/android/), a mobile phone handset based telemonitoring solution has become possible (Roberts, 2006).

In this chapter, we propose an electrocardiogram signal monitoring and analysis system utilizing the computation power of mobile devices. This system has good extensibility and can easily incorporate other physiological signals to suit various teleehalth scenarios. The system can be carried by both users, e.g., chronic patient, and the service providers, e.g., the medical doctors. Java™ based software running on the mobile phones performs computation intensive tasks like raw ECG data compression and decompression, encryption and detection of pathological patterns. The system can automatically alert medical service providers through Short Message Service (SMS) and Multimedia Message Service (MMS), when medical assistance is deemed crucial for the user based on the analysis results. Furthermore, in order to ensure the data interoperability and support further data mining and data semantics, a new XML schema is designed specifically for ECG data exchange and storage on mobile devices. This XML schema is named mECGML. The ECG data in mECGML format is tested in this application as a pilot study.
The rest of the paper is organized as follows. In the next section, the system architecture of the mobile phone based ECG analysis system is given. Section 3 presents a new XML schema specifically designed for ECG data storing and processing on mobile devices. In Section 4, the implementation of ECG R-R peak detection algorithms is described. Section 5 discusses the ECG signal visualization and transmission on mobile phone handset. The last section is a discussion on future work and conclusion.

2. System architecture and programming environment

2.1 J2ME

The core communication of the ECG monitoring system is done through the mobiles carried by both user and telemonitoring service provider. As our telemonitoring system targets on plain mobile phone handsets rather than iPhone or other high end handsets, the popular Nokia91 is chosen for this development. Most recent mobile phones support execution of miniature programs that utilize the mobile processing power. Java 2 Micro Edition (J2ME), .Net Compact Framework, Binary Runtime Environment for Wireless (BREW), Carbide C/C++ are some of the programming environments for mobile phone application development. J2ME is basically a subset of the Java platform designed to provide Java APIs for applications on tiny, small and resource-constrained devices such as cell phones, PDAs and set-top boxes. Among these languages J2ME is pervasively used, since the compact Java runtime environment, Kilobyte Virtual Machine (KVM), has been supported by a wide range of mobile phone handsets already. One major advantage of choosing Java is that a single program written in J2ME can be executed on a variety of mobile phones that support Java. Apart from the basic computation framework provided by KVM, each of the mobile phone also supports additional Java libraries for supporting additional functionalities such as Bluetooth connectivity, camera functionality and messaging services, etc. These additional libraries expose Application Programming Interfaces (APIs) to the programmer of the handset. J2ME architecture is composed of configuration and profile. Connected Limited Device Configuration (CLDC) defines the minimal functionalities required for a range of wireless mobile devices, e.g., mobile phone, PDA, Pocket PC, home appliances etc. Mobile Information Device Profile (MIDP) further focuses on a specific type of device like mobile phone or pager. MIDP also describes the minimum hardware or software requirement for a mobile phone. To the mobile application developer, both CLDC and MIDP expose Application Programming Interfaces (APIs) and functionalities supported by the KVM.

Since the computational powers of the mobile phone handsets are expanding rapidly, current mobile phones possess considerable computation powers which can perform runtime complex tasks such as 3D games, MP3 and MPEG encoding and decoding. Even, Optical Character Recognition (OCR) software was tested on current mobile phones (Graham-Rowe, 2004). It is feasible to utilize the processors inside the mobile phone to process, compress, and transmit data in realtime for various telehealth applications. The realtime availability is of great importance for the sake of life saving. In principle, by careful design or selection of the proper computational algorithms, many complicated medical data processing and analysis tasks such as compression, decompression, encryption, correlation and transformation, feature extraction, and pattern recognition, can be implemented. However, the mobile phone platform supporting Java™ language is subject to some software and hardware specific limitations. Unlike a Java runtime for PC, the KVM on mobile devices is a miniature version that can only run a subset Java APIs. Compared with a desktop PC, mobile phones based CLDC and MIDP restrict the usage of floating point operations, which means all the floating point must be removed before performing any operations on the mobile devices. Multi dimensional arrays are not supported as well; hence, any algorithm performing matrix based calculation needs to find an alternative approach. Luckily, those difficulties have been all successfully solved by sophisticated program skills employed in this project.

2.2 System block diagram

The architecture of our system is illustrated in Fig. 1. The mobile phone is the core part of this ECG telemonitoring system. The system is composed of total five subsystems, namely the patient's unit, the doctor's unit, the telephony network, the web based database system, and the server-side deployed intelligent analysis engine.

2.3 Sub-systems

Patient's Unit

This unit connects the biological acquisition device with the patient's mobile unit. Our own developed biosignal acquisition device with ECG, Oximetry, skin impedance and blood pressure sensors connects to the MIDlet software running on the patient's mobile via Bluetooth streaming. For the Bluetooth connectivity, JSR-82 (JSRS: Jave Service Request, 2008) specification was used. Third party Bluetooth enabled ECG monitoring device such as Alive Heart Monitor (www.alivetec.com) also can be used by this system.

Recently, a very new wireless interconnection technology, Near Field Communication (NFC) is being researched and on its way to be commercialized (NFC Forum web site, 2008). Study shows that the new generation NFC-Enabled phone will be widely available within next four years (Near Field Communications, 2008). Like Bluetooth, NFC based communication can easily be implemented to the proposed system, since the support for NFC with J2ME is already in progress through JSR-257 (JSRs: Java Service Requests, 2008). Third party sensors can also be supported for serving specialized purposes. Even sensors embedded with future generation mobile can be efficiently used through JSR-256 (JSRs: Java Service Requests, 2008).

Doctor's Unit

This unit is the specialized MIDlet software running on doctor's mobile handset. It serves the medical service provider's request of patient information as well as provides doctor with

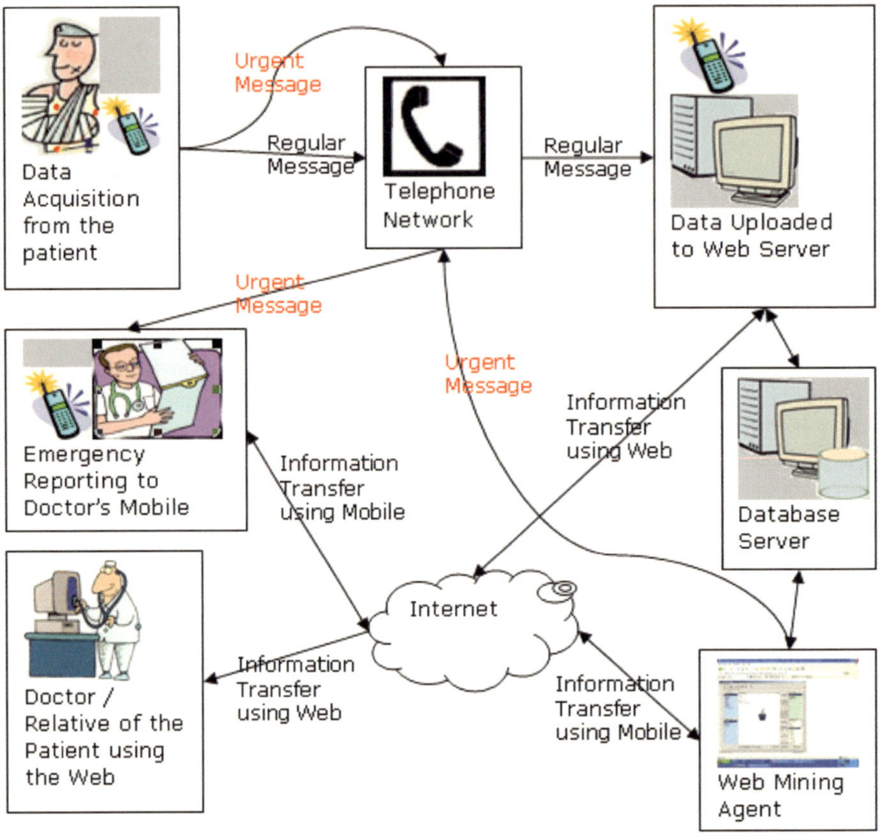

Fig. 1. System architecture of a mobile phone based ECG analysis system

the transmitted medical information and notifies the doctor in case of an emergency situation, where medical help is required the most. Custom reporting, charting and analysis of patient's condition for the selected period can be performed by the doctor's unit.

Web Server and Database

This unit provides restricted information to the authorized medical personnel or even relatives in case of elderly monitoring. All the biological signals from the patent's unit are stored here permanently. For implementation purposes we have chosen SQL Server 2000, a relational database, because of its support of data mining techniques (like, Clustering, Decision tree etc.) with Online Analytical Processing (OLAP) module. Intelligent Analysis Engine A web mining agent has been implemented. This agent is responsible for providing requested information to the doctor's mobile. Since our system is designed as a generic system it supports all the phones supporting Java™. Again, each phone (doctor's unit) is different in their display size, supported colors or even some operations. Web mining agent automatically analyses these information and presents formatted information to the doctor's mobile suitable for proper display. Moreover, web mining agent performs background data mining operations to analyze the stored information of patient. A feature database for various arrhythmia patterns has been created. The agent will perform a feature matching operation for any incoming ECG recording and make classification. If it discovers some pattern demanding urgent diagnosis, it can inform the doctor via SMS on a timely way.

3. Mobile ECG data exchange standard

Extensible Markup Language (XML), a semi-structured data format, has been widely used for various data processing tasks such as text based data permanent storage, data exchange, and Web service. In order to enhance the data processing capability of conventional mobile devices for the sake of extensibility and interoperability, the adoption of XML is inevitable. Currently, there is no XML standard specifically designed for mobile devices from World Wide Web Consortium (W3C). The standard XML specification for ECG such as HL7's aECG and DICOM waveformat is too complicated and unnecessary to be fully implemented on mobile computing platforms. As a pilot study, we propose here a light-weighted XML Schema, named as mECGML, to facilitate the manipulation of ECG Data on mobile devices. There are a few XML parsers have been developed under J2ME environment (Knudsen, 2002). Among them, KXML 2.2 is chosen for its simplicity of use and compact size (only 9 K).

3.1 Existing ECG file formats

There are many proprietary ECG data formats designed by different vendors for different applications. For example, PhysioNet uses a plain human readable text format containing signal, header, and annotation three components for physiological data including ECG. The PhysioNet format is not designed for machine operation. HL7 aECG is an annotated ECG format developed by HL7 Consortium. Its XML Schema is quite complicated. The ECG recording encoded in this format is a verbose file. SCP-ECG developed by European Union, is now approved as an international standard by ISO. SCP-ECG is not based on XML. It generates binary ECG files which are not human readable. Furthermore, DICOM, a standard for medical images, also proposed an auxiliary waveformat to integrate diagnostic ECG recordings. The DICOM waveforamt isn't based on XML either.

In many cases, the mobile devices are used for data transferring purpose rather than a data analysis platform. However, with the increasing power of the mobile devices, they can be further exploited to deal with complicated data processing tasks with sophisticated compact algorithms and proper programming skills. It is even possible to be used for data mining tasks. XML has been widely accepted as a standard for data exchange, storing and manipulation in a variety of application domains. Nevertheless, the use of XML in mobile devices is still limited due to aforementioned many computational constraints. Bearing this in mind, our newley designed light-weighted mECGML can be parsed by small or "tiny" XML parsers, such as KXML, in J2ME environment. The mECGML is designed to keep the essential information of the measured ECG data and has the capaibility to optionally keep pre-identified features for later intelligent data handling, such as data mining.

3.2 The hierarchical representation of mECGML and the mECGML schema

The design aim of mECGML is to provide an open standard for the storage, exchange and integration of ECG data among different mobile devices and other involved devices, e.g., acquisition devices, in an ambulatory monitoring applications. Normally, a remote or ambulatory monitoring system is an integrative system hence many incoming data are heterogeneous in nature. Table 1 shows the hierarchical representation of mECGML.

Element/ Attribute	Description	Required/ Optional	Data type	Example
mECG	Root element	Required	Element	
RecordTime	The time when the contained ECG data was recorded; the sampling rate and the recording duration are given here as well	Required	Element	<RecordTime> <SamplingRate> 350 </SamplingRate> <StartingTime> 2002-05-30T09:00:00 </StartingTime> <Duration> PT160S </Duration> </RecordTime>
RecordingDeviceDetail	The description of the recording device	Required	Element	<RecordingDeviceDetail SerialNo=”168312”> <DeviceManufacturer model=”MAC501”>GE </DeviceManufacturer> <CalibrationTime> 2008-06-30T10:00:00 </CalibrationTime> <Location> 10.7.18 </Location> </RecordingDeviceDetail>
PatientDetail	The description of patient	Required	Element	<PatientDetail FirstName=”John” LastName=”Smith” PatientID=”453212” />
RecorderDetail	The description of the acquisition unit operator	Required	Element	<RecorderDetail FirstName=”John” LastName=”Smith” EmploymentID=”44326” />
EcgData	The recorded raw data; up to 12 leads ECG data can be stored	Required	Element	
Feature	The pre-identified feature; the popular features including QRS complex, P wave, ST segment, T wave, etc.	Optional	Element	
Annotation	The annotation made by cardiologist	Optional	Element	

Table 1. Description of mECG element based on the hierarchical representation

The detailed mECGML Schema (partial) is listed in Figure 2.

```
  <?xml version="1.0" encoding="UTF-8" ?>
- <xs:schema xmlns:xs="http://www.w3.org/2001/XMLSchema">
  - <xs:element name="mECG">
    - <xs:complexType>
      - <xs:sequence>
        + <xs:element name="RecordTime">
        + <xs:element name="RecordingDeviceDetail">
        - <xs:element name="PatientDetail">
            <xs:attribute name="FirstName" type="xs:string" />
            <xs:attribute name="LastName" type="xs:string" />
            <xs:attribute name="PatientID" type="xs:string" />
          </xs:element>
        + <xs:element name="RecorderDetail">
        + <xs:element name="RecordMethod">
        - <xs:element name="ECGData" maxOccurs="12" minOccurs="1">
          - <xs:complexType>
            - <xs:sequence>
                <xs:element name="EncryptionType" type="xs:string" />
                <xs:element name="CompressionType" type="xs:string" />
                <xs:element name="LeadNo" type="xs:string" />
                <xs:element name="RawData" type="xs:hexBinary" />
              </xs:sequence>
              <xs:attribute name="Size" />
            </xs:complexType>
          </xs:element>
        - <xs:element name="Feature" type="xs:string" minOccurs="0">
            <xs:attributes name="type" type="xs:string" />
            <xs:attributes name="LeadNo" type="xs:string" />
          </xs:element>
          <xs:element name="Annotation" type="xs:string" />
        </xs:sequence>
        <xs:attribute name="recordId" />
      </xs:complexType>
    </xs:element>
  </xs:schema>
```

Fig. 2. The XML Schema of mECGML

4. Wireless ECG transmission

Mobile devices are predominantly used as a means of wireless transmission of signals (Jamemin et al, 2005). Earlier researchers used WAP gateways to transmit still images to the mobile phones (Zhao et al 2005). Since image files are generally larger than the text file files, WAP based technologies incur high usage of network bandwidth and slow transmission speed. We demonstrate here the possibility to transmit and receive biosignals in short text based messages and large binary files such as compressed ECG recordings via SMS and MMS using J2ME respectively. Graphical representation and image processing tasks can be performed by these J2ME miniature programs as well.

4.1 SMS and MMS

SMS is predominantly used to send short text only messages containing a maximum of 160 characters. SMS supports two operations, Message Originating (MO) and Message Terminated (MT). MO is for sending SMS and MT is for receiving SMS. Once an SMS is sent from a mobile phone, the message arrives at Short Message Service Center (SMSC). SMSC generally follows Store & Forward rule, which means message is stored inside SMSC until it reaches the recipient. Hence, an SMSC constantly tries to transmit the SMS until it is received by the recipient. Some SMSCs are guided by Forward & Forget rule which means after sending the SMS, the SMSC deletes the message from the server. Therefore receipt of the SMS is never guaranteed. Both text and binary data of limited length can be transmitted by SMS.

MMS utilizes the concept of other messaging services like SMS, Mobile Instant Messaging and Mobile E-Mail. Once a sender sends an MMS message, the receiver is notified via an SMS, followed by establishment of a WAP connection to download the MMS message. Unlike SMS, MMS provides support for transmission of text, audio, video and image files. A typical MMS file has a MMS header and MMS body. MMS body contains one or more Mulitpart Messages. Each of those Multipart Messages is composed of their own header and body. MMS supports emailing the message to multiple recipients (to, cc, bcc). The crucial benefit of MMS over SMS is the message length. But some of the telecommunication service providers impose a limitation in file size to reduce their network congestion. Mobile handsets also have regulated file size restrictions. It is possible to transmit larger files through MMS with minimal restrictions, e.g., each of the message part containing texts should be less than 30 Kb.

4.2 System design and implementation

To serve our purpose of automated sending and receiving of biosignals through SMS and MMS, we used JSR-205 library, which was included with our Mobile Phone Platform (Nokia N91). JSR-205 (Wireless Messaging API 2.0) is the update of JSR-120 (Wireless Messaging API 1.1). JSR-120 only supports CBS/SMS with text or binary input. But JSR-205 enhanced its support to Multipart MMS Messages. For drawing curves and graphic display on Mobile handset screen, the J2ME Graphic Library was utilised.

In a practical remote monitoring scenario, the patient is connected with an ECG monitor as well as devices for other physiological signals such as blood pressure, pulse and SpO2. The acquisition system transmits data to the patient's mobile phone via Bluetooth Connectivity. Different types of third party physiological acquisition systems with different data output formats can be used. The Mobile phone parses those input data in proprietary format and wraps the ECG data together with metadata into mECGML format. The generated mECGXML file is further compressed to reduce the transmission overhead. Then the mobile handset sends SMS and MMS packets, which will be forwarded to the SMS Center (SMSC) and MMS Center (MMSC). From SMSC and MMSC the biosignals (Blood pressure, Pulse & ECG) will disembark at the doctor's mobile phone. As soon as the SMS/MMS packets reach the doctor's mobile phone, the Java software installed in the doctor's mobile phone decompresses and parses the ECG recording, followed by the creation of graphs, curves and other signal processing tasks. Fig. 3 illustrates the whole telemonitoring scenario. For our experiments we developed a pair of J2ME based Java software (Called MIDlet), which were running in both patient's & doctor's mobile phone.

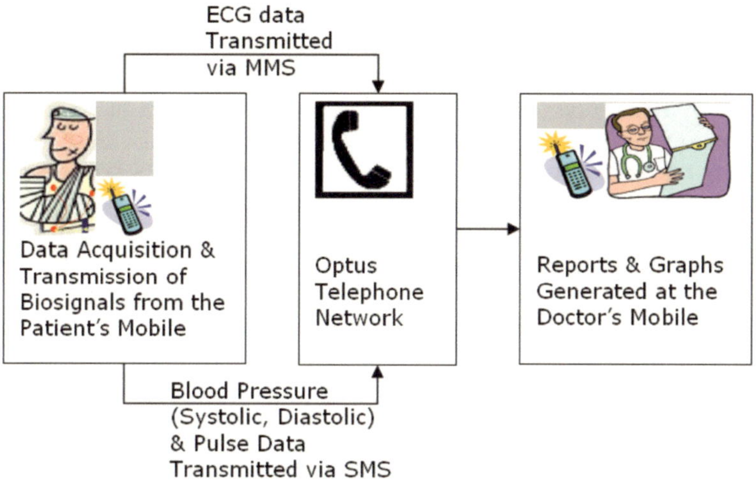

Fig. 3. Biosignal transmission via SMS and MMS

4.3 Patient's mobile phone

The MIDlet for patient's mobile phone is responsible for sending blood pressure and pulse data via SMS and compressed ECG data via MMS. SMS packets were created using the format presented in Fig. 4. as comma separated values. Because of the SMS length restriction only 15 hourly data could be accommodated using this format. For each hour Systolic Blood Pressure (SBP), Diastolic Blood Pressure (DBP) and Pulse (P) were sent via SMS. In the trial experiment, Siemens C75 hand set was utilised as the patients' handset to send SMS to the Doctors Mobile phone.

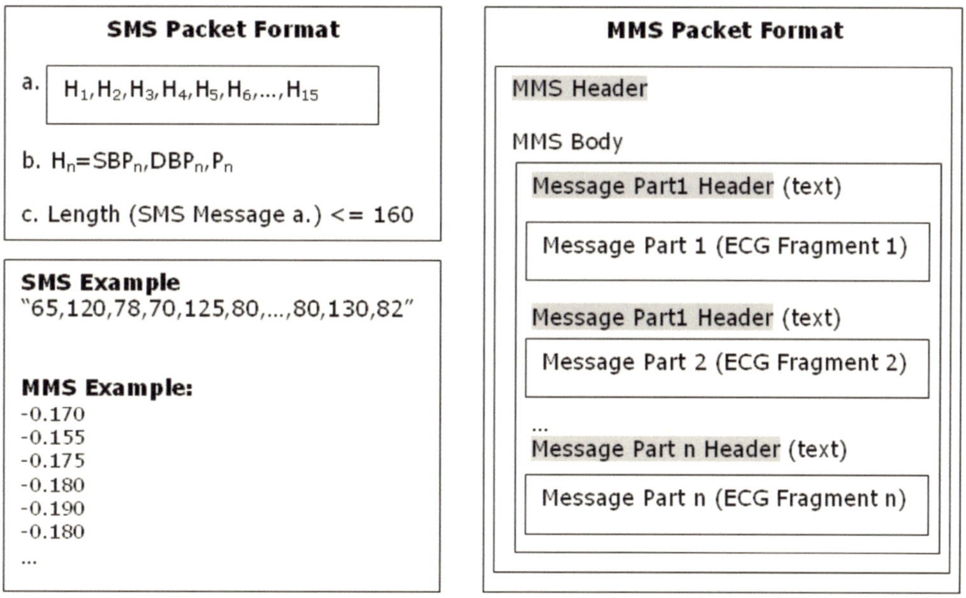

Fig. 4. SMS and MMS Packets (H= Hourly Data, SBP = Systolic Blood Pressure, DBP=Diastolic Blood Pressure, P= Pulse)

Meanwhile, for ECG data via MMS, it is possible to send files in bigger size, since our mobile phone supports up to 330 Kb of MMS data and the telephony network (Optus, Australia) doesn't impose any file size restriction. However, from our development platform (NetBeans IDE 5.5) a size restriction of 30k was imposed for each of the Message Part (for text data). Hence, to accommodate 1 minute data, which was about 157 K, we created 6 Message Parts by the segmentation of the ECG file. Following this procedure each of the 6 ECG segments became 10 second long ECG message part (text). Nokia N91 handset was used to send MMS message, since it supports JSR 205. Siemens C75 couldn't be exploited for sending MMS because of its lack of support for JSR 205 (it only supports JSR120).

4.4 Doctor's mobile phone

In the doctor's mobile phone, listeners were installed for listening to both SMS and MMS messages. To distinguish between messages sent from the patient and normal messages (sent from family, friends or colleagues) specific ports (for SMS) and Application ID (for MMS) was exploited. Hence, the patient's handset needs to send SMS and MMS messages to those predefined ports and application IDs. If messages without specifying any ports are sent from the patient's mobile, the server connection of the doctor's mobile phone would not be able to process those messages, instead, the mobile's own message handler (Inbox) will receive those messages. Port 5000 was used for sending and receiving of SMSs and Application ID com.ecg.mms was used for sending and receiving MMSs.

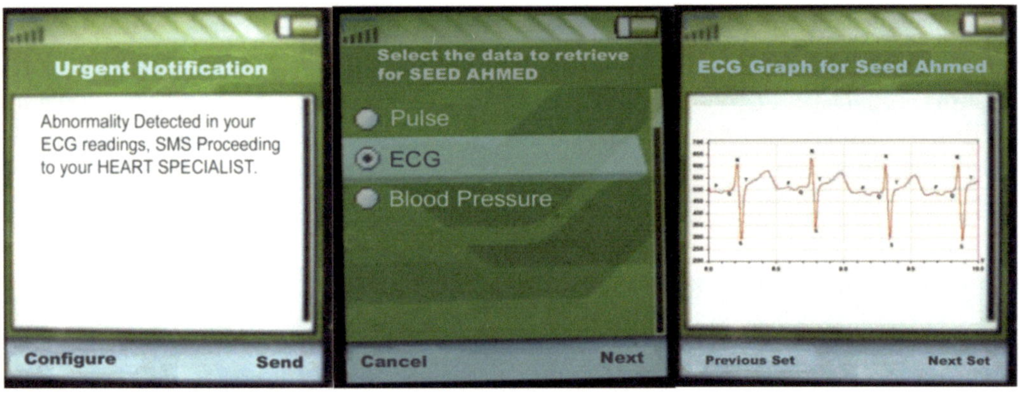

Fig. 5. Screen shot of the User Interface of Doctor's mobile

Once the messages containing biosignals are received and identified by the doctors mobile phone, Canvas class of J2ME is instanced and graphics are drawn on the doctor's mobile phone in realtime. Before the actual drawing of the curves and graphs, the text based SMS and MMS messages are transformed to multiple integer values. From those integer values appropriate coordinate system is generated, since mobile phone's origin of coordinate is located at the upper left corner of the screen. Therefore, generating curves and graphs of biosignals needs proper calculation and translation before drawing then on to the mobile phone's screen. Fig. 5. is the screenshot taken from a doctor's handset which shows the end result of menu and graphing.

4.5 Results

We successfully demonstrated that biosignal transmission via SMS and MMS using J2ME is a realistic solution. Mobile software can be programmed to automate the process of biosignal collection, noise identification, noise reduction, message packet creation and message transmission. On the other hand, realtime generation of curves and visual displays provide assistance for prompt medical decision. During our experimentation, we generated 12 SMSs and 9 MMSs. SMS Messages sent by the sender were always received by the receiver within one minute (12 out of 12 times). However, for only 2 cases of MMS messages, more than 1 minute time was consumed by the network operator. This result implies the fact that for monitoring less serious patient's, SMS and MMS transmission can be adopted, since these messaging techniques do not assure timely and dependable delivery.

5. ECG R-R peak detection

5.1 R-R peak and HVR

Electrocardiogram or ECG is the record containing electrical activities of the heart. ECG is widely used to diagnose different heart abnormalities. Different patterns of a normal ECG graph are denoted by P, Q, R, S and T. Detection of ECG RR interval and QRS complex from the recorded ECG signal is crucial for a sustainable health monitoring scenario, since a wide range of heart diseases like tachycardia, bradycardia, arrhythmia, palpitations etc. can be efficiently diagnosed utilizing the resultant RR interval. Many different RR interval calculation algorithms have been proposed. We selected a few preferred algorithms, which were previously executed only on PC environment for realtime RR detection, and deployed them in mobile phones to ascertain their suitability and performances. The experiment results suggest that mobile phones do possess the computation power to detect the RR peak in realtime. By knowing the RR peak, it is easy to further calculate the Heart Rate Variability (HRV). HRV is the rhythmic alteration in heart rate. Although there have been many researches conducted on HRV, the understanding of HRV is still not completed. It is generally accepted that HRV is an important index for heart condition in two aspects: the high frequency part (0.18-0.4Hz) is correspondent to respiration and the low frequency part (0.04-0.15 Hz) is related to vagus and cardiac sympathetic nerves. The fact that HRV is of great prediction value to heart attack survivors has been evidenced by a reported correlation between reduced HRV and the patient death []. There are many different approaches to assess the HRV. The tachogram is used in this study.

Fig. 6 shows an abnormal ECG recording representing the first 899 samples (2.5 seconds) of entry 232 of MIT-BIH arrhythmia database (MIT-BIH Arrhythmia Database, 2007). 12 ECG entries each with 60 seconds measurement from MIT-BIH arrhythmia database were used for our experimentation. MIT-BIH database has been extensively used in literature for performance monitoring and comparison of different algorithms that perform ECG signal processing (Friesen, 1990). In this research three fundamental QRS and RR interval detection algorithms namely Amplitude Based, First Derivative Based and Secondary Derivative Based techniques, have been chosen as a pilot study to implement ECG R-R peak detection on mobile phone.

5.2 Amplitude Based Technique (ABT)

The Amplitude based technique (ABT) performs very simple comparison where the ranges of sample ECG points falling beyond an amplitude threshold are determined to be a QRS complex candidate. For Fig. 6, the amplitude threshold can be 0.2. After the QRS complex is detected, the highest amplitude of the detected QRS is ascertained to be R peak. Equation (1)-(4) generalizes the amplitude based method. The original ECG signal, x_n, from the patient body is given by (1).

$$\mathbf{x}_n = x_1, x_2, ..., x_N \tag{1}$$

where, $n = 1, 2, ..., N$ and N is the length of the signal.

$$(x_r, x_{r+1}, x_{r+2}, ..., x_{r+k}), ..., (x_l, x_{l+1}, x_{l+2}, ..., x_{N-c}) > amplitude\,threshold \tag{2}$$

where, $1<r<l<N$, x_{N-c} is the last value greater than the threshold and both x r+k+1 and x nc+1 are less than the amplitude threshold.

Each of the section enclosed by the parenthesis of (2) (left side of the equation) is QRS complex candidate.

$$R\ peak = Max(QRS\ Complex) \tag{3}$$

$$RR\ Interval = \frac{n_r}{f} \tag{4}$$

where, n_r is the number of samples between two corresponding R peaks and f is the sampling frequency of the ECG.

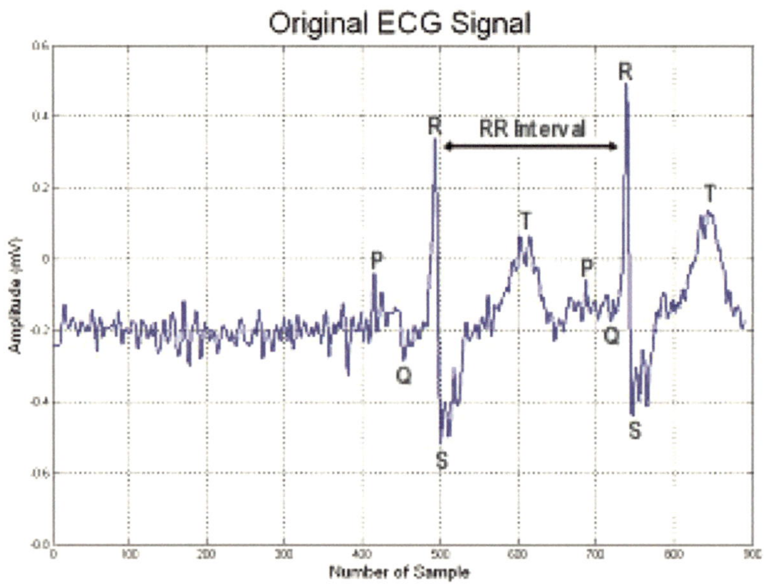

Fig. 6. An original abnormal ECG sginal

5.3 First Derivative Based Technique (FDBT)

This method is also called Hamilton-Tompkins method. The QRS detection is achieved by performing first derivatives of the ECG samples. This is because the QRS complex generally

has the steepest slope and has the maximal magnitude as well. RR interval can be measured by several first derivatives based QRS detection techniques described in the literature (Mahoudeaux, 1981; Menrad et al., 1981; Hosinger et al, 1971) followed by the application of (3)-(4).
To measure the performance of FDBTs in mobile phone platform, slightly modified version of [4] was adopted. The first derivative, y n was calculated at each sample point of x_n such that

$$y_d = x_{n+1} - x_{n-1} \qquad (5)$$

where, $d = 1, 3, \dots, N\text{-}1$
A QRS complex is detected whenever three consecutive first derivative values are greater than a positive slope threshold, followed within next ten samples by two consecutive first derivative values less than a negative slope threshold. Equation (6)-(8) describes the process

$$y_i, y_{i+1}, y_{i+2} > 0.1375 \qquad (6)$$

$$y_j, y_{j+1} < -0.2 \qquad (7)$$

$$j - \mathrm{i} < 10 \qquad (8)$$

After the detection of the QRS complex Eq. (3-4) is used to derive the RR interval.

5.4 Second Derivative Based Technique (SDBT)

Previous research reveals several second derivative based QRS detection algorithms [8, 9]. For performance comparison, a modified version of [8] was used. At first, Eq. (9-10) was used to evaluate the absolute values of first (y^0) and second (y^1) derivative.

$$y0_d = ABS\,(x_{n+1} - x_{n-1}) \qquad (9)$$

$$y1_s = ABS(y0_{n+2} - 2 * y0_n + y0_{n-2}) \qquad (10)$$

where, $s = 1, 2, 3\dots, N\text{-}3$
A scaling value, $y2$ is obtained from Eq. (11).

$$y1_s = ABS(y0_{n+2} - 2 * y0_n + y0_{n-2}) \qquad (11)$$

For all values exceeding a threshold, are determined to be the start of a QRS candidate (Eq. (12)).

$$y2_d \geqslant 0.9 \qquad (12)$$

Values from x_{d-3} to x_{d+3} is passed to Eq. (3) as the QRS Complex to compute R peak and finally Eq. (4) is used to calculate the RR interval. After locating a single R peak the next seven $y2_d$ values are ignored, since most of time there are few $y2_d$ values greater than the threshold surrounding a single R peak.

5.5 Algorithm implementation and results

Since, plain mobile phones are constrained with various hardware and software limitations and capable of executing only 3000 to 10000 operations per second, selection of RR detection algorithms was focused mainly on lower complexity level in this study. Three different RR detection algorithms representing three pioneering classifications namely amplitude based, first derivative based and second derivative based RR detection algorithms, were selected for running inside the mobile phones. The RR detection algorithms were then programmed for Java based mobile phones. Sun Java Wireless Toolkit 2.5 was used for programming MIDlets in regular mobile phones. Performances were compared for three different mobile phones (Nokia 91, Nokia 6280 and Siemens C75) using 12 randomly selected ECG entries from MIT-BIH Arrhythmia database. These three models are all popular and regular mobile phones within middle price range.

The ECG entries of MIT-BIH were kept inside the mobile phones during the testing and performance monitoring of the RR detection algorithms. Therefore, during that period Bluetooth was not used for sending ECG to the mobile phone from the acquisition device.

The ECG signal has single channel, 11 bit resolution with 360 Hz sampling frequency and yields a step size of 5 RV. They contained 60 seconds ECG signal meaning each of the selected MIT-BIH entries had total 21600 (360*60) samples.

Table 2 demonstrates the processing time requirement for different RR detection algorithms using different randomly selected ECG files on three different mobile phones. A realtime factor, Rf was calculated using (13).

MIT BIH Entry	Nokia N91			Siemens C75			Nokia 6280		
	ABT (ms)	FDBT (ms)	SDBT (ms)	ABT (ms)	FDBT (ms)	SDBT (ms)	ABT (ms)	FDBT (ms)	SDBT (ms)
100	6	8	8	5	6	6	1	1	2
102	6	7	7	5	6	6	1	1	1
105	6	6	8	5	5	6	1	1	1
114	6	7	7	5	6	6	1	1	1
117	7	8	7	6	6	6	1	1	1
201	6	7	7	4	5	5	1	1	1
213	7	7	8	4	5	6	1	1	1
219	6	7	7	4	6	6	1	1	1
222	6	7	7	5	5	6	1	1	1
228	7	7	8	6	6	6	1	1	1
231	6	7	7	5	6	6	1	1	1
234	7	7	7	5	5	6	1	1	1

Table 2. Performance Comparison of The RR Interval Algorithms Among 3 different Mobile Phone Handsets.

$$R_f = \frac{P_t}{Measurement \quad window} \tag{13}$$

where, Pt is the processing time needed to run the RR detection algorithm for an individual ECG entry within one measurement window and the window is 60 seconds in this study. Pt is measured by time stamps embedded in the beginning and the ending of the implementation codes. Whenever (14) is true, the algorithm is classified as realtime for mobile phone based processing.

$$R_f \langle\langle 1 \tag{14}$$

Equation (14) basically exemplifies the simple fact that to operate the algorithm in realtime, the processing time required to process 1 seconds ECG data must be much less than 1 second.
By using Eq. 14, the realtime factor can be calculated for all three RR detection algorithms implemented on three different mobile devices. It is shown that the value of Rf ranged from 1.6x10-5 to 13.3x10-5 which are much less than 1 during the entire experimentation process. Therefore, for all the mobile phones tested, realtime operations were achieved based on the criteria set in this study and Nokia 6280 was found to consume the least processing time. Though the data acquisition time isn't taken into account in this detection program, it will unlikely affect the experiment result due to multi-thread supporting of J2ME. The research of realtime RR peak detection on mobile phone is the foundation step for the future research of mobile phone based abnormality monitoring and identification from realtime acquired ECG recordings. Mobile phones based RR detection is certainly a cheaper solution since expensive PCs are not required for data processing tasks anymore. In addition, a mobile phone based system provides a true ambulatory and wireless connectivity for the patient and other needed user groups. The monitoring and pre-analysis results can be easily transmitted to remote locations using 3G, GPRS, SMS, CBS, MMS, Email, HTTP etc. or even it can be simply displayed on the mobile phone screen.

6. Conclusion and future work

We propose in this chapter a mobile phone based intelligent ECG telemonitoring system with good extensibility. The vital ECG signal can be acquired, analyzed locally, transmitted, and analyzed remotely in a quasi-realtime sense. The computation power of mobile handset is extensively harnessed to identify major ECG morphological abnormalities and activate the early warning mechanism via both SMS and MMS. We also designed a light weighted ECG data format, mECGML, to facilitate the seamless data integration within the system. The ECG data is also stored natively in this format in the server side.
The proposed system makes it easy to change the functionalities or telemonitoring applications, just by updating the program by Over-the-Air (OTA) deployment (Yuan 2004) of MIDlets to the mobile. So, the system can be adopted for different application with minimal effort. Most of all, J2ME based system reveals standard and different third party APIs for performing complex computations like, compression, encryption, steaming

multimedia for the service of telehealth within the mobile phone. The proposed platform provides flexibility in terms of wireless communication, from the ECG signal acquisition device to mobile through Bluetooth and from the patient to service provider communication via 2.5 G or 3 G network.
The proposed system enables the doctor to receive/analyse the patient report and also, deliver doctor's treatment and specialist advice to remote patient. The doctor doesn't need to be sitting in front of a stationary computer within the medical facility. The proposed system uses smart client technology instead of thin client technology used by some WAP based system (Hung & Zhang, 2003). So, it can use the network bandwidth much more efficiently. Moreover, it doesn't need any physical wired internet connection like some systems (Chen 2004; Jin-gang et al, 2005; Braecklein et al, 2005; Hung & Zhang, 2003; Shieh et al, 2005; Glaros et al, 2003), making the proposed system a true wireless solution. In addition, it doesn't have any restricted coverage area. It is accessible within the global mobile coverage area. The sending of physical parameters from the acquisition device is automated by the MIDlet running in patient's mobile, making the whole system less error prone compared to some existing system (Zhou et al, 2005). Finally the proposed system is based on generic mobile phone (costing 100s of dollars) supporting Java KVM, instead of expensive Pocket PC, Smart phone or iPhone (1000s of dollars) based solution. According to some recent studies (Baker 2006), cost of home monitoring unit is needed to be drop below 1000 USD to overcome the limited usage of telemonitoring devices. In this respect, cost effectiveness is another crucial advantage that the proposed system provides.
During our experimentation we used both SMS and MMS for transmission of medical information in both text format and binary format. At this stage, only compression ECG data is wrapped into MMS format, in the future, we will try on the transmission of different medical images files such as CT, MRI, X-ray and ultrasound images, using MMS on mobile. The implementation of DICOM standard will also be test on mobile device.
As a summary, the presented ECG telemonitoring system is a cost effective, flexible and robust solution supporting a unique mobile based computational platform where compression, detection and even encryption are some of the possibilities.

7. References

Access Economics Pty Limited (2005) The shifting burden of cardiovascular disease in Australia, A report of Heart foundation. [Online]. Available: www.heartfoundation.com.au/ media/nhfa_shifting_burden_cvd_0505.pdf

Baker, M.L. (2006) Study: Medicare, Insurers Reluctant to Pay for Telehealth. [Online]. Available: http://www.eprescribingnews.com/archives/2006/04/study_medicare.html

Braecklein, M. et al (2005). Wireless Telecardiological Monitoring System for the Homecare Area, *Proceedings of the 27th Annual Conference of IEEE Engineering in Medicine and Biology*, September 2005

Chen, Y. Y. et al (2004). Development of wireless blood glucose meter and diabetes selfmanagement system, Proceedings of the 26th Annual International Conference of the IEEE EMBS, September 2004, pp. 3384-3386

Friesen, G. et al (1990). A Comparison of the Noise Sensitivity of Nine QRS Detection Algorithms. *IEEE Transactions on Biomedical Engineering*, Vol. 37, No. 1, pp. 85-98

Glaros, C. et al (2003). A wearable intelligent system for monitoring health condition and rehabilitation of running athletes, *Proceedings of 4th IEEE Conf. on Information Technology Applications in Biomedicine*, pp. 276-279, 2003

Graham-Rowe, D. (2004). Camera phones will be high-precision scanners, NewScientist.com news service. [Online]. Available: http://www.newscientist.com/article.ns?id=dn7998

Hosinger, W.P. et al.(1971). A QRS pre-processor based on digital differentiation. *IEEE Trans. Biomed. Eng.* Vol. 8, pp. 212-217, 1971

Hung, K. and Zhang, Y. T. (2003). Implementation of a WAP-based telemedicine system for patient monitoring. *IEEE Transactions on Information Technology in Biomedicine*, Vol. 7, No. 2, pp. 101- 107

Knudsen, J. (2002). Parsing XML in J2ME. [Online]. Available: http://developers.sun.com/mobility/midp/articles/parsingxml/

Jin-gang, W. et al (2005). Remote Heart Sound Monitoring System, *Proceedings of the 27th Annual Conference of IEEE Engineering in Medicine and Biology*, September 2005

JSRs: Java Service Requests (2008). Java Community Press Web Site. [Online]. Available: http://www.jcp.org/en/jsr/overview

Mahoudeaux, M. (1981). Simple microprocessor based system for online ECG analysis, *Med. Biol.Eng. Comput.*, Vol 19, pp. 497-500

Menrad, A. et al. (1981). Dual microprocessor system for cardiovascular data acquisition, processing and recording, Proc, 1981 *IEEE Int. Conf. Industrial Elect. Contr. Instrument*, pp. 64-69

MIT-BIH Arrhythmia Database (2007). [Online]. Available: http://www.physionet.org/cgibin/ rdsamp

Near Field Communications (NFC) (2008). Simplifying and Expanding Contactless Commerce, Connectivity, and Content. ABI Research, Oyster Bay, NY, 4Q2005

NFC Forum web site (2008). [Online]. Available: http://www.nfc-forum.org/

Roberts, R. (2006). Use of Remote Monitoring Devices Increases, Telemedicine Information Exchange, (Original Source: Wall Street Journal, April 18, 2006). [Online]. Available: http://tie.telemed.org/legal/news.asp

Shieh, J. S. et al (2005). Web-Based Remote Monitoring Health of the elderly via mobility changes using frequency and rank order statistics, *Proceeding of the IASTED International Conference of Telehealth*, July 2005

Yuan, M. J. (2004). Enterprise J2ME: developing mobile Java, Upper Saddle River, NJ: Prentice Hall PTR, c2004

Zhao, E. and Cui, L. (2005). EasiMed: A remote health care solution, *Proceedings of the 27th Annual Conference of IEEE Engineering in Medicine and Biology*, September 2005

Zhou, H. et al (2005). A Real-Time Continuous Cardiac Arrhythmias Detection System: RECAD, Proceedings of the 27th Annual Conference of IEEE Engineering in Medicine and Biology, September 2005

Data Mining in Biological Research

13

A New Definition and Look at DNA Motif

Ashkan Sami[1,2] and Ryoichi Nagatomi[2]
[1]*Department of Computer Science and Engineering; Shiraz University; Shiraz 71348;*
[2]*Graduate School of Biomedical Engineering; Tohoku University; Sendai 980-8575;*
[1]*Iran*
[2]*Japan*

1. Introduction

Genetics is the main source of life. The more insights added to the knowledge of genetics, the more accurate prediction and even diagnosis of diseases may become. In genetics, a **sequence motif** is a nucleotide or amino-acid sequence pattern that is widespread and has, or is conjectured to have, a biological significance. Sequence motifs are short, recurring patterns in DNA that are presumed to have a biological function. Often they indicate sequence-specific binding sites for proteins such as nucleases and transcription factors (TF). Others are involved in important processes at the RNA level, including ribosome binding, mRNA processing (splicing, editing, polyadenylation) and transcription termination.

In this study we first concentrate on promoter motifs; however the discussions can easily be extended to other type of sequences. Promoter is a fragment of DNA sequence that is responsible for the transcription from DNA to RNA. Through the study on promoter, it can be found out which DNA sequence will be transcribed into RNA, and even transcription of any DNA sequence which is intended to study into RNA. In bacteria, the target sequence for RNA polymerase attachment is called the promoter. However, in eukaryotes, the term 'promoter' is used to describe all the sequences that are important in initiation of transcription of a gene.

Although no clear definition of motif exist (Pisanti et al., 2005), some define motifs based on statistical representations in the form of PSSM (Position Specific Scoring Matrix) (Gribskov et al., 1987; Hertz & Stormo, 1996; Lawrence & Reilly, 1990; Lawrence et al., 1993). Another school of thought defines a motif as a consensus (Brazma et al., 1998; Vanet et al., 1999). A motif is therefore a pattern that appears repeatedly in a sequence or set of sequences of interest.

The sequences that make up the E-coli promoter were first identified by comparing the regions upstream of over 100 genes. It was assumed that promoter sequences would be very similar for all genes and so should be recognizable when the upstream regions are compared. These analyses showed that the E. coli promoter consists of two motifs described as -10 box - TATA-box or 5'-TATAAT-3'and -35 box - TTG-Box or 5'-TTGACA-3' (Brown, 2002).

Most of the patterns known to biologist are contingent. In other words, nucleotides that these motifs have are located in consecutive positions. These patterns give more insight to understanding of DNA.

In this chapter, a need to a new definition for motif will be provided due to two kind of mentality. First of all by use of a very standard dataset and known concept of independence in statistics, it will be shown why TTG, a very well-known pattern in promoter, is not actually a "valuable pattern". This illustration leads us to a new direction of defining what actually a motif or pattern is in a DNA sequence like promoter. A measure to find significance based on shape distribution for two-item and multi-item patterns are presented. Later on limitation of the motif evaluation measure to patterns that lead to classification capabilities will be presented. The chapter concludes with summary and future research.

2. Why TTG is not a valuable pattern

Before entering the technical details of the chapter some very simple definitions just to avoid further confusions will be provided.

Frequency: The number of sequences having a specific pattern or property divided by number of all the sequences. Support and frequency are used interchangeably and have the same meaning in this chapter. 'F' is used as symbol for frequency. Its subscript presents the type or item. As an example, F_A means frequency of item A and F_{Exc} means 'excess' frequency (explained later in this chapter).

Position: position is presented by letter 'p' and afterwards an integer follows. The number represents the position with respect to a specific place. Positive integers present the position after the specific place and negative numbers present number of nucleotides prior. For example, in case of the promoters p-36 means the 36th nucleotide prior to Transcriptional Start Site. When p-36 = T is stated, it means at the mentioned position a Thymine exists.

E. coli promoter sequences in UC Irvine – Machine Learning Repository (UC-Irwin MLR) are used. The reason to use the dataset was familiarity of data mining community with the data and ease of access. There are 106 instances of 57 sequential DNA nucleotides (strings consisting of Adenine, Guanine, Cytosine and Thymine) that half of them are sample promoter sequences and the rest are non-promoter sequences. The range of a promoter sequence is starting at p-50 and ending at p7 relative to the Transcriptional Start Site (TSS). It is important to note that position zero does not exist. In other words, the position after position p-1 is p1.

Based on the definition of -35 box motif it is a six nucleotide motif TTGACA. An exact match for the pattern may not exist at position -35 of TSS. However here it will be shown that even for highly observed TTG pattern the pattern is not a valuable pattern. In other words, it is not TTG pattern that presents functionality.

By observing the promoter sequences of the dataset, we will notice that TTG pattern at position -35 occurs with %49.1 frequency. A closer look, although painstaking, reveals patterns with their respected frequencies at Table 1.

Calculation of the previous frequencies by simply counting the occurrence is very difficult. One of the methods to calculate the frequencies of different patterns in data is to convert a sequence to a graph and use of graph-data mining algorithms (Matsuda, et al., 2002). Matsuda et al. use BGI which is a greedy algorithm. Due to its greedy nature some of the pattern may be missed. Use of complete graph data mining algorithms (Yan & Han, 2002; Kuramochi & Karypis, 2001) solves the problem. However, due to NP-completeness of graph-isomorphism checking, the computational complexities of complete graph data mining algorithm are high. In the following section, a much simpler method of finding and calculating the patterns will be presented.

2.1 A simple method of finding patterns and their frequencies

A very simple and effective method of finding all the patterns and their corresponding support in DNA sequences is to use FAF (Sami, 2006; Sami & Takahashi, 2005a). FAF (Finding All Features) uses a special mapping that allows regular Frequent Itemset Mining or Apriori type algorithm (Hipp et al., 2000) be applied to Genetic sequences.

Position -36	*Position -35*	*Position -34*	*Frequency*
T			%81.1
	T		%81.1
T	T		%66.0
		G	%79.2
	T	G	%64.2
T		G	%60.4
T	T	G	%49.1

Table 1. The frequency of patterns in the promoter sequence

Mapping or pre-processing is one of the main issues that can be treated based on number of main factors. The main purpose of mapping is to come up with a number for each nucleotide in the record that can uniquely represent all the information regarding that main factors of the sequence. The FAF mapping is performed in 5 stages. However before the definition of the mapping, some formal definitions are presented.

A gene in the data set is a sequence R_m, an ordered collection of nucleotides and is represented as $R_m=\{x_1, x_2, \dots ,x_q\}$, where indexes are arranged with regarding to a specific position like transcriptional start site. The alphabet Alpha={A, C, G, T} is used for symbols (x). Each sequence in the data set can be treated as a string. The index of x is of high importance. Records have a class label C is also fixed and known in advance. The class labels are $C = \{C_1, C_2, \dots ,C_t\}$. $|C|$ presents the cardinality of set C. Even though here treated cases had $|C|$ equal to two, the formula is given for generalization purposes. Patterns like $P_i = \{p_1,p_2, \dots ,p_n\}$ are desired, where each p_i represents a specific alphabet and i is the index of x that belongs to a unique C_k within the same sequences with a frequency above a given threshold. Now the mapping is as follows:

1. First $|R|$, $|Alpha|$ and $|C|$ should be considered. In other words, to decide a mapping first the number of outcomes, types, positions, and etc must be calculated.
2. Secondly for $|R|$, $|Alpha|$ and $|C|$, k's should be obtained through calculations
   - $k_R = 10^n$ such that $10^{n-1} \leq |R| < 10^n$
   - $k_A = 10^m$ such that $10^{m-1} \leq |Alpha| < 10^m$
   - $k_C = 10^p$ such that $10^{p-1} \leq |C| < 10^p$
3. After calculating the k's, the results based on k_i and $|i|$ where i can be R, A or C must be sorted. As an example, we assume that $k_R > k_A = k_C$,and $|R| > |Alpha| > |C|$ regardless of the fact that the change in order can be easily generalized.
4. Now each value of records, x_i being a_j and belonging to C_t class the mapping is calculated based on Equation 1.

$$p_i = i + j * k_R + t * k_A * k_R \tag{1}$$

5. For each record in the database a unique number will be assigned that can be its order in the database.

The mapping should be done in a sense that each mapped member represents the type, position and class of the nucleotide in the sequence.

2.2 Observation of patterns based on process-oriented mentality

Meaningful patterns should present a combination that the combination by itself presents a functionality or identification. To present the mentality a process-oriented methodology is deployed. Considering occurrence of each nucleotide at specific position as a process, significance of co-occurrence of more than one nucleotide simultaneously at different positions will be will be judged based on the notion of independence. In other words, when two processes are independent of each other, their co-occurrence does not show any specific property.

Co-occurrence of p-36=T and p-35=T is not valuable. Based on Table 1, 66% of sequences have p-36=T and p-35=T, so why is this pattern not valuable or significant? At p-36 and p-35 more than 81% of all sequences have T. The occurrence of each T is completely independent of the other. In more details, two processes a and b are independent if p(ab)=p(a)p(b), where p(a) is the probability of occurrence of a. In case of p-36=T or p-35=T taking frequency directly as probability, it can be seen that 0.81*0.81=0.658 which is almost equal to 0.66. Stated differently, even though 66% of the sequences have T at position p-35 and p-36, considering process oriented mentality reveals that this is not a valuable pattern because the co-occurrence of two T's is independent of each other.

Other combinations of two nucleotides like TG at position -35 and -34 lead to same results (0.811*0.792=0.642). The conclusion can be drawn that no two-nucleotide pattern in TTG is a pattern but is occurring statistically due to high frequency of each of its components..

Since each single two-nucleotide motifs are just statistically occurring patterns due to high frequency of T or G, the discussion can further be extended to conclude that TTG is not a pattern by itself but a pattern due to high frequency of each single nucleotide. In other words, the high frequency of T at position -36 and -35 and G at position -34 lead to the observed co-occurrence of TTG. Having T alone at positions -36 or -35 or G at position -34 is a better indicator of a promoter.

It was shown by use of statistical concept of independence TTG (regardless of its high frequency) is not a significant or valuable pattern. There are several other statistical measures to present interestingness. For a review of the measures refer to (McGarry, 2005; Geng and Hamilton, 2006). Some researchers (Ohsaki et al., 2007) showed that these measures can fairly represent expert needs in a specific domain. It can be shown that deployment of some other measures will also lead to insignificance of TTG.

Next section will discuss another model of finding patterns that can be considered motifs. The main mentality of the new measure basically is based on ideas presented in (Sami, 2006). The measure uses the ranges of values that pattern may have and defines significance and value based on how close the actual value is compare to highest and lowest probable frequencies. By this view, it is the shape of distribution that presents knowledge not purely statistical parameters. In other words, instead of the statistical concepts shape distribution is used.

3. The need for evaluation measure of motifs

In the previous section use of process oriented observation of the frequencies of co-occurrence lead to show that TTG is not an actual pattern. Here a method to evaluate valuableness of the motif with the same mentality but different view is presented.

Basic mentality of the proposed method is based on the idea that the patterns that their support or frequency is comparable to support of single constituents are interesting. In other words, the frequency of each itemset should not be explainable based on the distribution of frequencies of the two categories that constitute the itemset. As an example: if A and B are two items where: F_A=30%, F_B=35% and F_{AB}=25%

Pattern AB is interesting, since 25% distribution is not explainable based on 30 and 35% (support of A and B). Illustration of frequent pattern evaluation measure is shown in Figure 1 (Good Example) and Figure 2 presents a pattern which is not a valuable pattern.

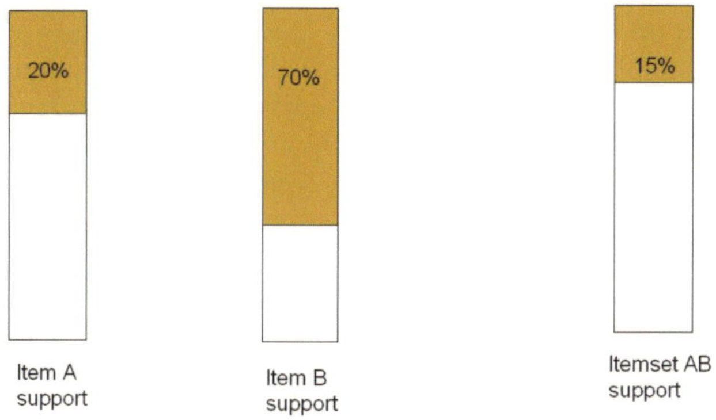

Fig. 1. Illustration of frequent itemset which is valuable

Figure 1 presents a valuable pattern since the frequency of the pattern AB is comparable to the frequency of the lowest frequent item of the pattern. In other words, it could have been possible to have item B's distributed in a sequences that no occurrence of AB existed. However, 15% of 20% of item A co-occur with item B which makes a valuable pattern. In contrast in Figure 2, item B is highly frequent and due to high frequency of item B it is impossible to have items A and B occur together less than 15%.

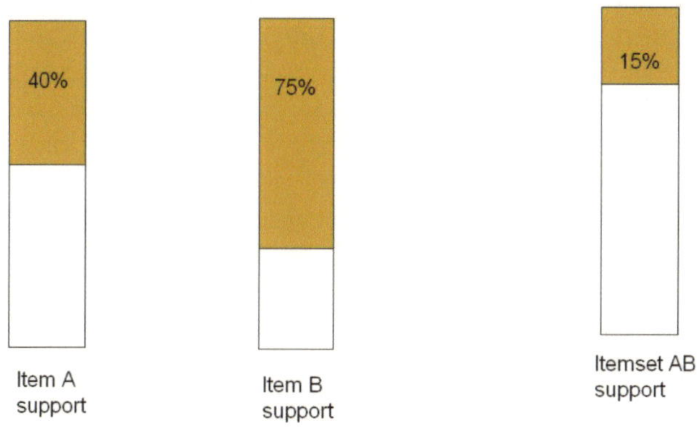

Fig 2. Illustration of frequent pattern which is not significant

In the following section evaluation measure for two-item patterns will be presented.

4. Evaluation measure for two-item patterns

As illustrated in section 3 of this chapter, lowest frequency of occurance of A or B should be comparable to frequency of sequences containing AB. The closer the frequency of sequences

containing AB to the minimum frequency of sequences having A or B, the more valuable the pattern.
In case of having two items their frequencies summation can be more than unit, below than one or exactly one. With respect to this summation, a two-item pattern that frequencies of its items add up to be more 100% is defined as having excess frequency. In contrast, two-item itemsets that the summation of frequencies of each item add up to less than one will be defined as a pattern without excess frequency. If the frequencies of the two constituantes of two-item pattern add up to one, the case can be categorized as either of the two. To deeply understand the derivation of the measure based on shape distribution the cases of having excess frequency and not having an excess frequency will be treated separately.

4.1 Evaluation measure for two-item patterns with excess frequency

As a definition for itemset AB, excess frequency exists if summation of frequencies of A and B exceeds 100%. Now a detail discussion on how to reach the measure is presented by an example. Considering the pattern presented in Figure 2, frequency of A is 40% and B is 75%. Since $F_A+F_B = 0.4+0.75 = 1.15$ (the summation of the frequencies exceeds 100%), excess frequency exists. The excess frequency is equal to 15%. Due to having excess frequency, at least 15% of the sequences will have pattern AB. It is impossible to have a sequence that has only A or B exclusively. At least 15% of the sequences have AB in their sequences. Stated differently, regardless of shape of distribution of A and B among sequences at least 15% overlap exists. Therefore 15% support is least significant value for the itemset.
In contrast, the pattern is most prominent if AB occurs with its highest possible frequency or near the minimum frequency of its constituants. Since minimum of the frequency of A and B is 40%, pattern AB would have been most meaningful if AB had occured with 40%. It is obvious that frequencies more than 40% is not possible. This is a knowm property in KDD community and was first introduced by Agrawal and Srikant (Agrawal and Srikant, 1994) as "downward closure property".
Due to downward closure property of co-occuring patterns, maximum frequency would be equal to the lowest frequency of the two items. Minimum of each item in the itemset frequencies is the frequency of A which is 40%. In other words, the maximum frequency of sequences that have both A and B cannot be more than 40%. The closer the F_{AB} to 40%, the more significant the pattern.
Since the relationship is based on shape of distribution of A and B, a linear form can be considered suitable. The evaluation measure would rank pattern with frequency of excess as not significant and with frequency of lowest frequency of the two items as the most valuable. Zero presents not valuable and one most valuable. So by a linear relationship the degree of significance in the relationship is assessed.
More specifically, if the excess frequency is presented as F_{Exc}, minimum of frequencies of A and B is presented as F_{Max}, ($F_{Max} = \min(F_A, F_B)$). Minimum of the frequencies is called max frequency since this is the highest possible value for AB support. The probable values of frequency of itemset AB may start from minimum value of F_{Exc} and reaches the maximum of F_{Max}. Therefore interestingness or significance of two-item pattern of AB based on shape distribution is the position of the actual frequency of AB on a simple line connecting (0, F_{Exc}) to (1, F_{Max}) or:

$$S = (F_{AB} - F_{Exc}) / (F_{Max} - F_{Exc}) \qquad (2)$$

where F_{AB} is the actual value of support of AB.
Following the example, S=0 for 15% frequency for AB pattern
As another example, if F_A=50% and F_B=60% and F_{AB}=30%, it is clear 10% excess frequency exists. Thus,
S=(30-10)/(50-10) = 0.5, which makes sense since 30% is in the middle of F_{Max} and F_{Exc}

4.2 Evaluation measure for two-item patterns without excess frequency

In case of frequencies of items of an itemset that do not add up to more than 100%, the maximum will not differ. In other words, in a two-item itemsets the highest frequency will be equal to the frequency of the lowest frequent item, F_{Max}. However the minimum is definately equal to zero.
To develop the measure consider two cases. In case I, F_A = 30% and F_B = 32%. In case II F_A is the same as case I but F_B = 60%. In either case the frequeny of itemset AB ranges from zero to 40%. However it does make sense to consider pattern F_{AB} = 20% in case I more valuable than case II. In other words, higher frequncy of B in case II increases the likelihood of having sequences with AB occuring in them. Therefore a hypothetical chance of having negative frequency to compensate for the effect is considered. Negative frequency is the value need to make the summation of frequencies equal to one or 100%.

$$F_{Neg} = 1 - (F_A + F_B) \tag{3}$$

As an illustration, in case I from the previous paragraphs, F_{Neg} = 100-(30+32) = 38% and in case II, F_{Neg} = 100-(30+60) = 10%. Again a linear relationship is considered between the amount of negative frequency and maximum as significance for negative frequency equal to zero and maximum frequency as one. Significance is defined as the value of F_{AB} on the line connecting (0, F_{Neg}) to (1, F_{Max}). Thus,

$$S = (F_{AB} + F_{Neg}) / (F_{Max} + F_{Neg}) \tag{4}$$

Going back to the case I and II of previouse paragraphs,
Significance for case I: S = (20+38)/(30+38) = 0.853. Where significance for case II: S = (20+10)/(30+10) = 0.75. These numbers somehow present the fact that regardless of same motif frequency the pattern is more valuable in case I than case II.
Close observation of measures derived in section 4 reveals that we can use Equation 3 instead of Equation 4 if F_{Neg} was actually a negative number. Therefore, only one equation exists for two-item patterns.

5. Evaluation measure for patterns having more than two items

Again the mentality behind the measure is same as before. Significance is measured with respect of how unlikely it is to have the pattern. The lower the chance of having the pattern, the higher the significance.
Due to downward closure property, maximum value for frequency of pattern with several constituents is equal to the lowest frequency among all the items. It is intuitive to consider concept of F_{Neg} one more time. F_{Neg} presents the freedom of choices that may lead to no pattern. The same type of concept is extended to consider multiple factors involving a multi-item pattern, F_{NegMul}. Definitely the value that F_{Neg} type of parameter has should increase in magnitude as the number of items increases.

Let's start with an example, assuming A has frequency of 30%, B 40% and C 50%. How can a value be given to the significance of frequency of pattern ABC?
The maximum possible frequency would be the lowest frequency of the items. Thus, F_{Max} = 30%. What number should be assigned to present the lower possibility of having ABC?
First defining $F_{\sim A}$ as the frequency of sequences not having A. If BC occurs in ~A sequences, no ABC pattern would exist. Thus negate of a pattern provides a constraint on construction of the pattern. Obviously the greater the $F_{\sim A}$, the less likely existence of ABC. On the same token, ABC is more valuable when F_A, F_B and F_C are all small. So, ~A, ~B and ~C are profound factors. To present significance value as a linear relationship as before, the lower bound must be calculated in a way that increase of number of items departs it further away from F_{Max}. A simple extension of negative frequency would be based on linear assumption of increasing chance that is presented as follows; if F_{Xi} presents the frequency of x_i, where x_i is *i*-th item of an n-item pattern (*i*=1,…,n) and

$$F_{x_k} = \min\left(F_{x_1},\ldots,F_{x_n}\right) \quad (5)$$

$$F_{NegMul} = \sum_{i=1\&i\neq k}^{n} F_{\sim x_i} - F_{x_k} = \sum_{i=1}^{n} F_{\sim x_i} - 100 \quad (6)$$

Then the significance based on linear relationship would be evaluated based on where pattern frequency on the line of connecting (F_{NegMul},0) and (F_{Max}, 1) lies or:

$$S = (F_{Pattern} + F_{NegMul}) / (F_{Max} + F_{NegMul}) \quad (7)$$

Going back to our example, instead of x_i's, A, B, and C exist.

$$\begin{aligned} F_{NegMul} &= \sum_{i=1}^{n} F_{\sim x_i} - 100 \\ &= (100-30)+(100-40)+(100-50)-100 = 80 \end{aligned} \quad (8)$$

In case of TTG box;

F_{NegMul} = (100-81.1)+(100-81.1)-79.2 = -41.4
S= (49.1-41.4) / (79.2-41.4) = 0.20

Thus, TTG pattern is not significant even based on a more relax measure of shape distribution in comparison to regular independence in statistics.

6. Motif based on functionality

It is important to note that all that has been said was with respect to a specific sequence namely promoter in E. Coli. The purpose of viewing the motif in other situations can lead to different definitions. In other words, the distinction between sequences was not considered. All the evaluation measures discussed so far are not suitable for classification purposes. Viewing motifs with classification capabilities may lead to different motifs. This issue has been addressed to some extend by some researchers in graph data mining community (Geamsakul et al., 2003a and 2003b). As stated before graph data mining algorithms are either greedy and fast or complete and very slow. Another approach to motif discovery with classification capability is based on the mapping of FAF discussed (Sami & Takahashi, 2005b).

7. Conclusions and future research

In this chapter a close look at genetic motifs especially TTG-box or -35 box was provided. Based on statistical measure of independence it was shown that TTG box is not actually a significant pattern. Based on statistical notion of independence, it was shown that in TTG if occurrence of each nucleotide is considered as a process are completely independent of each other. Afterwards, another view that focused on shape distribution was deployed. Again after developing the model and measure, it was shown that the TTG pattern is not valuable. Even though TTG has near 50% support; it has a low frequency with respect to its constituents' frequencies.

In addition to use of bigger datasets, this research can be extended in two major ways. As suggested in the chapter, deployment of other interestingness measures to reach the same results or similar is one direction. Secondly, devising non-linear measures of significance based on shape distributions that form in high dimensional space of multi-item patterns.

8. References

Agrawal, R. and Srikant, R. (1994). Fast algorithms for mining association rules. In Proc. of *the 20th Int'l Conf. on Very Large Databases (VLDB' 94),* Santiago, Chile.

Brazma, A.; Jonassen, I.; Eidhammer, I. and Gilbert, D. (1998). "Approaches to the Automatic Discovery of Patterns in Biosequences," *Journal of Computational Biology,* vol. 5, pp. 279-305, 1998.

Brwon, T.A., (2006). *Genomes.* Garland Science, Taylor & Francis Group, May 2006, ISBN: 9780815341383

Geamsakul, W.; Matsuda, T.; Yoshida, T.; Motoda, H. and Washio. T. (2003a). Classifier construction by graph-based induction for graph-structured data. *In PAKDD'03: Proc. of 7th Pacific-Asia Conference on Knowledge Discovery and Data Mining,* LNAI2637, pp. 52--62.

Geamsakul, W.; Matsuda, T.; Yoshida, T.; Motoda H. and Washio, T. (2003b). Constructing a Decision Tree for Graph Structured Data, *Proc. of First International Workshop on Mining Graphs, Trees and Sequences (MGTS-2003), 14th European Conference on Machine Learning (ECML'03) and 7th European Conference on Principles and Practice of Knowledge Discovery in Databases (PKDD'03),* pp.1–10.

Geng, L. and Hamilton, H.J. (2006). Interestingness measures for data mining—a survey, *ACM Comput Surveys,* Vol. 38, No. 3, pp. 1-32.

Gribskov, M., McLachlan, A. and Eisenberg, D., (1987). Profile Analysis: Detection of Distantly Related Proteins, *Proc. Nat'l Academy of Sciences,* vol. 84, no. 13, pp. 4355-4358.

Hertz, G.Z. and Stormo, G.D. (1996). "Escherichia Coli Promoter Sequences: Analysis and Prediction," *Methods in Enzymology,* vol. 273, pp. 30-42.

Hipp, J.; Güntzer, U. and Nakhaeizadeh, G. (2000). Algorithms for Association Rule Mining A General Survey and Comparison, *SIGKDD Explorations,* vol. 2, no. 1, July 2000, pp. 58-64.

Kuramochi, M. and Karypis, G. (2001). Frequent Subgraph Discovery, *Proceedings of the 2001 IEEE International Conference on Data Mining,* November 29-December 02, 2001, pp. 313-320.

Lawrence, C.E.; Altschul, S.F.; Boguski, M.S.; Liu, J.S.; Neuwald, A.F. and Wooton, J.C. (1993). "Detecting Subtle Sequence Signals: A Gibbs Sampling Strategy for Multiple Alignment," *Science*, vol. 262, pp. 208-214, 1993.

Lawrence C.E. and Reilly A.A., (1990). "An Expectation Maximization (EM) Algorithm for the Identification and Characterization of Common Sites in Unaligned Biopolymer Sequences," *Proteins: Structure, Function, and Genetics*, vol. 7, pp. 41-51, 1990.

McGarry, K. (2005). A survey of interestingness measures for knowledge discovery, *The Knowledge Engineering Review*, Vol. 20 No. 1, March 2005, pp.39-61.

Matsuda, T. Motoda, H. and Washio. T. (2002). Graph-based induction and its applications. *Advanced Engineering Informatics*, Vol. 16 No. 2, pp:135–143, 2002.

Ohsaki, M., Abe, H., Yokoi, H., Tsumoto, S., Yamaguchi, T. (2007). Evaluation of rule interestingness measures in medical knowledge discovery in databases. *Artificial Intelligence in Medicine*, Vol. 41, No. 3, pp. 177–196.

Pisanti, N.; Crochemore, M.; Grossi, R. and Sagot, M.F. (2005). Bases of Motifs for Generating Repeated Patterns with Wild Cards. *IEEE/ACM Transaction on Computational Biology and Bioinformatics*, Vol. 2, No. 1, JANUARY-MARCH 2005

Sami, A. (2006). *Knowledge Discovery in Biomedical Sciences Based on Shape Distribution Methods*. Ph.D. Thesis; August 2006; Tohoku University; Sendai, Japan.

Sami, A. and Takahashi, M. (2005a). "FAF: Finding All Features Relating to Different Gene Sequences" *Workshop on Knowledge Discovery and Data Management in Biomedical Sciences, (KDDMBS 2005) in conjunction with PAKDD*, pp. 4-13; 18 May 2005; Hanoi, Vietnam.

Sami, A. and Takahashi, M. (2005b). Decision Tree Construction for Genetic Applications based on Association Rules, *IEEE TENCON 2005*, Melbourne, Australia, November 2005, pp.21-25.

UC-Irwin MLR., University of California at Irwin – Machine Learning Repository; http://www.ics.uci.edu/~mlearn/MLRepository.html, Last visited March 2006.

Vanet, A.; Marsan, L. and Sagot, M.F. (1999). "Promoter Sequences and Algorithmical Methods for Identifying Them," *Research in Microbiology*, vol. 150, pp. 779-799, 1999.

Yan X. and Han, J. (2002). "gSpan: Graph-Based Substructure Pattern Mining," *Proc. Int'l Conf. Data Mining,* (ICDM 2002), December 2002, pp. 721-724.

14

Data Mining Applications in the Post-Genomic Era

Eugenia G. Giannopoulou[1] and Sophia Kossida[2]
[1]*University of Peloponnese, Department of Computer Science and Technology,*
[2]*Biomedical Research Foundation of the Academy of Athens,*
Greece

1. Introduction

The post-genomic era involves the experimental and computational efforts that aim to address the challenge of clarifying and understanding the function of the genes and their products. In particular, functional genomics intends to exploit the great wealth of data produced nowadays by high-throughput methods, in order to describe gene and protein functions and their interactions.

Proteomics, playing a significant role in this endeavour by complementing other functional genomics approaches, encompasses the large-scale analysis of complex mixtures, including the identification and quantification of proteins expressed under different conditions, the determination of their properties, modifications and functions. Although the term proteomics was initially defined as the large-scale study of the functions of all expressed proteins within an organism, it now also evokes the set of all protein isoforms and modifications as well as the interactions between them. In other words, proteomics expanded to the point that it now integrates all information that could be characterized "post-genomic" (Tyers & Mann, 2003). Therefore, the area of proteomics can be broadly divided into two subcategories: protein expression mapping and protein interaction mapping (Palzkill, 2002).

The protein expression mapping area uses separation and identification methods, such as 2-Dimensional Gel Electrophoresis (2DGE) and Mass Spectrometry (MS) respectively, to perform differential analysis of proteome expression levels (e.g., normal versus diseased cells, diseased versus treated cells and so on). Also known as *differential proteomics,* its basic aim is to discover reliable biomarkers for different biological states, to be used for diagnostic or therapeutic purposes, by identifying proteins that are up- or down-regulated or modified in a disease-specific manner (Monteoliva & Albar, 2004).

The protein-protein interaction mapping (also known as functional proteomics) includes the determination of protein interactions that exist in a proteome and aims at inferring unknown functions of specific proteins. Through these interactions, proteins carry out most of the processes in cells, such as gene regulation, intracellular communication and others. By exploiting protein interactions, it is feasible for the researcher to deduce the unknown function of a protein from the known functions of its interaction partners (i.e., proteins that participate in the same interaction). For example, if protein A with unknown function is found to participate in an interaction with proteins B and C, which are known to be involved in cellular process X, then protein A could be inferred to play a part in X as well. Thus, protein-protein interaction maps of the cell assist in the comprehension of its biology.

High-throughput technologies are widely used in proteomics, in order to achieve the analysis of thousands of proteins. These technologies generate high-dimensional proteomics data which require the application of different data mining approaches for efficient and accurate analysis of the proteomics results. More specifically, the application of data mining techniques on large-scale proteomics data sets can assist in many ways the data interpretation; it can reveal protein-protein interactions, improve the protein identification, evaluate the experimental methods used and facilitate the diagnosis and biomarker discovery, to name a few.

This chapter aims to: (a) familiarize the user with the most commonly used proteomics analysis methods, (b) present data mining techniques that have been used in the broad field of proteomics and (c) demonstrate indicative examples that highlight the importance of these methods in biological research.

In this chapter we will proceed as follows. In Section 2, we familiarize the reader with the typical proteomics workflow, introduce proteomics definitions and explain the benefits of applying mass spectrometry-based proteomics. In section 3, we discuss basic data mining methods, their characteristics and application to proteomics studies. Section 4 presents outstanding application paradigms, which confirm that data mining approaches are needed at all levels of proteomics analysis to provide a wealth of information. Finally, in the conclusion section, we summarize the chapter and discuss possible future research directions in this field.

2. Proteomics basics

2.1 Mass spectrometry-based proteomics workflow

A proteomic analysis includes two basic steps: application of a separation method (e.g., 2-Dimensional Gel Electrophoresis (2DGE), Liquid Chromatography (LC)), followed by a mass spectrometry (MS)-based identification method (Liebler, 2002). As far as the separation step is concerned, it is important to note that although two-dimensional electrophoresis (2DGE) is the separation technique most frequently used in proteomics, lately Liquid Chromatography (LC) is gaining momentum due to its ability to detect low abundance proteins and peptides (Garbis et al., 2005; Neverova & Van Eyk, 2004).

More specifically, 2DGE is applied to a complex protein mixture in order to separate its proteins in the highest possible degree. The protein mixture is inserted into a polyacrylamide gel and is resolved in two dimensions, the isoelectric point (pI) (i.e., the pH at which a particular molecule carries no net electrical charge) and the molecular weight (MW). As a result, proteins move to certain places in the polyacrylamide gel and after staining, they form the well-known gel spots. The outcome of this technique, a 2D-gel image, is then subjected to image analysis so as to detect and extract the spots from the gel. At this point, several statistical and quantitative methods (e.g., Mann-Whitney test, Student's t-test, volume fold factor criterion) are applied in order to perform differential expression analysis and detect the spots that discriminate the biological states.

After the extraction of the gel spots and their enzymatic digestion, the resulting peptides are inserted into a mass spectrometer, which produces spectra of their mass-to-charge (m/z) ratio. Using *peptide mass fingerprinting* (PMF) method, the information that the spectra carry for every peptide mass that appears in them (i.e., the m/z and the intensity), is used from software tools to achieve protein identification. In particular, search engines (e.g., Mascot, Sequest) compare and match the measured masses with already known theoretical masses in protein databases and provide identification results which show the protein most likely contained in each gel spot.

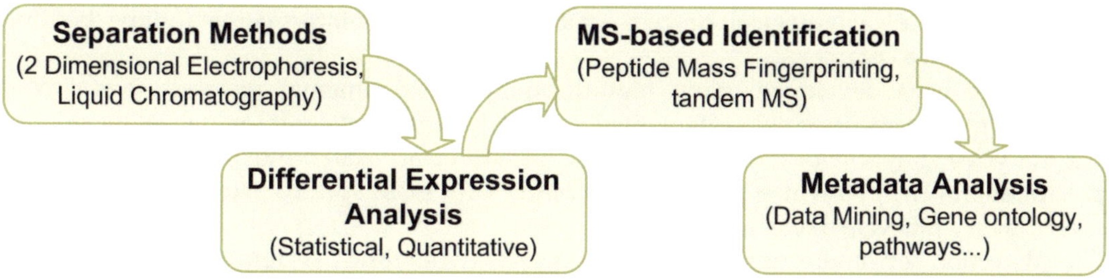

Fig. 1. Steps of a typical MS-based proteomics workflow.

In the case of LC coupled to tandem MS (LC-MS/MS), the mixture of many different proteins is digested to yield peptides, which are then resolved into fractions by two- or multi- dimensional liquid chromatography. The peptide fractions can then be processed by *tandem Mass Spectrometry* (MS/MS) to generate amino acid sequence information. This amino acid sequence can be used for protein database searching to identify the protein of interest (Liebler, 2002). As it is obvious, the most important benefit of the tandem mass spectrometry compared to peptide mass fingerprinting, apart from increasing selectivity and specificity in protein identification, is that the amino acid sequence information of the peptides is more precise for the protein identification than the peptides masses.

Differential proteomics is a powerful approach since it offers the ability to measure the relative abundance of proteins between two or more different biological states. A variety of quantitation approaches have been recently introduced, most of which use methods of stable isotope labeling (e.g., iTRAQ, ICAT, SILAC) that determine accurately, through the mass spectrometer, the relative changes in the two (or more) states of the proteome (Flory et al., 2002; Griffin et al., 2003; Gygi et al., 1999; Zieske, 2006).

The MS-based identification and quantitation is not the last step in a proteomic analysis workflow. Meta-data analysis follows and includes several methods that assist in the interpretation of the high-dimensional proteomics results. Several data mining and statistical methods (e.g., clustering, classification, ANOVA and so on) have been used extensively to facilitate the proteomics results interpretation (Beer et al., 2004; Bensmail et al., 2005; Cannataro et al., 2007; Hilario et al., 2006; Ventoura et al., 2008). Moreover, matching the identified proteins to their corresponding Gene Ontology annotations (i.e., molecular function, biological process, cellular component) is a task that places the protein results in a global perspective (Halligan et al., 2007). Lately, it has also become of immense importance to retrieve pathway information from databases (Krishnamurthy et al., 2003), in order to discover the biological pathways and molecular networks, that the proteins participate in. In summary, meta-data analysis includes using different methods and tools which focus on inferring protein-protein interactions, understanding how proteins are organized into biological networks and generally speaking, perceiving proteomics data from a "systems biology" point of view. Figure 1 summarizes the steps of a proteomics workflow, as described above.

2.2 Protein-protein interactions discovery

The proteome-wide scale discovery of physical interactions among proteins, plays a key role in the functioning of cells, since it assists in understanding the function of each protein. The integration and visualization of such interactions in protein networks, provides interesting hints for the unknown functions of proteins (Schwikowski et al., 2000) and new insights into the mechanism of a biological process by offering detailed information for the binding partners within a complex.

There have been developed many high-throughput experimental methods that aim at detecting thousands of protein interactions per study. The most commonly used techniques are the yeast 2-hybrid (Y2H) (Uetz et al., 2000; Ito et al., 2001) and the tandem affinity precipitation (TAP) (Gavin et al., 2002) combined with mass spectrometry or tandem mass spectrometry (Shevchenko et al., 1996).

The detection of interactions using the yeast two-hybrid system is based on the reconstruction of transcription factors by exploiting the modular properties of site-specific transcriptional activators (Fields & Song, 1989). For example, hybrid proteins composed of a DNA binding domain fused with protein A and a transcriptional activation domain fused with protein B, are produced in yeast. If proteins A and B interact, it reconstitutes the transcription factor and leads to the expression of a reporter gene. The main drawback of this method is that it allows the detection of interactions in the nucleus of the cell only.

The TAP method combined with mass spectrometry, a powerful approach for the comprehensive analysis of protein–protein interactions, involves identifying the components of protein complexes. First, the complexes are isolated from cells using affinity-based methods, which demand the identification of at least one protein in the complex. Then, after this protein has been tagged with an affinity handle, it can be over-expressed in cells and affinity purified so that its interaction partners co-purify. The complex is then subjected to a typical proteomics analysis using mass spectrometry, so that individual proteins can be identified.

Computational methods have also been developed and used widely, in order to infer protein-protein interactions, not from physical proteins binding, but indirectly from properties that are related to interacting protein pairs. Some of the most known computational methods for discovering protein interactions are the domain fusion or Rosetta Stone method (Marcotte et al., 1999), the phylogenetic profiles (Pellegrini et al., 1999), the correlated expression of gene pairs (Grigoriev, 2001; Deng et al., 2003) and the gene neighbor method (OverBeek et al., 1999).

The domain fusion method is based on the observation that some pairs of interacting proteins have homologs in another organism that are fused into a single protein chain. For instance, the interacting proteins A and B in the fly genome might be found as a single longer protein C in the worm genome. If such proteins or protein domains unrelated in the fly, are fused together in worm, it suggests that they are likely to function or interact together in the fly. The fused protein C is called Rosetta Stone Sequence (Marcotte et al., 1999; Ng et al., 2003). Thus, this computational method entails searching through genomic sequences for two proteins, A and B, which in some other species are expressed as a fused protein, A-B.

Phylogenetic profiles encode patterns of presence or absence of genes across genomes, and are used to assign functional relationships to non-homologous pairs of proteins (Pellegrini et al., 1999). This method is based on the hypothesis that proteins which are functionally linked (i.e., participate in a common structural complex or biochemical pathway) evolve in a correlated way and, thus, they have homologs in the same subset of organisms. In other words, it is very unlikely that two proteins would always be both present (or absent) to a new species unless they were functionally linked. Thus, if homologs to a pair of proteins are found in the same subset of organisms, the proteins are functionally linked.

The correlated gene expression methods (Grigoriev, 2001; Deng et al., 2003) detect protein-protein interactions based on the assumption that genes with correlated gene expression levels are more likely to encode interacting proteins.

Last but not least, the idea behind the gene neighbor method (Overbeek et al., 1999) is that if the genes encoding proteins A and B are neighbours on the chromosomes of several genomes, then A and B could participate in the same interaction or be involved in a similar function.

3. Data mining in proteomics

3.1 Classification

Classification is a data analysis task in which individual items are placed into groups based on one or more quantitative characteristics inherent in the items (also called "variables") and is based on a training set of previously labeled items. This means that classification is a supervised technique, since the prediction results fall in classes which are known beforehand. The algorithms used for classification are numerous. Here, we mention only the k-nearest-neighbour (k-NN) and the Support Vector Machines (SVMs), two algorithms that have been extensively used in proteomics.

The k-nearest-neighbour algorithm is amongst the simplest and mostly used algorithms for classification. In k-NN, an object is assigned to the class most common amongst its k nearest neighbours, where k is a typically small positive integer. If k = 1, then the object is simply assigned to the class of its nearest neighbor. In binary classification problems (i.e., two classes), it is helpful to choose k to be an odd number as this avoids tied votes. The neighbours are taken from a set of objects for which the correct classification is known. This can be thought of as the training set for the algorithm, though no explicit training step is required. In order to identify neighbours, the objects are represented by position vectors in a multidimensional feature space. In k-NN several distance measures can be used, such as the Euclidean, Manhattan or Mahalanobis distance. In proteomics, k-NN has been used to classify mass spectra data (Taguchi et al., 2007), as well as jointly with a genetic algorithm approach, first introduced for microarray data, in order to discover biomarkers of chemical exposure and disease (Li et al., 2004).

The Support Vector Machines define a hyperplane (i.e., a linear decision boundary) that separates the classes under study. The hyperplane maximizes the distance (also called margin) between the two sample groups. By using the margin optimization only a small set of data points, called support vectors are critical for the separation, while the dimensions unnecessary for the separation of the classes are penalized. Thus, the problem of model overfit can be handled using SVMs. As a result, the SVM is a robust classification technique which is suitable for datasets with many features and a relatively small sample size, such as the microarrays and the proteomics datasets. Applications of SVM-based classifiers in proteomics include identifying significant differences between patients and healthy individuals from mass spectra (Willingale et al., 2006), as well as producing prediction models for the classification or annotation of biological function of novel protein sequences (Yang & Chou, 2004).

Other classification methods are the decision trees as well as the artificial neural networks. An extensive and more detailed description of many classification algorithms used in proteomics is provided in (Mavroudi et al., 2007).

3.2 Clustering

Clustering is the unsupervised (i.e., not available class labelling of the training patterns) classification of objects into different groups. Clustering techniques have found many applications in many fields, such as machine learning, pattern recognition, image analysis, bioinformatics and so on. In order to perform a clustering analysis task, one should follow the steps of (a) features selection, (b) choosing the appropriate proximity measures and clustering criteria, (c) running the clustering algorithm, (d) validating and interpreting the results. During the first step, features must be properly selected so as to encode as much information as possible regarding the dataset and the given problem, and possibly undergo preprocessing. In the next step, the measure which quantifies the similarity or dissimilarity of feature vectors is chosen and the clustering criteria of a specific algorithm are selected. Once the results of the clustering algorithm have been obtained, it is important to validate their correctness by comparing the scores of different results using validity indices (e.g., Silhouette, Dunn, Daves-Bouldin). The results interpretation is of great importance since an expert in the application field integrates the clustering results with other experimental evidence in order to draw the right conclusions.

According to the final representation of the results, data can be clustered either in a hierarchical or in a non-hierarchical way. Hierarchical clustering is a widely used data analysis method which tries to reveal the underlying structure of a dataset at many levels, based on the idea of building iteratively a tree by successively merging groups of data points, starting from the most similar ones. In other words, hierarchical clustering algorithms produce a hierarchy of nested clusters. They require as input a metric for measuring the distance between data points, and a linkage method, which defines how the distance between two already formed clusters is estimated. These methods are appropriate for the recovery of both elongated and compact clusters. Hierarchical clustering is very popular due to its simplicity and has been applied in various scientific fields, including functional genomics using DNA micro-arrays (Eisen et al., 1998; Heyer et al., 1999).

A very representative example of a non-hierarchical clustering algorithm is k-means. K-means is a greedy iterative algorithm, which assigns each data vector to the cluster the center of which (also called "centroid") is nearest to it. Unlike hierarchical clustering algorithms, k-means requires as input the number of clusters (k) to be formed. Furthermore, the user should specify a distance metric, a centroid initialization method and a stopping criterion. As a data partitioning algorithm, it has also found many applications in genomics (Tavazoie et al., 1999). The reasons for its popularity are its implementation simplicity, performance scalability, convergence speed and adaptability to sparse data.

Clustering algorithms have been widely used in functional genomics (Bolshakova et al., 2005) in order to group genes based on their relative expression levels in a sample. In proteomics, clustering methods have been recently introduced for LC-MS/MS spectral analysis (Beer et al., 2004), as it has been observed that they can contribute to peptide identification, comparison of peptide mixtures, prediction of retention time and so on. Moreover, as a recent review indicates (Hilario et al., 2006), for data extracted from 2D gels, clustering the peptide mass fingerprinting spectra can divulge the similarity of spots without even knowing their protein identity.

3.3 Association rules

The aim of association rules mining is to reveal underlying interactions in large sets of data items. This data mining method was initially used in "market basket analysis" for discovering regularities between products in large scale transaction data recorded in supermarkets. The output from this analysis consists of association rules, which describe groups of items that are frequently purchased together.
In general, an association rule is of the form of:

$$\{X\} => \{Y\} \quad (1)$$

where Y, represents the items that consist the Left Hand Side (LHS) of the equation, and X represents the items included in the Right Hand Side (RHS) of it. A rule states that whenever the LHS items are present in a transaction, the RHS items are likely to be present as well.
To evaluate the importance of an association rule, "interestingness measures" have been established and used. The *support* of rule (1) is the probability of a transaction in the dataset to contain both X and Y. In other words, support describes how frequently the rule occurs among transactions. The *confidence* of rule (1) shows its accuracy and is defined as the number of transactions with both the X and Y items, divided by the number of transactions with X items. Confidence shows the number of transactions in which the rule is correct, relative to the number of transactions in which it is applicable. An interesting rule must at least have support and confidence values greater than the user-specified minimum thresholds. *Leverage* is another measure which shows the percentage of additional cases covered by both the X and Y, above those expected if X and Y were independent of each other, and represents the unexpectedness of the rule. *Coverage* is the proportion of the transactions in the dataset which have the X items. Finally, the *lift* is a measure of the association's importance, which is independent of coverage, and is the confidence divided by the proportion of all transactions which have the Y items.
A number of approaches and methods have been proposed for association rules extraction, the main idea of which is based on the concept of frequent itemsets (i.e., sets of values in the same tuple). Some well known algorithms are Apriori (Agrawal & Srikant, 1994), Eclat (Zaki, 2000) and FP-Growth (Han et al., 2000).
Data mining based on association rules has also been applied in biomedical research. For instance, in the medical domain, association mining has been used to discover rules that relate patient symptoms, diagnosis and procedures performed on patients (Doddi et al., 2001), as well as to detect hidden and previously unknown patterns on large public health datasets, which can provide surveillance warnings (Giannopoulou et al., 2007), to name a few. Association mining has been also applied to the analysis of gene expression data, in order to reveal biologically relevant associations among different genes or between environmental effects and gene expression (Creighton & Hanash, 2003), as well as to proteomics, where it is important to discover rules that relate protein properties (e.g., functional annotation, sequence motifs) to protein-protein interactions (Kotlyar et al., 2006; Oyama et al., 2002).

4. Application examples

4.1 Sample classification from protein mass spectra

The study described in (Tibshirani et al., 2004) suggests a novel algorithm for pattern classification from protein mass spectra, which is a slight variation of the "nearest centroid" classiffication. In particular, when applied to spectra from both diseased and healthy patients, the proposed "Peak Probability Contrast" (PPC) technique provides a list of all common peaks among the spectra, their statistical significance, and their relative importance in discriminating between the two groups. Compared to other statistical approaches for class prediction, this method performs as well or better than several methods that require the full spectra, rather than just labeled peaks. The algorithm consists of six sequential steps, shown in Figure 2.

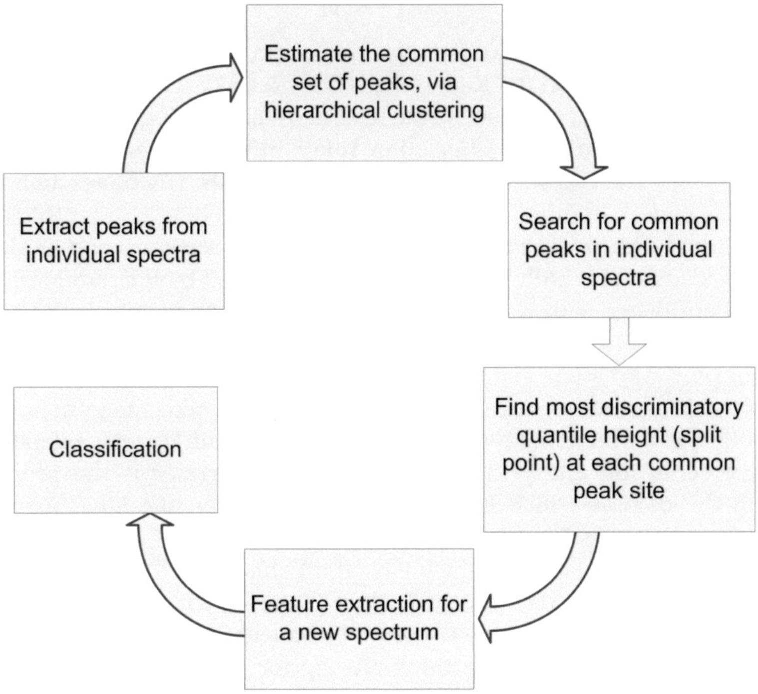

Fig. 2. Flow chart of the Peak Probability Contrast classification analysis. Figure adapted from (Tibshirani et al., 2004).

The step of peak extraction looks for mass-to-charge ratio (m/z) values the intensity of which is higher than that at the ±s m/z value surrounding it, and higher than the estimated average background at that m/z.

The next step estimates the common set of peaks using complete linkage hierarchical clustering. The clustering is one dimensional, using the distance along the log m/z axis. The idea is that tight clusters should represent the same biological peak that has been horizontally shifted in different spectra. Then the mean position (centroid) of each cluster is extracted, to represent the "consensus" position for that peak across all spectra.

Searching for common peaks in individual spectra is the step to follow. In particular, given the list of common peaks from clustering in previous step, the individual spectra are searched in order to record whether each spectrum exhibits each of these common peaks. A peak in the individual spectra is considered to be one of the common peaks if its center lies within a specific distance from the estimated center position of the common peak. If it is present, the height of the individual peak in the spectrum is also recorded.

From the previous steps, the spectrum peak heights are estimated for all observations and for all m/z values. As mentioned before, these heights are the centroids from the hierarchical clustering of all individual spectra peaks. If there is no peak at a specific m/z value, then the corresponding height is zero. During this step, the algorithm "cuts" each peak height at some quantile, in such a way so as to maximally discriminate between the healthy and normal samples in the training set.
The final step involves the class prediction of new mass spectra. A spectrum from a new patient has a binary feature vector of peak heights, with a component equal to one if the spectrum has a peak above the cutpoint height at that m/z value, and zero otherwise. Then, this binary profile is compared to each of the probability centroid vectors of the two classes (e.g., health vs. cancer) and classified to the class that is closest in overall squared distance (or some other metric).
The application of this method, so as to find a relative small number of peak clusters for class prediction, is expected to facilitate the identification of biologically significant and relevant proteins for specific biological states, such as tumor development and progression.

4.2 Clustering mass spectra peak-lists

In the study presented in (Ventoura et al., 2007) clustering algorithms are applied to proteomics data, in an attempt to group proteins based on their spectral similarities. Moreover, clustering validation methods are used to find the clustering method which most faithfully captures the underlying distribution of the samples. This work also shows that the application of clustering algorithms in proteomics can assist in (a) identifying peak features responsible for categorizing samples, (b) formulate hypotheses on the possible function and role of unidentified proteins and (c) reveal proteins which act jointly as biomarkers in a concrete biological state.
The proteomics data on which clustering is performed are the mass spectra peak-lists (not the raw mass spectra) which derive from a mass spectrometer. A mass spectrum peak-list is the intensity as a function of mass-to-charge ratio (m/z) profile of a sample (e.g., a protein spot) that has undergone mass spectrometry analysis. In order to apply cluster analysis, these peak-lists are represented as vectors in a multidimensional space, where each vector element is a feature of a specific mass (e.g., its intensity) or a group of masses. To deal with the high dimensionality of the generated peak-list vectors mass "bins" (i.e., contiguous non-overlapping regions in the m/z axis) can be defined before analyzing the samples of an experiment. The process of binning performs dimensionality reduction by grouping consecutive masses and selecting a representative feature of those masses for each group (e.g., mean, log, maximum intensity value). Moreover, one can preprocess the peak-lists vectors by performing scaling or normalization.
The suggested clustering algorithms for these data are the hierarchical as well as the k-means clustering. For a better comprehension of the clustering results several visualization methods are also exploited (i.e., dendrograms, heatmaps and cluster sets). In the clustering results that derive from this method, not only well separated protein clusters can be easily discerned, but also the spectral bins that are most influential in partitioning the proteins into clusters (Figure 3).
Furthermore, the presented method offers the option of integrating the identification results for the proteins - members of each cluster, as well as their Gene Ontology annotation. By exploiting both the identification and the Gene Ontology classification information for most

proteins in each cluster, one can attempt to infer the role of unidentified proteins. This can be based on the already known functions of the proteins which are identified with high confidence and are found to be close to unidentified proteins in the same cluster.

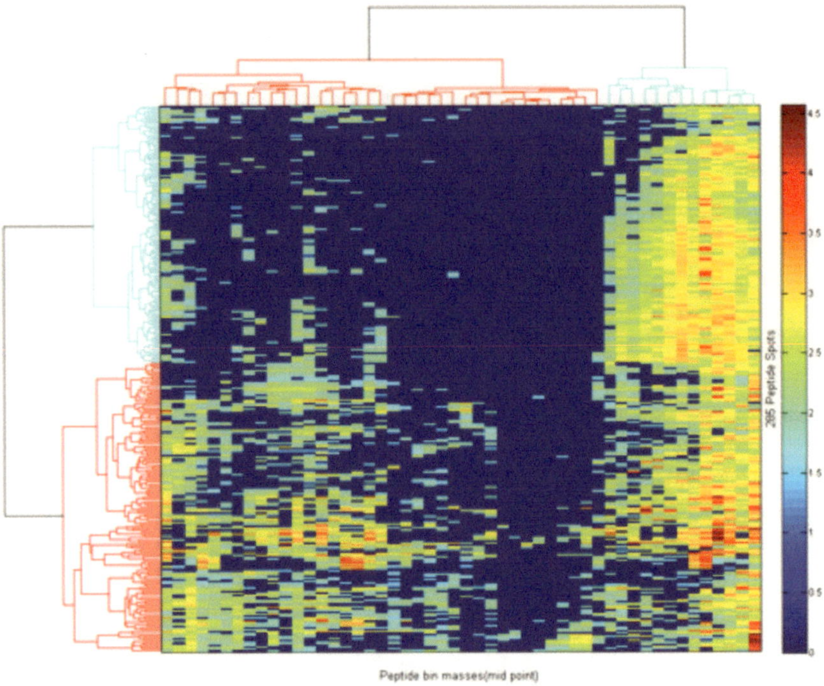

Fig. 3. Heatmap visualization of a hierarchical clustering result. Two well separated protein clusters (horizontal dendrogram) and two well separated bin clusters (vertical dendrogram) can be observed at the top-level. Figure adapted from (Ventoura et al., 2007).

4.3 Protein-protein interactions prediction using association rules

The work by (Kotlyar et al., 2006) is a very recent attempt that uses association rules not only to discover protein-protein interactions, but also to predict whether a given pair of proteins interacts. Predicting interactions with association mining can be viewed as a classification problem where the RHS part of the rule consists of a single item only, the class variable. After the application of association mining, the rules are ranked according to a measure of "interestingness" (e.g., confidence, support) and used for prediction as follows: a given protein pair is predicted to interact if its attributes include the LHS items of any rule. The presented approach is based on the idea that both direct and indirect evidence (e.g., data coming from experimental and computational methods) could be used to predict interactions reliably and on a proteome-wide scale. In particular, datasets that consist of interacting and non-interacting protein pairs annotated with different types of evidence are first constructed. Then, with the help of association rules, patterns that discriminate the interacting and the non-interacting proteins are detected. Lastly, using these patterns the prediction of interactions is achieved, assigning a confidence level to each interaction. The three steps followed in this approach to predict protein-protein interactions will be further described (Figure 4).

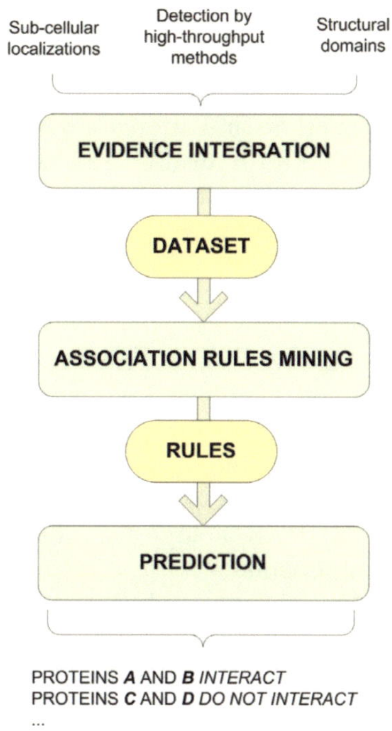

Fig. 4. Predicting protein-protein interactions using association rules. The reliability of interactions is increased if different types of evidence (direct and indirect) are jointly considered.

The first step in the suggested approach refers to the creation of datasets which integrate evidence from (a) high-throughput interaction detection methods, (b) gene expression microarrays and (c) protein annotation projects. This step seems to be of immense importance since previous studies have shown that by integrating data the reliability of protein-protein interactions can be improved (Goldberg & Roth, 2003; Zhang et al., 2004). Thus, a dataset is generated from protein pairs annotated with various attributes (e.g., detection by high-throughput methods, sub-cellular localizations, structural domains and so on). Since the aim of this work is to be able to decide if protein pairs interact (classification problem of 2 classes), the datasets deliberately include both protein pairs that represent true interactions, as well as randomly chosen non-interacting protein pairs.

During the association mining step, the Extended FP-Growth algorithm is chosen for creating association rules, due to its ability to succeed short run times in these large datasets. It is important to note that in the protein-protein interaction prediction problem, the vast majority of the rules are associated with non-interacting protein pairs that may not be very informative, and that significant rules may have very low support relative to the size of the dataset. These observations can be explained by the very low ratio of interacting to non-interacting protein pairs that has been observed in organisms (e.g., 1 interaction pair to 600 non-interacting pairs in the yeast).

After the rules are determined, they are ranked based on confidence. Rules having the same confidence are ranked by support. To predict if a given protein pair interacts, its attributes should match the LHS items of any rule. Then, the confidence of this prediction is the confidence of the highest ranked rule that is matched.

To conclude, with this approach, different types of evidence for interaction are integrated in order to create rules that act as a classifier for new interaction pairs. Thus, association mining is used to search thoroughly in large datasets for predictive patterns. However, to evaluate the performance of this method and strengthen its applicability, it is important to incorporate additional evidence, perform testing and validation using already known interactions from specific organisms and compare the results to those of other interaction detection methods.

5. Conclusion

Proteomics, the large-scale study and analysis of proteins, is a field of powerful techniques which offer significant experimental knowledge to experts in drug design and clinical applications (Fountoulakis & Kossida 2006; Simpson et al., 2008; Ge et al., 2008). Several studies and reviews available in the literature (Bachi & Bonaldi, 2008; Feng et al., 2008) also indicate that proteomics is of great value and significance to the analysis of complex biological model systems and to systems biology (i.e., the systems-level understanding of correlations among molecular components).

Using data-mining techniques in the large volumes of data obtained either by high-throughput differential expression proteomics analyses or by large-scale protein interaction experiments, serves as a powerful and promising mechanism for extracting useful knowledge and reaching interesting biological conclusions. This research area is rapidly growing and enriched with new applications which focus on detecting previously unknown protein functions and relations. However, the future directions should concentrate on developing novel methods and algorithms so as to improve the proteomics mining results in terms of validity, scientific soundness and verification.

6. References

Agrawal, R. & Srikant, R. (1994). Fast algorithms for mining association rules in large databases. *Proceedings of the 20th International Conference on Very Large Data Bases*, pp. 487-499, ISBN 1-55860-153-8, Santiago Chile, September 1994, Morgan Kaufmann

Bachi, A. & Bonaldi, T. (2008). Quantitative proteomics as a new piece of the systems biology puzzle. *J Proteomics*. (July 2008)

Beer, I.; Barnea, E.; Ziv, T. & Admon, A. (2004). Improving large-scale proteomics by clustering of mass spectrometry data. *Proteomics*, Vol., 4, (February 2004) 950– 960

Bensmail, H.; Golek, J.; Moody, M. M.; Semmes J. O. & Haoudi A. (2005) A novel approach for clustering proteomics data using Bayesian fast Fourier transform. *Bioinformatics*, Vol., 21, (March 2005) 2210-2224

Bolshakova, N.; Azuaje, F. & Cunningham, P. (2005). An Integrated Tool for Microarray Data Clustering and Cluster Validity Assessment. *Bioinformatics*, Vol., 21, (February 2005) 451–455

Cannataro, M.; Guzzi, P. H.; Mazza, T.; Tradigo, G. & Veltri P. (2007). Using Ontologies for preprocessing and mining spectra on the Grid. *Future Generation Computer Systems*, Vol., 23, (January 2007) 66-60

Creighton, C. & Hanash, S. (2003). Mining gene expression databases for association rules. *Bioinformatics*, Vol., 19, (January 2003) 79–86

Deng, M.; Sun, F. & Chen, T. (2003). Assessment of the reliability of protein-protein interactions and protein function prediction. *Pac Symp Biocomput*, 140–151

Doddi, S.; Marathe, A.; Ravi, S. S. & Torney, D. C. (2001). Discovery of association rules in medical data. *Med Inform Internet Med*, Vol., 26, (January/March 2001) 25–33.

Eisen, M. B.; Spellman, P. T.; Brown, P. O. & Botstein, D. (1998). Cluster analysis and display of genome-wide expression patterns. *Proc. Natl. Acad. Sci.*, Vol., 65, (December 1998) 14863–14868

Feng, X.; Liu, X; Luo, Q. & Liu, B. F. (2008). Mass spectrometry in systems biology: An overview. *Mass Spectrom Rev.* (July 2008)

Fields, S. & Song, O. (1989). A novel genetic system to detect protein–protein interactions. *Nature*, Vol., 340, (July 1989) 245–246

Flory, M. R.; Griffin, T. J.; Martin, D. & Aebersold, R. (2002). Advances in quantitative proteomics using stable isotope tags. *Trends in Biotechnology*, Vol., 20, (December 2002) 23-29

Fountoulakis, M. & Kossida, S. (2006). Proteomics-driven progress in neurodegeneration research. *Electrophoresis*, Vol., 27, (April 2006) 1556-1573

Garbis, S.; Lubec, G. & Fountoulakis M. (2005). Limitations of current proteomics technologies. *Journal of Chromatography A*, Vol., 1077, (May 2005) 1 - 18

Gavin, A. C.; Bosche, M.; Krause, R.; Grandi, P.; Marzioch, M.; Bauer, A.; Schultz, J.; Rick, J. M.; Michon, A. M.; Cruciat, C. M.; Remor, M.; Hofert, C.; Schelder, M.; Brajenovic, M.; Ruffner, H.; Merino, A.; Klein, K.; Hudak, M.; Dickson, D.; Rudi, T.; Gnau, V.; Bauch, A.; Bastuck, S.; Huhse, B.; Leutwein, C.; Heurtier, M. A.; Copley, R. R.; Edelmann, A.; Querfurth, E.; Rybin, V.; Drewes, G.; Raida, M.; Bouwmeester, T.; Bork, P.; Seraphin, B.; Kuster B.; Neubauer, G. & Superti-Furga, G. (2002). Functional organization of the yeast proteome by systematic analysis of protein complexes. *Nature*, Vol., 415, (January 2002) 141–147

Ge, X.; Wakim, B. & Sem, D. S. (2008). Chemical Proteomics-Based Drug Design: Target and Antitarget Fishing with a Catechol-Rhodanine Privileged Scaffold for NAD(P)(H) Binding Proteins. *J Med Chem.* (July 2008)

Giannopoulou, E. G.; Kemerlis, V. P.; Polemis, M.; Papaparaskevas, J.; Vatopoulos, A. C. & Vazirgiannis, M. (2007). A Large Scale Data Mining Approach to Antibiotic Resistance Surveillance. *Proceedings of 20th IEEE International Symposium on Computer Based Medical Systems*, pp. 439-444, ISBN 0-7695-2905-4, Maribor Slovenia, June 2007, IEEE Computer Society

Goldberg, D. S. & Roth, F. P. (2003). Assessing experimentally derived interactions in a smallworld. *Proc Natl Acad Sci*, Vol., 100, (April 2003) 4372–4376

Griffin, T. J.; Lock, C. M.; Li, X.; Patel, A.; Chervetsova, I.; Lee, H.; Wright, M. E.; Ranish, J. A.; Chen, S. S. & Aebersold, R. (2003). Abundance ratio-dependent proteomic analysis by mass spectrometry. *Analytical Chemistry*, Vol., 75, (January 2003) 867–874

Grigoriev, A. (2001). A relationship between gene expression and protein interactions on the proteome scale: analysis of the bacteriophage T7 and the yeas Saccharomyces cerevisiae. *Nucleic Acid Res*, Vol., 29, (July 2001) 3513-3519

Gygi, S. P.; Rist, B.; Gerber, S. A.; Turecek, F.; Gelb, M. H. & Aebersold, R. (1999). Quantitative analysis of complex protein mixtures using isotope-coded affinity tags. *Nature Biotechnology*, Vol., 17, (October 1999) 994-999

Halligan, B. D.; Mirza, S. P.; Pellitteri-Hahn, M. C.; Olivier, M. & Greene, A. S. (2007). Visualizing Quantitative Proteomics Datasets using Treemaps. *Proceedings of 11th International Conference Information Visualization*, pp. 527-534, ISBN 0-7695-2900-3, Zurich Switzerland, July 2007, IEEE Computer Society

Han, J.; Pei, J. & Yin, Y. (2000). Mining frequent patterns without candidate generation. *Proceedings of the 2000 ACM SIGMOD International Conference on Management of Data*, pp. 1–12, ISBN 1-58113-218-2, Dallas Texas, May 2000, ACM

Heyer, L. J.; Kruglyak, S. & Yooseph S. (1999). Exploring Expression Data: Identification and Analysis of Coexpressed Genes. *Genome Research*, Vol., 9, (November 1999) 1106–1115

Hilario, M.; Kalousis, A.; Pellegrini, C. & Muller, M. (2006). Processing and Classification of Protein Mass Spectra. *Mass Spectrometry Reviews*, Vol., 25, (February 2006) 409– 449

Ito, T.; Chiba, T.; Ozawa, R.; Yoshida, M.; Hattori, M. & Sakaki, Y. (2001). A comprehensive two-hybrid analysis to explore the yeast protein interactome. *Proc Natl Acad Sci*, Vol., 98, (March 2001) 4569–4574

Kotlyar, M. & Jurisica, I. (2006). Predicting protein-protein interactions by association mining. *Inf Syst Front*, Vol., 8, (February 2006) 37-47

Krishnamurthy, L.; Nadeau, J. H.; Ozsoyoglu, G.; Ozsoyoglu, Z. M.; Schaeffer, G.; Tasan, M. & Xu, W. (2003). Pathways Database System: An Integrated System for Biological Pathways. *Bioinformatics*, Vol., 19, (May 2003) 930-937

Li, L.; Umbach, D. M.; Terry, P. & Taylor, J. A. (2004). Application of the GA/KNN method to SELDI proteomics data. *Bioinformatics*, Vol., 20, (July 2004) 1638-40

Liebler, D. C. (2002). *Introduction to Proteomics*, Humana Press, ISBN 978-089603-991-9, Totowa New Jersey USA

Marcotte, E. M.; Pellegrini, M.; Ng, H. L.; Rice, D. W.; Yeates, T. O.; & Eisenberg, D. (1999). Detecting protein function and protein-protein interactions from genome sequences. *Science*, Vol., 285, (July 1999) 751-753

Mavroudi, S.; Papadimitriou, S.; Kossida, S.; Likothanassis, S. D. & Vlahou, A. (2007). Computational Methods and Algorithms for Mass-Spectrometry Based Differential Proteomics. *Current Proteomics*, Vol., 4, (December 2007) 223-234

Monteoliva, L. & Albar, J. P. (2004). Differential proteomics: An overview of gel and non-gel based approaches. *Briefings in Functional Genomics and Proteomics*, Vol., 3, 2004, (November 2004) 220-239

Neverova, I. & Van Eyk, J. E. (2004). Role of chromatographic techniques in proteomic analysis. *Journal of Chromatography B*, Vol., 815, (December 2004) 51 - 63

Ng, S.K.; Zhang, Z.; Tan, S. H. & Lin, K. (2003). Interdom: A database of putative interacting protein domains for validating predicted protein interactions and complexes. *Nucleic Acids Res.*, Vol., 31, (October 2002) 251–254

Overbeek, R.; Fonstein, M.; D'Souza, M.; Pusch, G. D. & Maltsev, N. (1999). The use of gene clusters to infer functional coupling. *Proc Natl Acad Sci*, Vol., 96, (March 1999) 2896-2901

Oyama, T.; Kitano, K.; Satou, K. & Ito, T. (2002). Extraction of knowledge on protein-protein interaction by association rule discovery. *Bioinformatics,* Vol., 18, (May 2002) 705-714

Palzkill, T. (2002). *Proteomics,* Kluwer Academic Publishers, ISBN 0-792-37565-3, USA

Pellegrini, M.; Marcotte, E. M.; Thompson, M. J.; Eisenberg, D. & Yeates, T. O. (1999). Assigning protein functions by comparative genome analysis: Protein phylogenetic profiles. *Proc. Natl. Acad. Sci.*, Vol., 96, (April 1999) 4285-4288.

Shevchenko, A.; Jensen, O. N.; Podtelejnikov, A. V.; Sagliocco, F.; Wilm, M.; Vorm, O.; Mortensen, P.; Shevchenko, A.; Boucherie, H. & Mann, M. (1996). Linking genome and proteome by mass spectrometry: large-scale identification of yeast proteins from two dimensional gels. *Proc Natl Acad Sci,* Vol., 93, (December 1996) 14440-14445

Simpson, R. J.; Bernhard, O. K.; Greening, D. W. & Moritz, R. L. (2008). Proteomics-driven cancer biomarker discovery: looking to the future. *Curr Opin Chem Biol.,* Vol., 12, (February 2008) 72-77

Taguchi, F.; Solomon, B.; Gregorc, V.; Roder, H.; Gray, R.; Kasahara, K.; Nishio, M.; Brahmer, J.; Spreafico, A.; Ludovini, V.; Massion, P. P.; Dziadziuszko, R.; Schiller, J.; Grigorieva, J.; Tsypin, M.; Hunsucker, S. W.; Caprioli, R.; Duncan, M. W., Hirsch, F. R.; Bunn, P. A. & Carbone D. P. (2007). Mass spectrometry to classify non-small-cell lung cancer patients for clinical outcome after treatment with epidermal growth factor receptor tyrosine kinase inhibitors: a multicohort cross-institutional study. *J Natl Cancer Inst.,* Vol., 99, (June 2007) 838-846

Tavazoie, S.; Hughes, J. D.; Campbell, M. J.; Cho, R. J. & Church G. M. (1999). Systematic determination of genetic network architecture. *Nat Genet,* Vol., 22 (July 1999) 281-285

Tibshirani, R.; Hastiey, T.; Narasimhanz, B.; Soltys, S., Shi, G.; Koong, A. & Le, Q. (2004). Sample classification from protein mass spectrometry, by "peak probability contrasts". *Bioinformatics,* Vol., 22, (November 2004) 3034-3044

Tyers, M. & Mann, M. (2003). From genomics to proteomics. *Nature,* Vol., 422, (March 2003) 193-197

Uetz, P.; Giot, L.; Cagney, G.; Mansfield, T. A.; Judson, R. S.; Knight, J. R.; Lockshon, D.; Narayan, V.; Srinivasan, M.; Pochart, P.; Qureshi-Emili, A.; Li, Y.; Godwin, B.; Conover, D.; Kalbfleisch, T.; Vijayadamodar, G.; Yang, M.; Johnston, M.; Fields, S. & Rothberg, J. M. (2000). A comprehensive analysis of protein–protein interactions in Saccharomyces cerevisiae. *Nature,* Vol., 403, (February 2000) 623–627

Ventoura, S.; Giannopoulou, E. G. and Manolakos, E. S. (2008). ProtCV: A Tool for Extracting, Visualizing and Validating Protein Clusters Using Mass Spectra Peak-Lists. *Proceedings of 21st IEEE International Symposium on Computer Based Medical Systems,* pp. 221-223, ISBN 978-0-7695-3165-6, Jyvaskyla Finland, June 2008, IEEE Computer Society

Willingale, R.; Jones, D. J.; Lamb, J. H.; Quinn, P.; Farmer, P. B. & Ng, L. L. (2006). Searching for biomarkers of heart failure in the mass spectra of blood plasma. *Proteomics,* Vol., 6, (November 2006) 5903-14

Yang, Z. R. & Chou, K, C. (2004). Bio-support vector machines for computational proteomics. *Bioinformatics.* Vol., 20, (March 2004) 735-741

Zaki, M. J. (2000). Scalable algorithms for association mining. *IEEE Transactions on Knowledge and Data Engineering*, Vol., 12, (May/June 2000), 372-390

Zieske, L. R. (2006). A perspective on the use of iTRAQ reagent technology for protein complex and profiling studies. *Journal of Experimental Botany*, Vol., 57, (March 2006) 1501-1508

Zhang, L.V.; Wong, S. L.; King, O. D. & Roth, F. P. (2004). Predicting co-complexed protein pairs using genomic and proteomic data integration. *BMC Bioinformatics*, Vol., 5, (April 2004) 38

15

Topological Analysis of Cellular Networks

Carlos Rodríguez-Caso and Núria Conde-Pueyo
ICREA-Complex Systems Lab, Universitat Pompeu Fabra (GRIB-PRBB).
Dr Aiguader 88, 08003,
Barcelona, Spain

1. Introduction

The description of the molecular world conforming living cells has been a long standing enterprise since Biochemistry foundation. The elucidation of biochemical pathways in the early-middle twenty century gave way to a more complete picture of genes, proteins and metabolites by the beginning of Molecular Biology. Nowadays, the ultimate deciphering of such a molecular world is now becoming to be reality by the huge biotechnological advance on high throughput analysis. Genomic, proteomic and metabolomic tools have provided a revolution of the molecular biology and biomedicine expectations in very few years, as well as, the emergence of novel disciplines such as Systems and Synthetic Biology.

One of the first conclusions of such large-scale analyses is that molecular species are networked in giant interconnected entities. The so-called *cellular networks,* -consisting of protein maps, metabolism, and gene regulatory networks- but also other systems such as food webs, internet, or social relations constitute a sort of complex networks. Contrasting with the initial thought, it was observed that their organisation strongly departs from simple random homogeneous metaphors. Interestingly, their internal organization reveals common traits that can be analysed from the perspective of modern graph theory. In this theoretical framework, a graph is a mathematical abstraction of reality that can be tackled from statistical physics and computation science perspectives.

In this chapter we will present a repertoire of methods for a standard graph analysis, particularly oriented to the study of cellular networks. These tools allow us to measure and compare different networks in order to uncover their internal organization from a statistical point of view. We will show that the network approach provides a suitable framework to explore the organisation of the biomolecular world.

2. Graph theory approach

The aim of this chapter is not to present a collection of methods but an orientation about how is the network that we are studying by a description of the most relevant descriptors of a graph. We will start with describing those descriptors to define, in a topological way, an element within a network. In second place, we will provide global descriptors to define a network.

2.1 Graph concept

A *graph* (or *network*) G is defined by a set of N vertices (or nodes) $V=\{v_1, v_2,...,v_N\}$ and a set of L edges (or links), $E=\{e_1, e_2, ...,e_L\}$, linking the nodes. Two nodes are linked when they satisfy a given condition, such as two metabolites participating in the same reaction in a metabolic network. The graph definition does not imply that all nodes must be connected in a single component. A *connected component* in a graph is formed by a set of elements so that there is at least one path connecting any two of them. Graphs are *undirected* when the interaction between nodes is mutual and equal, as in the protein maps. On the contrary, the web is *directed* when the connection indicates that one element affect to the other but not the opposite. As we will see, this is the case of gene regulatory networks (Shen-Orr et al. 2002) and signal transduction pathways (Ma'ayan et al. 2005). Additionally, graphs can also be *weighted* when links have values according to a certain property. This is the case for gene regulatory networks, where weights indicate the strength and direction of regulatory interactions. Although graphs are usually represented as a plot of nodes and connecting edges, they can also be defined by means of the so-called *adjacency matrix*, i.e., an array A of NxN elements a_{ij}, where a_{ij}=1 if v_i links to v_j and zero otherwise. A is symmetric for undirected graphs, but not for the directed ones. For weighted nets a matrix W can be introduced, where w_{ij} indicates the strength and type of the link. The network can also be described using a list of pairs of connected nodes (edge-list), which has some computational advantages. Figure 1 summarizes the different ways of representing a graph.

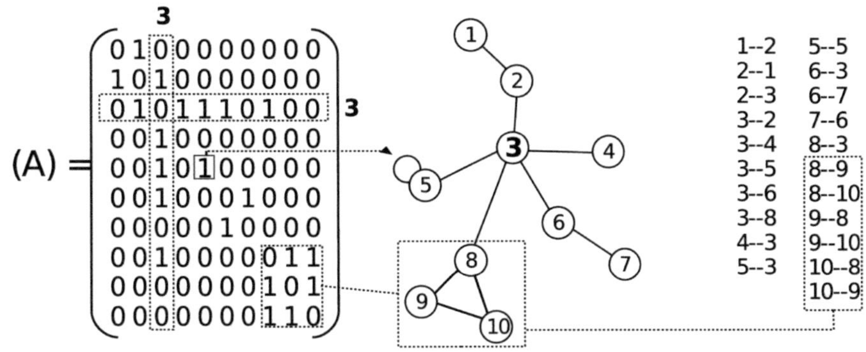

Fig. 1. Different ways of representation for a directed and unweighed graph. Left: Adjacency matrix (A). Centre: Drawn graph. Right: List of pairs (edge list). The triangle motif (in dashed box) is indicated for the three representations. The autoloop concept is represented in the vertex 5. Some examples of k, C and b values: for v_3, k_3=5, C_3=0, b_3=0.69; v_8, k_8=3, C_8=0.33, b_8=0.36; v_{10}, k_{10}=2, C_{10}=1,b_{10}=0.

2.2 Node attributes

Here we summarize the measures required to describe individual nodes of a graph. They allow identifying elements by their topological properties. The *degree* -or *connectivity*- (k_i) of a node v_i is defined as the number of edges of this node. From the adjacency matrix, we easily obtain the degree of a given node as

$$k_i = \sum_{j=1}^{N} a_{ij}$$

See examples of k values in figure 1. For directed graphs, we distinguish between incoming and outgoing links. Thus, we specify the degree of a node in its *indegree*, k_i^{in}, and *outdegree*, k_i^{out}.

The *clustering coefficient* C_i is a local measure quantifying the likelihood that neighbouring nodes of v_i are connected with each other. It is calculated by dividing the number of neighbours of v_i that are actually connected among them, n, with all possible combinations excluding autoloops, i.e., $k_i(k_i-1)$. Formally, we have:

$$C_i = \frac{2n}{k_i(k_i - 1)}$$

Notice that, auto-loops, i.e., links that starts and end in the same vertex (see figure 1), are not considered in this measure. Examples of C values are illustrated in figure 1.
The *betweenness centrality* b_m for a node v_m is the fraction of *shortest pathways* Γ for each pair of nodes (v_i, v_j) also containing v_m, that is

$$b_m = \sum_{i \neq j} \frac{\Gamma(i,m,j)}{\Gamma(i,j)}$$

The ratio $\Gamma(i,m,j)/\Gamma(i,j)$ indicates how crucial v_m is relating v_i and v_j. We introduce the term *pathway* (or simply *path*) as the string of nodes relating v_i and v_j (see graph and values for b in Figure 2). This concept is similar to the metabolic pathway describing a set of coupled reactions from one metabolite to another. The shortest path connecting v_i and v_j is the one where the lowest number of nodes are involved to connect them. Such topological descriptors are useful to identify particular nodes in the network. Under this point of view, such particularities can be mapped into relevant topological properties. For instance, high k_i for a node might relate to a relevant role, since many other nodes interact with it. Alternatively, high b_i can also indicate a relevant role since it tells us that many nodes are efficiently connected through it. It is noteworthy that, b_i usually scales with degree, although this is not always true (see figure 2).

2.3 Graph attributes

For a network of size N, global measures can be defined, each one providing very different, but complementary, sources of information. The *average degree*, defined as $\langle k \rangle = 2L/N$, indicates how sparse a graph is. Real networks are sparse, i.e. $\langle k \rangle \ll N$. In the case of networks with auto-loops the average degree must be corrected as $\langle k \rangle = (2L-A)/N$ where A corresponds with the number of auto-loops in the network.

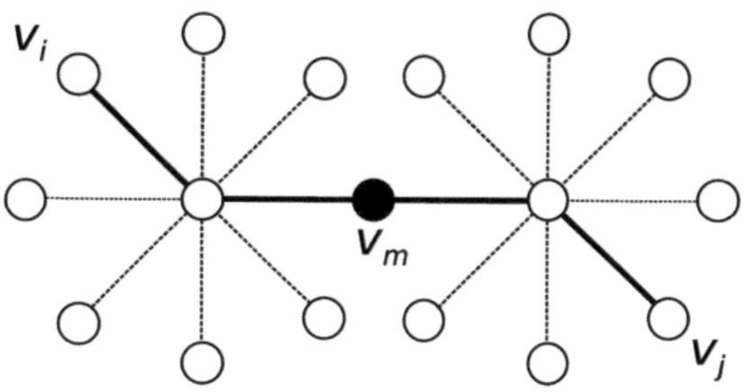

Fig. 2. Relation between degree and betweenness. The two-star graph shows a case where the two hubs support a high level of shortest pathways whereas the central node v_m shows the highest b of the graph keeping a low degree. The shortest path connecting v_i and v_j through v_m is indicated by solid lines.

The *average clustering*, $\langle C\rangle = 1/N\sum_i C_i$, provides a measure of local organization. High ⟨C⟩ indicates that neighbours of a node are likely to be linked between them. It actually gives the probability of finding triangles.
The *average path length* (*APL*) indicates the average length of the shortest pathways separating each node pair. If d_{min} is the length of the shortest path connecting nodes v_i and v_j, then *APL* is defined as:

$$APL = \frac{2}{N(N-1)}\sum_{i>j} d_{\min}(v_i, v_j)$$

Another measure is the *degree distribution* *p(k)*. It indicates the probability of a node having *k* links. Usually, because network size is restricted, the statistics are poor. It is rather difficult to get a good fitting for distribution degree from real data. A common problem in real networks is the fluctuations in the vertex abundance for very large degrees. One common solution, and in particular when we observe a power-law behaviour, is the cumulative distribution of degree frequency (Dorogovtsev & Mendes 2003), formally, $P_{cum}(k) = \sum_{k'=k}^{\infty} p(k')$.
Real networks are usually associated with the term of *scale-free*. They exhibit a degree distribution following a power-law decay, $p(k) \sim k^{-\gamma}$. Here, γ is a positive parameter that for real networks is usually in the range $2<\gamma<3$ (Albert et al. 2002). Notice that for cumulative distributions $P_{cum} \sim k^{-(\gamma-1)}$.
Scale-free (SF) graphs have a *p(k)* with a maximum at *k=1* (thus most elements have a single link) and rapidly decay at higher *k* values. Nevertheless, the tail of the distribution is very long and thus nodes with a very high degree are possible. Before the discovering of such an evidence, it was thought that real networks might follow a Gaussian distribution where the average degree represents a central position of a well confined distribution. The mathematical models describing this behaviour correspond with the Erdös-Renyi (ER) graph. ER graphs predict that very high *k* is exceedingly rare and unlikely to be observed at all. SF distributions have no humps and have extremely large standard deviations, which means that no confidence can be placed in a prediction of the number of links of any node sampled at random (Albert et al. 2002). Typically, real networks exhibit a mixed distribution, that is, a power-law with a sharp exponential cut-off determined by k_c in the expression $p(k) \sim k^{-\gamma} e^{-k/k_c}$ indicating that arbitrarily high degrees are not allowed (Amaral et al. 2000).
The *clustering distribution* *C(k)* represents C_i against *k*. ER and pure scale-free webs do not exhibit any dependency between C_i and *k*. By contrast, in so-called *hierarchical networks*, it has been associated with a decay of *C(k)* with inverse of the degree ($C \sim k^{-1}$) (Barabasi et al. 2004). This type of network exhibits modularity (nodes are preferentially linked inside clusters or modules). A *module* can be defined as a set of nodes in a connected component which tend to be more connected among them than with the rest of the network.
The *assortative mixing* (*r*) is a measure of the correlation among degrees in a graph, giving information about the likelihood to find linked nodes of a certain degree. This measure compares the correlation among degrees in the studied network (noted as G_R) with its *uncorrelated* counterpart. The expression for *r* can be obtained in (Newman 2002). Here we will only present an intuitive understanding of *assortativenness* concept. The value of *r*

ranges between -1 and 1. Here $r=0$ indicates no correlation among degrees, as it occurs for example in ER graphs. Otherwise, most complex networks have been found to be *disassortative*, i.e., $r<0$, where higher degree nodes tend to be connected with lower degree ones rather than nodes with the same k (see Figure 3A). These networks display hubs that are not directly connected among them. It has been suggested that this situation confers network robustness (Maslov et al. 2002). When $r>0$, nodes with the same degree tend to be linked among them (see figure 3B) and the graph is called *assortative*.

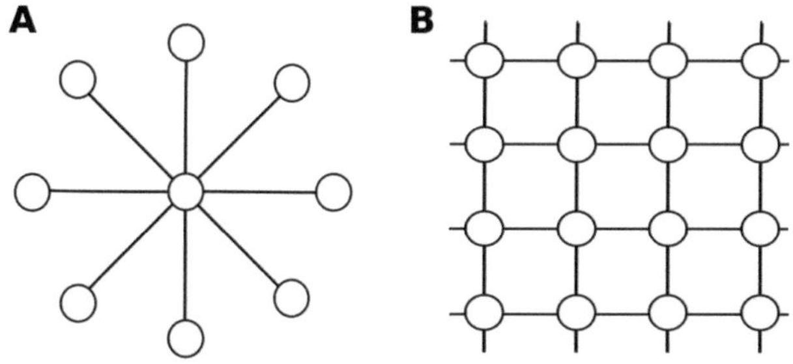

Fig. 3. Illustration of *assortativenness*. Panel A, a star graph, showing a correlation among highly connected nodes with poorly connected ones ($r<0$). Panel B, a lattice where all nodes have $k=4$. It is the extreme case where nodes with the same degree tend to be linked among them ($r>0$).

Small world pattern is a qualitatively property that exhibit most real networks. A small world criterion compares the clustering coefficient and *APL* of a real network with the respective ER model with the same average degree and size. ER graph constitutes a null model for comparison with real data. It captures the properties of a network derived from a purely random process of connection. The probability P, defines the likelihood that two vertices are linked among them. For ER graphs, $\langle k_{ER} \rangle = PN$, where N is the size of the network and $\langle C_{ER} \rangle = k/N$. *APL* follows the expression $APL_{ER} = \log N / \log \langle k \rangle$. When a graph G_R fulfils the conditions $APL_R \cong APL_{ER}$ but $\langle C_R \rangle << \langle C_{ER} \rangle$ then it is said that G_R exhibits a *small world* (SW) *pattern*. These networks keep their local order (high C) but also allow a very efficient communication (low *APL*) (Watts & Strogatz 1998).

2.4 Graph analysis and visualization software

For general purposes, the most popular visualization software is Pajek (http://vlado.fmf.uni-lj.si/pub/networks/pajek/), which is free for Windows operating systems. Pajek provides a graphic interface and a set of algorithms for graph analysis. Graphviz package (http://www.graphviz.org/) is another generic free package but it only provides visualization tools. Interestingly, a number of command line tools for complex network analysis for Linux/Unix platform can be found at http://www.lsi.upc.edu /~pfernandez/ software-networks.html.

Within the biological context, many databases offer a graph visualization of their content, for example KEGG database, or Transfac (http://www.biobase.de/) and Ingenuity (http://www.ingenuity.com) commercial databases.

The most interesting software for cellular network visualization and analysis is Cytoscape (http://www.cytoscape.org/). This software is supported by an open community where computer scientists can develop plugins for specific purposes: visualization methods, algorithms and the integration of the information from biological databases.

3. Cellular networks

Cellular network is the term commonly used for the current interacting molecular sets within cells (Albert, 2005; Barabasi & Oltvai, 2004). It includes mainly protein-protein interactions, metabolism, gene transcriptional regulatory networks and signal transduction pathways. All of them are different subsets of a single large-scale cellular network, since they are eventually cross-linked.

3.1 Protein-protein interaction networks

Protein-protein interaction (PPI) networks, interactomes and protein maps make reference to the collection of proteins interacting by physical contact. Proteins are the nodes and physical interactions among them are the links in the graph.

PPI networks are undirected graphs where two connected proteins are mutually affected. They exhibit a power-law decay with an exponential cut-off and small world behaviour. Interestingly, as it occurs in most cellular networks, vertices do not represent an individual but a molecular species. For this reason the appearance of auto-loops is justified since they represent the ability to make homo-multimers.

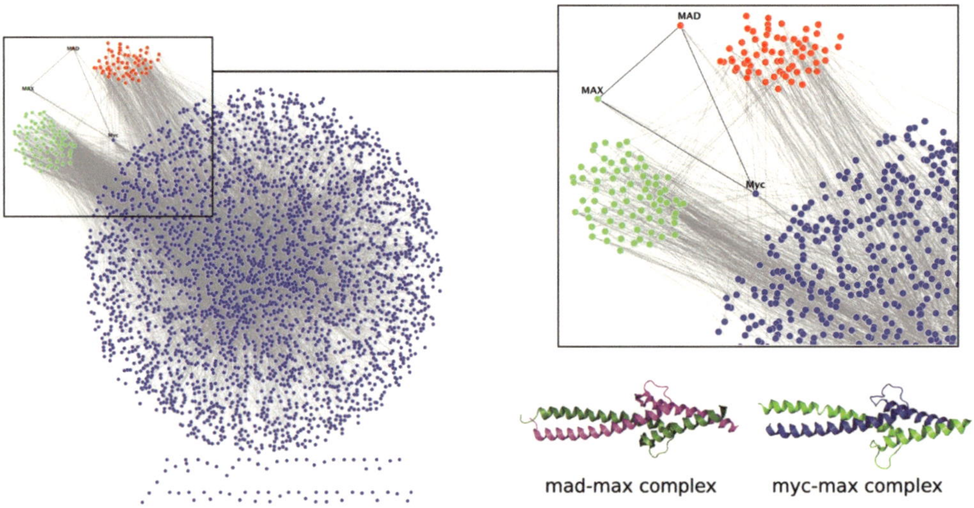

Fig. 4. Fraction of human PPI network filtered by nuclear localization criteria using Gene Ontology annotation (http://www.geneontology.org/). All proteins and interactions are expected to be in the nucleus. In red are represented those proteins marked as transcriptional co-suppressors. In green, transcriptional co-activators. As an example of interaction, the relation between mad/max and myc/max transcriptional cancer related protein complexes are depicted. Notice that databases may contain artefacts not observed in nature (e.g. myc/mad interaction). Below zoom box, protein complex representation from crystal structure. Data obtained from HPRD database. Graph generated with Cytoscape.

Measures such as clustering coefficient or average degree do not consider such a circumstance. This can be a source of errors in our analysis depending on how the measures have been implemented. To be consistent with the theory we must avoid auto-loops for such measures.

At low scale, *cliques*, i.e. full connected subgraphs within the network, constitute a way to complex protein detection (Yu, et al. 2006). The smallest clique that can be observed is the triangle, suggesting a possible hetero-trimer complex. However, the biological conclusions derived from a specific network configuration at the scale of a very few number of elements must be contrasted with different information sources. In general, this approximation must be considered as a methodology for the inference of potential biological relations among proteins to be tested experimentally. We must remain that, in spite of the analysis of different PPI networks reveals robust results in their global parameters, database information can contain artefacts. This is relevant when our aim is to focuss on functional/biological relations of a particular part of the network. After a first identification by automatic filters, a manual curation of the database for our study system is recommended (see figure 4).

To this day, large-scale studies have explored the proteome structure in viruses (McCraith et al., 2000), yeast (Uetz et al., 2000; Ito et al., 2001; Ptacek et al., 2005), the worm *Caenorhabditis elegans* (Walhout et al., 2000; Li et al., 2004), *Helicobacter pylori* (Rain et al., 2001), Drosophila melanogaster (Giot et al., 2003) and more recently in humans (Rual et al., 2005; Stelzl et al., 2005). Protein map elucidation is obtained mainly by two large-scale experimental approaches, namely, the yeast two-hybrid (Y2H) (Uetz & Hughes, 2000) and the tandem affinity purification (TAP) followed by mass spectroscopy (Gavin et al., 2002). Such information is collected in annotated databases. Different databases such as MIPS (http://mips.gsf.de/), DIP (http://dip.doe-mbi.ucla.edu/), Intact (http://www.ebi.ac.uk/intact/site/index.jsf) and in particular for humans HPRD (www.hprd.org/) are the main repositories commonly used for the acquisition of current protein maps.

3.2 Gene transcriptional regulatory networks

The assembly of regulatory interactions linking transcriptions factors (TFs) to their target genes constitutes the first level of a multilayered network of gene regulation; the so called gene transcriptional regulatory networks (GTRN) (Babu et al. 2004). Genome scale approaches have provided a reliable picture of the regulatory maps for the prokaryote *Escherichia coli* (Thieffry et al. 1998; Shen-Orr et al. 2002) and the eukaryote *Saccharomyces cerevisiae* (Lee et 2002; Balaji et al. 2006). Directed graphs are the mathematical abstraction of GTRNs (Babu et al. 2004, Albert et al. 2005). The regulatory effect of a TF gene (let's say A) on a specific target gene (B) is depicted by ($A \rightarrow B$). In graph theory, A y B are vertices linked by an arrow. TFs are easily identified in the graph since they exhibit outgoing arrows. In turn, non TF genes -the target ones- only receive arrows from the TF set. The number of outgoing links of a vertex is known as *outdegree* (denoted by k^{out}) whereas the number of incoming edges corresponds with *indegree* (k^{in}). Interestingly, as a TF can be a regulatory target of other TFs, they can exhibit both incoming and outgoing arrows.

As it is occurs with PPI networks, we can find auto-loops. In this case, it means that a gene product causes a regulatory effect in its own promoter. Interestingly, the identification of network motifs in GTRN remarks the view of minimal genetic circuits as the building blocks of the networks (Shen-Orr et al. 2002; Milo et al. 2002). However, the Achilles heel of this approach is that motif analysis is restricted to previous selection criteria by the investigator which specifically must define the subgraph to be detected.

3.3 Metabolic networks

Metabolism is the best described cellular network so far. However, a global topological view of metabolism was not available until recently (Jeong et al., 2000; Ouzounis & Karp, 2000). Metabolic pathways are composed by two types of molecular species: enzymes and metabolites. In this case, one or more than one metabolites (substrates) are transformed (in products) by enzyme mediation. The resulting graph is known as *bipartite graph*, since one type of vertices (metabolites) is always related through the other type of elements (enzymes). Therefore, no enzyme-enzyme and metabolite-metabolite interactions are found. This network definition allows defining an arrow from substrates to enzymes and from enzymes to products for irreversible reactions. However, arrow definition is not possible for reversible reactions. In spite of this graph definition is the most informative, its topological treatment results more complicated, and the graph is usually *projected* over a single type of vertex. As figure 5 shows, two types of projections can be done (Wagner & Fell, 2001). One way is considering the *substrate graph*, where each metabolite is a vertex that will be linked with those metabolites participating in the same reaction. Alternatively, a *reaction graph* is made by considering reactions as nodes and metabolites as links. This mathematical treatment has permitted to uncover the scale free (Jeong et al. 2000), small world behaviour and the hierarchical and modular organization of metabolic networks (Wagner & Fell 2001, Ravasz et al. 2002). Metabolic pathways can be found in KEGG (http://www.genome.jp/kegg/) and Reactome database (http://www.reactome.org/).

3.4 Cell signalling networks

These networks depict those processes allowing cells integrating responses to external stimuli. They are a combination of metabolic reactions and protein interactions that trigger specific changes in gene expression. Protein modifications such as phosphorylation, acetylation and ubiquitination, among others, lead to conformational changes allowing ligand-protein recognition and functional protein complexes assembling. At the present, kinases and phosphatases relations constitute the best described signalling pathways. Bibliographic sources provide the current information to reconstruct this kind of networks (Ma'ayan et al. 2005). Additionally, several databases compile this information such as the *Kinbase* (http://kinase.com/) and Reactome databases. Interestingly, this kind of networks presents a diverse type of vertices and type of connections. By this reason, its biological interpretation of topological analysis is not trivial.

3.5 Filtered networks

Network analysis can be focussed on a sub-part of the system. Figure 4 illustrates an example of this. Gene ontology annotation provides biological information about function and localization of genes. However, depending on the particular process to be considered, the heterogeneity in the quality of the gene annotation constitutes a bias. In agreement with this philosophy, several works have provided relevant biological insights about the biological meaning of the network organization (Rodríguez-Caso et al. 2005, Ravazs et al. 2002).

3.6 Feature based networks.

As we have seen, several cellular networks offer a picture that captures the biological machineries within a living cell. We observe that all of them are constructed by a well defined type of interaction. The link features that two elements are involved by physic contact (PPI and GTR networks) or transformation process (metabolism).

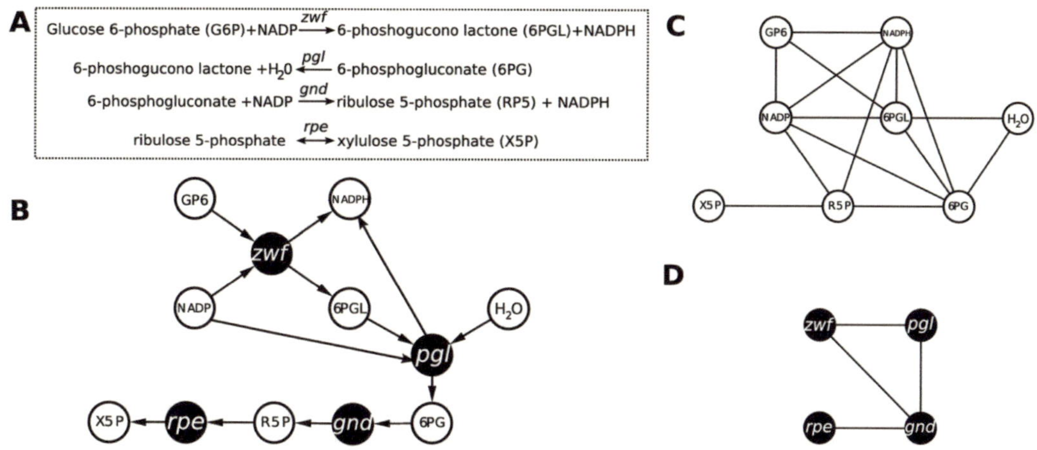

Fig. 5. Metabolic network representations (picture modified from Wagner & Fell 2001). Panel A, description of the reactions. Panel B, bipartite graph representation. Panel C, substrate projection. Panel D respective reaction projection. White vertices represent metabolites whereas black vertices represent enzymes.

Recently, network approach has been applied to define a sort of networks that captures relations in a broader sense. The purpose of these networks is not to describe truly molecular machinery but to offer a global view of some type of biological property, function or consequence. This is the case of the human disease network (Goh et al. 2007) that relates the diseases contained in OMIM database with their responsible genes. As it occurs with metabolic networks, this constitutes a bipartite graph with two kinds of entities, genes and diseases. This network, more than recovering a biological process, give us a conceptual picture of the relation between genes and diseases.

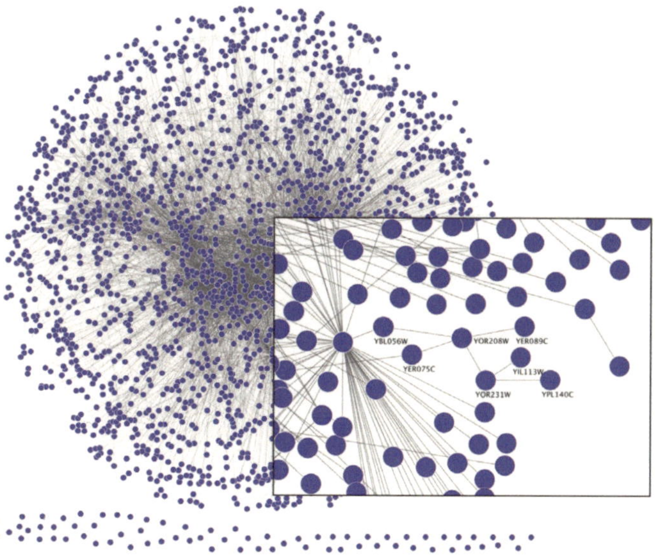

Fig. 6. Example of a feature based network. Yeast synthetic lethal network obtained from BioGRID database (http://www.thebiogrid.org/). Graph generated with Cytoscape.

In this direction, the same group goes beyond, constructing a bipartite graph composed of US Food and Drug Administration–approved drugs and proteins linked by drug–target binary associations. This drug-target protein network does not capture any biological machinery but offer a global picture of the relation between drugs and targets by the conceptualization of the problem in a graph. As another example, figure 6 illustrates the case of Synthetic Lethal network in yeast (Tong et al. 2001), that recovers the information of those pair of gene that simultaneously mutated lead to lethality but not when they are individually mutated.

4. Topological analysis of cellular networks

Since cellular networks are in constant change, here we present the *state of the art* of different cellular networks. The topological analysis is based on the previously described estimators. Table 1 summarizes the topological analysis of PPI, metabolic and gene regulatory networks. In addition, we have included the yeast synthetic lethal network as an example of featured base networks. All these networks present a single giant component and a number of very small subgraphs. The statistics are provided for the giant components. In general, these networks are sparse graphs. Remarkably, all the networks are dissasortative *($r<0$)*, i.e, high degree tends to be connected with lower degree. Small world behaviour is clearly evidenced in yeast and human PPI networks. Interestingly, these two networks differ in their size but present a high similarity in their organization. The two available GTRN present a very small *APL*. The explanation if found in the biology, since only a small fraction of genes are TFs. The major fraction of vertices corresponds with terminal genes linked to one of these factors. These gene regulatory networks differ in their <C>, in other words, in their local organization.

	N	*L*	<*k*>	<*C*>	(<C_{ER}>)	*APL* (APL_{ER})	*r*	**Source Data**
Human PPI *	9048	34876	7.71	0.16	($8.52\ 10^{-3}$)	4.26 (4.46)	-0.04	HPRD
Yeast PPI *	4842	17119	7.07	0.10	($1.46\ 10^{-2}$)	4.14 (4.34)	-0.13	DIP
E.coli GTRN **	1589	4030	5.07	0.43	($3.19\ 10^{-2}$)	2.68 (4.54)	-0.26	RegulomDB6.0
Yeast GTRN **	4441	12864	4.79	0.08	($1.08\ 10^{-2}$)	3.49 (5.36)	-0.59	Balaji *et al.* 2006
Human metabolism	2827	5988	4.23	0.00	($1.5\ 10^{-3}$)	4.55 (5.50)	-0.12	KEGG
Yeast SL *	2287	9616	8.34	0.30	($3.67\ 10^{-2}$)	3.75 (3.65)	-0.19	BioGRID

Table 1. Global descriptors for the giant component of cellular networks. Notice that, for all the cases, giant component represents almost the total number of interactions. Parenthesis shows the <C> and APL values are showed for respective ER counterparts (calculated according definition described in the text). (*) It indicates a small world pattern. (**) Notice that APL is revealed shorter than the expected in ER model. Human metabolism presents <C>=0 due to the bipartite nature of the graph. Graph descriptors were calculated by Gstats command line software available at http://www.lsi.upc.edu/~pfernandez/software-networks.html. Autoloops were eliminated for the topological analysis.

Metabolic network corresponds with the bipartite representation. This imposes a restriction on the clustering coefficient. Since two vertices of the same nature cannot be connected, $\langle C \rangle = 0$ by definition.

In spite of SL network has not a biomolecular machinery correlate, it reveals a small world pattern indicating that SL are not trivially organised. In this case, high clustering is interpreted as two synthetically lethal genes tend to make a synthetic interaction with a common third gene.

It is remarkable that some relevant properties of these examples can be explained by the consideration of the network definition. This suggests that a suitable knowledge of the study of the system besides graph theory approach provides the best system study comprehension.

5. Goals and pitfalls of network approach

Uncovering the molecular world constitutes the new frontier of biology. Large zoological and botanical expeditions at the end of nineteen century pursued the characterization of organism diversity and their relations. Nowadays, in a similar way, the molecular biologist explores the diversity inside the cell. Unfortunately, the current picture of the study system is only a sketch of the actual relations between elements and most of the biological details are still unknown. Precisely, the relations among elements are the target for graph theory approach that has been profusely applied in many real systems. During the last decade, graph view has been incorporated to a diverse number of disciplines. This approach opens the possibility of a global comprehension of the system, against the predominant reductionism of the current scientific thought. We can access to the study of very large systems even when we do not know the details. Pioneer works about scale-freeness in metabolism, proteome (see the review, Albert 2005), the diameter of the world wide web (Albert et al. 1999), well as the widely observed small world behaviour in real networks have demonstrated that the pattern of interactions encloses relevant constraints defining the internal organisation of networks.

Graph theory enables a systemic study through the statistical approximation from the collection of local interactions; nevertheless, a limitation of such a global understanding is precisely its own size. In general for any statistical approach, the larger size of our data the more reliable is the statistics. This is not an exception for the global estimators of graph theory such as degree distribution, or assortativeness. From a theoretical point of view, the graph properties derived from analytical models are established when graph size tends to infinite. Therefore, if our study system is not large enough, deviations from the theory are expected.

In any case, we must remain that the true understanding of our study system will be only successful if we exactly know what is the captured from the reality in our graph abstraction and what is not. A graph is constructed by considering some particular property that is used to link a set of elements. Both of them -elements and their relation type- must be clearly defined. Most probably, graph definition does not affect to the topological analysis but it is essential for its biological interpretation that is, in the last instance, the aim of the biologist.

6. Acknowledgements

This work has been supported by 6th EU framework SYNLET (NEST-043312), ComplexDis (NEST-043241) and NHI CA 113004 projects. We thank Dr Ricard Solé and Complex

Systems Lab members for successful comments. We thank Itziar Castanedo for her successful comments during the writing of this work.

7. References

Albert, R.; Yeong H. & Barabasi, A. L. (1999). Diameter of the world-wide web. *Nature* 401 (September 1999) 130.

Albert, R. & Barabasi, A. L. (2002). Statistical mechanics of complex networks. *Rev. Modern Phys,* 74, (January 2002) 47-97

Albert, R. (2005). Scale-free networks in cell biology. *Jcell Sci,* 118, (Pt 21) (October 2005) 4947-57.

Amaral, L.A.N.; Scala, A.; Barthél'emy, M. & Standley H.E. (2000). Classes of small-world networks. *Proc. Natl. Acad Sci.* USA, 97, 21, (September 2000) 11149-11152.

Babu, M.M.; Luscombe N.M.; Aravind, L.; Gerstein, M. & Teichmann, S.A. (2004). Structure and evolution of transcriptional regulatory networks. *Curr Opin Struct Biol* 14, (2004 Jun) 283-291.

Balaji, S.; Babu, M.M.; Iyer, L.M.; Luscombe, N.M. & Aravind, L (2006). Comprehensive analysis of combinatorial regulation using the transcriptional regulatory network of yeast. *J Mol Biol,* 360, (June 2006) 213-27.

Barabasi, A.L. & Oltvai, Z.N. (2004). Network biology: Understanding the cell's functional organization. *Nat. Rev. Genet,* 5, (February 2004) 101-13.

Dorogovtsev, S.N. & Mendes J.F.F. (2003). *Evolution of Networks. From Biological Nets to the Internet and WWW.* Oxford University Press ISBN 0-19-851590-1, Oxford UK.

Gavin, A. C.; Bosche, M & Krause, R. et al. (2002). Functional organization of the yeast proteome by systematic analysis of protein complexes. *Nature,* 415.; (January 2002) 141-147

Giot, L.; Bader, J.S & Brouwer, C. et al. (2003). A protien interaction map of drosophila melanogaster. *Science,* 302, 5651, (December 2003) 1727-1736

Goh, K. I.; Cusick, M.E.; Valle, D.; Childs, B.; Vidal, M and Barabási, A.L. The human disease network. *Proc Natl Acad Sci USA,* 104, 21, (May 2007) 8685-8690

Ito, T.; Chiba, T.; Ozawa, R.; Yoshida, M.; Hattori , M. & Sakaki, Y. (2001) . A comprehensive two-hybrid analysis to explore the yeast protein interactome. *Proc. Natl. Acad. Sci. USA,* 98, 8, (April 2001) 4569-4574

Jeong, H.; Tombor, B.; Albert, R.; Oltvai, Z. N. & Barabasi, A.L. (2000). The large scale organization of metabolic networks. *Nature,* 407, 6804, 651-654

Lee, T. I.; Rinaldi, N. J & Robert, F. et al. (2002). Transcriptional regulatory networks in saccharomyces cerevisiae. *Sciencie,* 298, 5594, (October 2002) 799-804

Li, S.; Armstrong, C.M.; Berint, N.; Ge, H.; Milstein, S.; Boxem, M.; Vidalain, P.O & et al. (2004). A map of the interactome network of the metazoan C.elegans. *Science,* 303, 5657, (January 2004) 540-543

Ma'ayan, A.; Jenkins, S.L.; Neves, S.; Hasseldine, A.; Grace, E.; Dubin-Thaler, B. & et al. (2005). Formation of regulatory patterns during signal propagation in a mammalian cellular network. *Science,* 309, 5737, (August 2005) 1078-1083

Maslov, S. & Sneppen K. (2002). Specificity and stability in topology of protein networks. *Science,* 296, 5569, (May 2002) 910-913

McCraith, S.; Holtzman, T.; Moss, B. & Fields, S. (2000). Genome-wide analysis of vaccinia virus protein-protein interactions. *Proc. Natl. Acad. Sci. USA,* 97, 9, (April 2000) 4879-4884

Milo, R.; Shen-Orr, S.; Itzkovitz, S.; Kashtan, N.; Chklovskii, D. & Alon, U. (2002). Network motifs: simple building blocks of complex networks. *Science,* 298, 5595 (October 2002) 824-7

Newman, M. E. (2002). Assortative mixing in networks. *Phys Rev Lett.* 89, 20, (Novembre 2002)

Ouzounis, C. A. & Karp P.D. (2000). Global properties of the metabolic map of escherichia coli. *Genome Res.* 10, 4, (April 2000) 568-576

Ptacek, J.; Devegan, G.; Michaud,; G. Zhu,; H. Zhu,; X. Fasolo,; J. & et al. (2005). Global analysis of protein phosphorylation in yeast. *Nature,* 438, 7068, (December 2005) 679-84

Ravasz, E.; Somera, A.L.; Mongru, D.A.; Oltvai, Z.N. & Barabasi, A.L. (2002). Hierarchical organization of modularity in metabolic networks. *Science,* 297, 5586, (August 2002) 1551-1555

Rodríguez-Caso, C.; Medina, M.A. & Solé, R.V. (2005).Topology, tinkering and evolution of the human transcription factor network. *FEBSJ* 272 (December 2005) 6423-34.

Rual, J. F.; Venkatesan, K.; Hao, T.; Hirozane-Kishikawa, T.; Crico, A.; Li, N.; Berriz, G. F. & et al. (2005).Towards a proteome-scale map of the human protein-protein interaction network. *Nature,* 437, 7062, (October 2005) 1173-1178

Shen-Orr, S.S.; Milo, R.; Mangan, S.; & Alon, U. (2002). Network motifs in the transcriptional regulation network of *Escherichia coli. Nat Genet.,* 31, 1, (April 2002) 64-68

Stelzl, U.; Worm, U.; Lalowski, M.; Haening, C.; Brembeck, F.H.; Goehler, H. & et al. (2005). A human protein-protein interaction network: a resource for annotating the proteome. *Cell,* 12, 6, 957-968.

Tong, A.H.; Evangelista, M.; Parsons, A.B.; Xu, H.; Bader, G.D.; Pagé, N.; et al.(2001).Systematic genetic analysis with ordered arrays of yeast deletion mutants. *Science.* 294, 5550 (2001 December) 2364-8

Thieffry, D.; Huerta, A.M.; Pérez-Rueda, E. & Collado-Vides, J. From specific gene regulation to genomic networks: a global analysis of transcriptional regulation in Escherichia coli. *Bioessays,* 20, 5, (1998 May) 433-40

Uetz, P. & Hughes, R. E. (2000). Systematic and large-scale two-hybrid screens. *Curr. Opin. Microbiol.* 3, 3, (June 2000) 303-308

Uetz, P.; Giot, L.; Cagney, G.; Mansfield,T.A.; Judson, R.S.; Knight, J.R.; & et al. (2000). A comprehensive analysis of protein-protein interactions in *Saccharomyces cerevisiae. Nature,* 403, 6770, (February 2000) 623-627

Wagner, A. & Fell, D. A. (2001). The small world inside large metabolic networks. *Proc. Biol. Sci.* 268, 1478, (September 2001) 1803-1810

Walhout, A.J.; Boulton, S. J. & Vidal, M. (2000). Yeast two-hybrid systems and protein interaction mapping projects for yeast and worm. *Yeast,* 17, 2, (June 2000) 88-94

Watts, D.J.; Strogatz, S.H.; Collective dynamics of 'small-world' networks. *Nature,* 393, 6684, (June 1998) 440-442

Yu, H.; Paccanaro, A.; Trifonov, V. & Gerstein, M. (2006). Predicting interactions in protein networks by completing defective cliques. *Bioinformatics*, 22, 7, (February 2006) 823-829

16

Biomedical Literature Mining for Biological Databases Annotation

Margherita Berardi[1,5], Donato Malerba[1] , Roberta Piredda[2],
Marcella Attimonelli[2], Gaetano Scioscia[3,4] and Pietro Leo[3,4]
[1]*Dipartimento di Informatica – Università degli Studi di Bari*
[2]*Dipartimento di Biochimica e Biologia Molecolare "E.Quagliariello" – Università degli Studi di Bari*
[3]*IBM Italia S.p.A. - Molecular Biodiversity Laboratory*
[4]*IBM Italia S.p.A. - GBS Innovation Centre*
[5]*Exhicon S.r.l., Bari*
Italy

1. Introduction

In biological research, there are thousands of specialized data repositories, focusing on particular molecules, organisms or diseases, which offer sets of richly annotated records. To ensure data of the highest quality, manual data entry and curation (annotation) processes are generally performed on these databases. Database curators are domain experts who search biomedical research literature for facts of interest, and manually transfer knowledge from published papers to the database. This helps experts to consolidate data about a single organism or a single class of entity, often in conjunction with sequence information. Most importantly, this process makes the information searchable through a variety of automated techniques, given that the curators use standardized terminologies or ontologies. However, as the volume of biomedical literature increases, so does the burden of curation, making annotation databases incomplete and inconsistent with the literature. It has been shown empirically that manual annotation cannot keep up with the rate of biological data generation (Baumgartner et al., 2007). Seemingly, simple tasks of gene annotation by means of a controlled vocabulary becomes very laborious since an expert is required to inspect carefully the whole literature associated to each gene, to identify the appropriate terms. On the other hand, the contribution of the manual annotation community is essential to the understanding of the ever more complicated biological landscape and it is widely accepted that it produces the most accurate annotations currently available. To reduce the cost of obtaining annotations, several initiatives for collaborative curation, such as community annotation projects (e.g., http://www.pseudomonas.com/) and wiki-based prototypes (e.g., http://www.wikiprofessional.org/) have been recently promoted. Nevertheless, there is not enough evidence to clearly assess if collaborative curation solves the problem (Lu et al., 2007). As of now, PubMed remains the richest and most updated source of information about biological data despite its unstructured nature. This motivates the upsurge of interest in text mining techniques which enable various degrees of automation in the analysis of scientific literature, such as identification of named entities, classification of documents, extraction of relevant facts (i.e., relationships between two or more named entities expressing a fact), and generation of hypotheses (Cohen & Hersh, 2005; Jensen et al., 2006; Krallinger et al., 2005). The fundamental challenge in the application of data mining to text data is the translation of text into such a structured form that should, intrinsically, encapsulate the data semantics.

Despite the fact that many text mining systems have been deployed in the biomedical context and reasonable levels of performances on gold standard data have been achieved (Hirschman et al. 2005; Cussens and Nedellec, 2005; Shatkay and Feldman, 2003), the actual contribution to database curation efforts is still unclear (Yeh et al., 2003; Rebholz-Schuhmann et al., 2005). Most of these systems have been developed to solve very specific problems on task-tailored data and very few of them have been concretely used to assist curators in the population of biological databases. An example in this direction is the PreBIND system (Alfarano et al, 2005) which serves to curate the BIND (http://bind.ca/) protein-protein interactions database. This uses a combination of statistical methods for relevant document retrieval and rule-based methods for bio-molecule name recognition with the aim to find statements about protein interactions. It is reported that the system is able to reduce the time necessary to perform a representative task by 70%, savings 176 person days thanks to its ability to suggest candidate additions. Similar example is the LSAT system (Shah and Bork, 2006) developed for the extraction of alternative transcripts to populate the ASD database (http://www.ebi.ac.uk/asd). The MuteXt system (Horn et al., 2004) extracts from literature point mutations useful for the maintenance of the GPCRDB (www.gpcr.org/7tm/mutation/) and the NucleaRDB (www.receptors.org/NR/mutation/) protein databases. LSAT performs automatic classification of sentences about transcripts and automatic role labelling of text tokens. MuteXt exploits manually encoded regular expressions to capture textual patterns. In both cases, a considerable additional effort is necessary since extracted knowledge requires to be manually combined with sequence and structural information. In fact, the nomenclature adopted for entries in a database often uses wording that is very different from what is explicitly stated in text passages; it is also possible that the information to be extracted has to be deduced from more than one portion of text. Links to entries on different databases should be disambiguated and added to make the annotation result useful for data analysis. These aspects further complicate the feasibility of involving completely automatic tools for database annotation. It appears clear that text mining technology can contribute to this field by operating together with curators to minimize their involvement and speed up the pace of research, but it will not completely substitute their role.

In this work, we tackle the problem of supporting biological database annotation through a data mining approach to Information Extraction (IE). IE is the discipline that aims to extract relevant information from natural language documents. The goal of an IE process is to map unstructured text into structured form, such as databases or knowledge bases, by filling pre-specified information templates describing objects of interest (i.e., entities such as a protein or, more specifically, a kinase) and facts about them (e.g., phosporylation or interaction relationships). This is achieved by supplying quite sophisticated language processing methodologies (e.g., taggers, chunkers, light semantic interpreters, information extraction rules) and domain-specific resource developments (e.g., dictionaries and ontologies). While significant progresses have been made in developing tools for IE from biomedical data, the difficulties encountered in adapting systems to new applications and domains remain the main barriers to their wider use. Thanks to their ability to analyse large volumes of unstructured data, data mining methods are promising candidates to alleviate the burden in developing and customizing IE systems to extract the required domain-specific knowledge. More precisely, we address the problem of mining extraction patterns for information template filling, i.e., to discover conditions to fill slots of templates of interest. Domain experts are asked to define annotation schema in terms of entities and templates (i.e., a set of properties characterizing each entity) and to provide examples of documents labelled with filled templates. Discovered patterns allow the IE system to automatically identify template instances occurring in new documents. We describe a strategy for extraction pattern mining which is based on an Inductive Logic Programming (ILP) approach to recursive theory learning from examples. It is implemented in the ATRE[1] system which works on logical representations of the textual content. Implemented methods are general and domain-dependency is limited to specific thesauri of the biomedical domain. We present a real-world case study concerning the annotation in HmtDB[2] of mitochondrial (mt) DNA. HmtDB stores human mt genomes from healthy or pathological phenotypes and their variability and clinical data associated to diseases are annotated (Attimonelli et al., 2005).

2. Background

Text mining tasks for biomedical literature mining can be grouped into some few main classes (Jensen et al., 2006; Shatkay & Feldman, 2003; Cohen & Hersh, 2005). First, *named entity recognition* aims to identify, within a collection of text, all of the instances of a name for a specific type of thing. The detection of biologically significant entities such as gene and protein names is a very important task for biological database curation since these constitute the main entry points for biological databases. Second, *text classification* attempts to determine automatically whether a document or part of a document discusses a given topic or contains a certain type of information. Accurate text classification systems can be especially valuable to database curators, who may have to review many documents to find a few that contain the kind of information they are collecting in their database. Third, *terminology extraction* aims to collect synonyms and abbreviations of biomedical entities to aid literature search engines and mining systems to be more precise. Fourth, *relationship extraction* systems detect occurrences of a pre-specified type of relationship between a pair of entities of given types. Finally, *hypothesis generation* (Srinivasan, 2004) attempts to uncover relationships that are not present in the text but may be inferred by the presence of other more explicit relationships (e.g., if "BRCA1" and "breast cancer" occur in the same sentence, a relationship between breast cancer and the BRCA1 gene might be assumed).
In the IE literature for biomedicine, little attention has been devoted to classic IE tasks of template filling (Gaizauskas and Wilks, 1998), despite the fact that these naturally fit in database annotation problems. For instance, considering the annotation schema adopted to develop and maintain the IARC TP53 database (http://www-p53.iarc.fr/Help.html#annotations) which compiles all TP53 mutations that have been reported in the

---

[1] http://www.di.uniba.it/~malerba/software/atre
[2] http://www.hmtdb.uniba.it

published literature since 1989, we can observe that main annotations (i.e., mutation, tumour, demographic information, reference and detection method) are structured in form of templates. Each template correlates some entities (e.g., the detection method is added to the database by collecting information on tissue processing, start material, pre-screening method, sequenced material, etc.). Instances of each template can be extracted from a paper pertaining TP53 mutations by analysing relationships implicitly expressed to link target entities. While in a named entity recognition task, the goal is to identify peculiar objects of interest, such as all the disease names occurring in a text, in a template filling task, conceptual relationships between named entities, such as the DNA position and the mutant base pairs characterizing a mutation, should be taken into account.

Several strategies ranging from hand-coded patterns to various machine learning based approaches have been employed to solve this class of problems (Nédellec, 2004). In this work, we follow a different strategy based on the remark that template filling tasks, which are generally based on the results of a named entity recognition task, can be simplified when tagging of named entities is, in its turn, performed by considering conceptual dependencies implicitly defined at either the syntactic or structural level (e.g., the type of mutation is normally reported before the DNA position). Therefore, we adopt a method to learn tagging models in the form of recursive logical theories which can naturally represent conceptual dependencies between named entities. We report results of a first tentative to annotate HmtDB data related to human mtDNA mutations in diseased phenotypes. Thus, the issue is to extract from relevant papers information regarding the mutation and the features associated to the phenotype.

3. Issues

Recursive theory learning falls within the class of supervised concept learning methods, which are supplied with information about objects whose class (or concept) membership is known (i.e., training examples) and produces from this a characterization of each class in some formal language. If U is a universal set of objects (or observations), a concept C can be formalized as a subset of objects in U: $C \subseteq U$. To learn a concept C means to learn to recognize objects in C.

Inductive concept learning. Given a set E of positive and negative examples of a concept C, find a hypothesis H, expressed in a given concept description language L, such that every positive example is covered by H and no negative example is covered by H.

In Inductive Logic Programming (ILP) (Muggleton, 1992; Nienhuys-Cheng and de Wolf, 1997) the formal languages for describing objects and concepts are typically based on Horn clausal logic. More precisely, concepts to be learned are represented by means of predicate symbols, and the result of the learning process is a logical theory. In the IE framework considered in this work, concepts to be learned correspond to entities involved in a template of interest and the logical theory includes clauses expressing the conditions to fill template slots.

The typical formalism adopted in ILP allows the representation of relational (or structural) patterns. In particular, classification rules can express conditions on both properties of single objects and relations between them. In addition classification rules can also express dependencies or relations between concepts. This is a main issue in information extraction from biomedical text since it is the typical application where examples, in addition to their inherent relational structure, present relations to other examples. Some authors have already

used ILP to construct theories for information extraction (Aitken, 2002; Goadrich et al., 2004). In particular, the work by Goadrich et al. (2004) tackles the problem of learning biomedical target relationships (i.e., protein-location) between items of text, namely multi-slot extraction (i.e., two-slot extraction). Our goal is to learn single-slot extraction rules that should take into account implicit relations expressed in the text between entities of the same template. For this reason, we resort to recursive theory induction as learning framework, since recursive theories can express well-defined mutual dependencies between predicates. A different IE problem is handled with ILP in (Ramakrishnan et al., 2007), that is automatic feature construction. The authors employ ILP to define new features given a logical representation of texts and some background knowledge. This is an important problem since one of the issues in IE concerns the definition of the appropriate representation of text. Afterwards, additional issues are raised by the complexity of text processing operations necessary to produce logical representations of textual content. Several sources of difficulties are peculiar of the biomedical language such as ambiguities occurring when the same term denotes more than one semantic class (e.g., p53 is used to specify both a gene and a protein) or when many terms lead to the same semantic class (abbreviations, acronym variations); continuous creation of new biological terms or evolutions of the same biological object (e.g., genes are renamed once their function is known); use of non standard grammatical structures as well as domain-specific jargon; gene symbol polysemy (i.e., a symbol can refer to more than one gene, both within a single species an disparate organisms). This makes the preparation of training data really difficult. A number of controlled vocabularies, lexicons and ontologies for biomedicine which can be exploited both in the data preparation and reasoning steps are available. This further motivates an ILP approach which can naturally handle external background knowledge.
In the rest of the chapter we briefly introduce the HmtDB resource and the information extraction problem involved in curation activities. Our approach to training data preparation and rule learning is proposed. A framework which integrates the proposed solution to support experts in the training of the mining module and to revise annotation results is described.

4. The HmtDB annotation case study

4.1 The biomedical problem

Mitochondrial DNA (mtDNA) has been widely studied both in population genetics and mitochondrial disease studies. In particular, the high mutation rate, absence of recombination, and maternal transmission all make this DNA different from its nuclear counterpart and suitable for evolutionary studies aimed at tracing the migrations which led to the colonization of the various geographic areas of the world. The mtDNA genome of two unrelated individuals may differ in the presence of about 50 mitochondrial Single Nucleotide Polymorphisms (mtSNPs) (Wallace D. C. et al. 1999; Smeitink J. et al., 2001). Study of these polymorphisms in various human populations has allowed us to group differing human mtDNAs in haplogroups, each containing a subset of mtDNA sharing characteristic mutations acquired from the same ancestral mtDNA molecule. Hence, various population lineages may be described by means of a phylogenetic network, in which the top nodes define haplogroups and the tips define haplotypes represented by the sequence of the entire mitochondrial genome in the best situation (Torroni A. et al., 2001). Nevertheless, mitochondrial DNA also plays an important role in the oxidative metabolism of the cell. Hence, mutations occurring in mitochondrial DNA can alter the oxidative phosphorylation, which seriously damages cells and tissues, causing mitochondrial diseases. Mitochondrial disorders - associated with dysfunctions of the Oxidative Phosphorylation (OXPHOS) system - are caused by genetic defects both in the mitochondrial and nuclear genome, leading to energy metabolism errors, and have an estimated frequency of 1 out of 10000 live births. Due to the important role played by the OXPHOS system in ATP production, the causes and effects of mitochondrial disorders are extremely heterogeneous and complex. This explains the pressing need for further research on this topic, despite the many studies on mitochondrial disorders published in the last 20 years. In this scenario HmtDB (Attimonelli M. et al., 2005) plays an important role, gathering all complete human mitochondrial genomes worldwide distributed and enriching sequence information with statistically validated variability data estimated through the application of specific algorithms implemented in an automatically running Variability Generation Work Flow (VGWF). Knowledge through HmtDB of the variability of specific position of the genome is highly informative, as shown in a recent study by Accetturo et al. (2006), which demonstrates that continent specific high variability values can act as haplogroup markers.

4.2 Database description

HmtDB consists of a database of Human Mitochondrial Genomes annotated with population and variability data, the latter estimated through the application of a new approach based on site-specific nucleotidic and aminoacidic variability calculation (Pesole & Saccone, 2001; Horner & Pesole, 2003). Currently, HmtDB stores data from entire human mt genomes only, while a great quantity of published data related to single human mtDNA mutations and associated to clinical studies available through PubMed are not annotated in HmtDB.
In particular, HmtDB

- collects and integrates the publicly available human mitochondrial genomes data;
- produces and provides the scientific community with site-specific nucleotide and aminoacid variability data estimated on all the collected human mitochondrial genome sequences;
- allows all researchers to analyse their own human mitochondrial sequences (both complete and partial mitochondrial genomes) in order to automatically detect the nucleotide variants compared to the revised Cambridge Reference Sequence (rCRS) (Andrews et al., 1999) and to predict their haplogroup paternity.

At present, HmtDB contains 4061 human mitochondrial genomes. They are stored and analysed as a whole dataset and grouped into continent-specific subsets (AF: Africa (347 mtGenomes), AM: America (216), AS: Asia (1493), EU: Europe (1233), OC: Oceania (133)); 729 genomes are unclassified as regards the geographic origin of individual donors of DNA. Human mtDNA is composed by 16569 nucleotides, of which 4542 (data from HmtDB) present variability values differing from 0.
HmtDB can be queried according to different criteria combined among them through the AND Boolean Operator. The most important selection criteria are listed in table 1.
Multi-alignment and site-variability analysis tools included in HmtDB are clustered in two workflows: the Variability Generation Work Flow (VGWF) and the Classification Work Flow (CWF), which are applied both to human mitochondrial genomes stored in the database and to newly sequenced genomes submitted by users, respectively.

Selection criteria in HmtDB	Meaning of criteria
Subjects' geographical origin	Continent and Country origin of the subject
Haplogroup Code	Code assigned by population genetists to human mtDNA genomes clustered according to common mtSNPs
SNP Position	Position of the genome where variation is sought
Variation type	Transition, trasversion, deletion, insertion
Subject Age (year)	Age of the subject when DNA was extracted
Subject Sex	Sex of the subject donor of the DNA
DNA source	Blood, tumor tissue, buccal swab, blood, etc
Individual type	Returns genomes correlated to the selected phenotype: Normal, Patient, Control or Disease Phenotype
References	Journal, Authors, Haplotype paper code, PubMedID

Table 1. Database search criteria

4.3 Database annotation

HmtDB currently stores data derived from the knowledge of complete mt genomes. 635 out of the 4061 genomes stored in HmtDB are related to disease phenotypes associated to 13 different diseases. This last datum highlights the real need of the experience presented here. The number of mt diseases is far higher than 13, and literature reports data from single mt mutations screened in families and populations to assess associations of mutation with mt diseases. This type of information is available through MITOMAP[3], but here the mtSNP is associated with the various phenotypes and literature data in a qualitative way and thus the data structure does not allow any quantitative estimate of the occurrence of the mutation in different phenotypes and different populations. Our goal is to include in HmtDB data extracted from the great quantity of papers available on the topic "mtDNA mutation and disease" and to integrate the data, structured and analysed with statistical tools, with the variability data derived from the human mt complete genomes already in HmtDB, thus allowing a comprehensive study of mtDNA variability related to population genetics and mt diseases. Until now, this has been partially carried out through manual inspection of mitochondrial literature. We are currently testing the text mining approach proposed in this work to perform automatic extraction of information from PubMed. Desired information concerns mutations, method of detecting mutations, and demographic details. More precisely, the nature of a mutation (e.g, insertion, deletion, transversion, etc.), mutant base (i.e. nucleotide), involved gene (i.e., locus), type of pathology, age, sex and nationality of patients/individuals, method and source of analysis (e.g., tissue, blood, etc.) are all categories of terms to be automatically identified in texts.

4.4 Literature preparation

Generating a reliable training set is a slow and labour-intensive task since there are no publicly available datasets about mtDNA annotation from the literature. For this aim,

[3] http://www.mitomap.org/

HmtDB curators have performed several steps: (1) retrieval of relevant literature, (2) definition of annotation schema, (3) collection of domain-dependent language resources, (4) manual annotation of text. The first and the last steps were the most demanding. To retrieve literature pertaining to the HmtDB scope, PubMed was queried for "mitochondrial disease", looking for papers published after 2000 concerning human mtDNA and where mutations involving mitochondrial genes were studied. Papers that do not report strictly clinical data were discarded. All papers in which mitochondrial mutations and diseases were associated on the basis of alternative information such as biochemical experiments, drug treatment or therapy, species different from the human type, etc. were also excluded from the dataset as well. Then, a suitable annotation schema was defined. Two main schema appear to meet the database annotation requirements: one to describe features reported on the *mutation* and the other describing *subjects* from whom the DNA comes. As shown in table 2, the mutation template includes ten categories of information, while the subjects template involves seven.

Template	Entity	Definition
mutation	heteroplasmy	Quantity of mutant mtDNA (%)
	locus	Gene where mutation is found
	novelty	Flag stating that mutation is published for the first time
	pathology	Disease or syndrome (phenotype)
	penetrance	Different pathological phenotype expression
	position	Nucleotide position in mtDNA where mutation is located
	risk	Probability of expressing a pathological phenotype
	substitution	Nucleotide changed, compared with reference sequence (rCRS)
	type	Type of mutation
	type_position	Type and position encoded by a single alphanumeric string
subjects	age	Age of the subject
	category	Single patient or pedigree
	gender	Gender of subject
	method	Biomolecular method to detect mutation
	nationality	Geographic origin
	number	Number of subjects affected
	source	Biological source of mtDNA

Table 2. Database annotation schema

Domain-dependent dictionaries to guide the annotation process are carefully selected by curators. Some dictionaries are obtained by directly extracting controlled vocabularies stored in the database, like methods, diseases, ethnic groups, locus and sources.

In the final step, selected papers were manually analysed to identify pieces of text satisfying the annotation schema. This was the most laborious phase, as curators are asked to perform manual tagging in the most homogeneous way by inevitably facing different difficulties due to the non-standard way of publishing information. A first problem is raised by gene referencing, since each gene typically has several names and abbreviations (e.g., the ATP6 mt gene can be also mentioned as "ATP synthase F0 subunit 6" or "MTATPase6" or "adenosine triphosphatase 6" as well) and sometimes authors and publishers do not agree on standards. A mt gene abbreviation dictionary has been prepared by curators to give direction to a locus annotation strategy. However, the most complex activity concerns the identification of the pathology associated with the mutation. This results to be very hard because many different clinical presentations of mitochondrial diseases are possible. Hence, the diagnosis is often not really established by the authors themselves, while one or more terms are used to describe a large collection of disorders. For instance, in the following abstract:

"The authors describe a novel pathogenic G5540A transition in the mitochondrial transfer RNA (tRNA)Trp gene of a sporadic encephalomyopathy characterized by spinocerebellar ataxia. Clinical features also included neurosensorial deafness, peripheral neuropathy, and dementia"

the pathological condition is defined by a standard "encephalomyopathy" disease with additional symptoms such as "spinocerebellar ataxia", "neurosensorial deafness", etc. In addition, typical mitochondrial disease names are obtained by grouping different symptoms (e.g., the "MELAS" syndrome is considered in the case of "mitochondrial myopathy, encephalopathy, lactic acidosis, and strokelike episodes") but a standard nomenclature of mitochondrial diseases is not available in the scientific community; in fact, there are also cases, as in the abstract reported below, where atypical combinations of symptoms are connected to the mutation.

"Mitochondrial cytochrome b mutations have been reported to have a homogenous phenotype of pure exercise intolerance. We describe a novel mutation in the cytochrome b gene of mitochondrial DNA (A15579G) associated with a selective decrease of muscle complex III activity in a patient who, besides severe exercise intolerance, also has multisystem manifestations (deafness, mental retardation, retinitis pigmentosa, cataract, growth retardation, epilepsy)".

To manage such cases, the MITOMAP annotation of diseases associated with mtDNA mutations from the perspective of phenotype was adopted as a reference. There are also some papers describing not only a patient but their family pedigrees, which lead to very heterogeneous clinical presentations also creating coreference resolution problems. E.g., *"The proband showed isolated, spastic paraparesis. A brother, who had suffered from a multisystem progressive disorder, ultimately died of cardiomyopathy. Another brother is healthy. The proband's mother showed truncal ataxia, dysarthria, severe hearing loss, mental regression, ptosis, ophthalmoparesis, distal cyclones, and diabetes mellitus. ... Sequence analysis of mtDNA showed a heteroplasmic mutation of the tRNA(Ile) gene (G4284A). ..."*

The curators decided to consider the abstract and the title of each article, since other mutations and populations that are not being studied are often cited in the introduction and discussion sections of papers. Indeed, selecting relevant portions of text is a prerequisite step for IE, since the sparseness of data and lack of robustness of IE methods makes them inapplicable to large corpora or irrelevant texts.

5. The approach

5.1 Problem definition

The problem we are addressing is the typical template filling task reported in the IE literature (Gaizauskas & Wilks, 1998). This means that, rather than learning one extraction pattern for each slot of interest, a single model for all slots of interest is learned. Dependencies among facts are also investigated in the context of template filling, since the pattern should link isolated facts in some way.

Let us consider the following example of a text fragment of the collection described in the previous section:
*"Cytoplasts from two unrelated patients with MELAS (mitochondrial myopathy, encephalopathy, lactic acidosis, and strokelike episodes) harboring an A-*G transition at nucleotide position 3243 in the tRNALeU(UUR) gene of the mitochondrial genome were fused with human cells lacking endogenous mitochondrial DNA (mtDNA)"*
Here "MELAS" is an instance of the *pathology* associated to the mutation in question, "A-*G" is an instance of the *substitution* that causes the mutation, "transition" is the *type* of the mutation, "3243" stands for the *position* in the DNA where the mutation occurs, "tRNALeU(UUR)" is the *gene* associated with the mutation, "two" is the number of *subjects* under study. An extraction pattern relating *type* and *substitution* items is exemplified by the following two Horn clauses:

```
substitution(X) ← follows(Y,X), type(Y)
type(X) ← distance(X,Y,3), position(Y),
             word_between(X,Y,''nucleotide position'')
```

The first clause states that a token X is recognized as the *substitution* (i.e., which nucleotide is substituted by which other, A in G in the specimen text) if it is followed by a token Y which has been recognized as mutation *type* (transition). The second clause states that X fills the mutation *type* (transition) slot if it is three words far from a token Y that has been associated with the mutation *position* (3243) slot and there is the intermediate word "nucleotide position".
It should be noted that, in the above example, some dependencies between slots of the same template (mutation) are shown. As previously mentioned, learning information extraction rules which express these dependencies may lead to more accurate models, which reflect some co-occurrence of named entities in the text. In addition, when automated annotation is performed, context-sensitive recognition of named entities is possible, thanks to learned models which reflect dependencies among annotation classes. A solution to the problem of searching for concept dependencies (i.e., mutual recursion) in the space of candidate patterns and to reason in the presence of relational knowledge is provided by the learning algorithm reported in Section 5.4.

5.2 Data preprocessing

Texts are preprocessed by means of natural language facilities provided in the GATE (General Architecture for Text Engineering) system (Cunningham et al., 2002). We exploit the ANNIE (A Nearly-New IE system) component which contains finite-state algorithms and the JAPE (a Java Annotation Patterns Engine) language which is also a finite-state transduction engine to recognize regular expressions. We use ANNIE to perform tokenization, sentence splitting, part-of-speech tagging, general purpose named-entity recognition (e.g., persons, locations, organizations) and mapping into dictionaries. We use both predefined dictionaries available with ANNIE (e.g., organization names, job titles, geographical locations, dates, etc.) and domain-specific dictionaries prepared by curators. General domain dictionaries are used to clarify some terms (e.g., places and geographical locations are useful in recognizing terms about the ethnic origin of the diseased sample). Domain-specific dictionaries are flat dictionaries of canonical forms and variants of names of mitochondrial genetics. Some general-purpose biological dictionaries were also considered e.g., those on enzymes, units of measurement, and nucleic acids. They are exploited to reduce data heterogeneity and to perform syntactic and semantic normalization, such as rough resolution of acronyms which, as already stated, are one of the sources of redundancy and ambiguity. JAPE grammars have been defined to identify appositions occurring in texts as well as some numeric and alphanumeric strings which are frequent in this domain. Lastly, stopwords (e.g., articles, adverbs, and prepositions) are removed and stemming is performed by means of the Porter's algorithm for English texts (Porter, 1997).

5.3 Data representation

In this work, the units of analysis are sentences, which are composed of tokens. Each sentence or token is given a unique identifier (in the context of an abstract or a title of selected papers) based on its ordering within the given text. The relational (or structural) representation of a sentence is described by a set of predicates expressing properties of occurring tokens and relations between them.

Properties, which are represented by unary function symbols (or descriptors), express statistical (e.g., token frequency), lexical (e.g., alphanumeric, capitalized token), structural (e.g., structure of complex tokens such as alphanumeric string, abbreviations, acronyms, hyphenated tokens), syntactical (e.g., singular/plural proper/not proper nouns, base/conjugated verbs) and domain-specific knowledge (e.g., an entity belonging to a dictionary). More precisely, the descriptor *class* specifies the category of the described text (i.e., abstract, title, results, etc.) and expresses information on the localization of annotations in documents. The descriptor *word_to_string* maps an identifier to the corresponding stemmed token, while *word_frequency* expresses the relative frequency of a token in the given text, and *type_of* refers to morphological features and takes values in the set {allcaps, mixedcaps, upperinitial, numeric, percentage, alphanumeric, real number}. Parts-of-speech are encoded by the descriptor *type_pos*, and semantics is added by the descriptor *word_category*.

Binary descriptors express structural properties such as the composition of sentences in passages of text and tokens in chunks or directly in sentences. Indeed, the following descriptors have been defined: *part_of*, which lists tokens composing a sentence, and *follows*, which relates a token to its direct successor. Complex tokens (e.g., A-*G) are described by some descriptors (e.g., *middle_is_char*, *first_is_numeric*) defining the morphological nature of an alphanumeric string. Another form of relational knowledge concerns domain dictionaries and expresses the distance between two categorized tokens in the context of a sentence (*distance_word_category*).

For the training data, only sentences containing at least a positive example of concepts to be learned are considered. Henceforth, they are called target sentences. No relation between target sentences is currently considered: that is, the extraction of slot fillers remains local to sentences.

An example of relational description generated for the target sentence reported in Section 5.1 is the following:

```
annotation(3)=no tag,
...
annotation(7)=pathology,
annotation(8)=no_tag,
```

```
...
annotation(13)=substitution,
annotation(14)=type,
annotation(15)=no_tag,
...,
annotation(17)=position,
annotation(18)=locus,
...,
annotation(30)=no_tag
                    ←
class(2)=abstract, part_of(2,3)=true, ..., part_of(2,30)=true,
word_to_string(3)=cytoplast, ..., word_to_string(14)=transition,
..., word_to_string(30)=cell,
type_of(3)=upperinitial, ..., type_of(29)=alphanumeric,
type_pos(3)=nnp, ..., type_pos(30)=nns,
word_frequency(3)=1, ..., word_frequency(30)=2,
word_category(7)=disease, ..., word_category(28)=nucleic_acid,
distance_word_category(7,9)=2, ..., distance_word_category(27,28)=1,
follows(3,4)=true, follows(4,5)=true, ..., follows(29,30)=true
```

It is in form of a multiple-head clause (Levi & Sirovich, 1976), where the body (left) part lists literals describing properties of the sentence and the head (right) part states annotations occurring in the sentence. Constant 2 denotes the described sentence, which belongs to an abstract of the collection. Constants 3, 4, ..., 30 denote identifiers of tokens in the described sentence.

We observe that the particular form of literal used in this work, namely $f(t_1, \ldots ,t_n)=Value$, where f is an n-ary descriptor, t_i's are constant terms, and *Value* is one of the possible values of f's domain, can be easily reported to the typical notation adopted in predicate calculus $p_{f=Value}(t_1, \ldots ,t_n)$, where $p_{f=Value}$ is the n-ary predicate associated to the pair $\langle f, Value \rangle$.

Background knowledge is also defined to support qualitative reasoning in the learning phase. This includes a number of Horn clauses such as the following, which express the synonymy between (stemmed) biological terms:

```
word_to_string(X)=transit ← word_to_string(X)=transversion
word_to_string(X)=substitut ← word_to_string(X)=replac
```

A transitive definition of the relation of "indirect successor" was also defined to unburden the representation language, which includes only the direct successor relation:

```
tfollows(X,Y)=true ← follows(X,Y)=true
tfollows(X,Y)=true ← follows(X,Z)=true, tfollows(Z,Y)=true
```

Lastly, a typified form of both direct and transitive successor relations is introduced to compact knowledge encapsulated in rules further. Some examples are reported in the following:

```
follows_string_jj(Y)=Z ← word_to_string(X)=Z, follows(X,Y)=true,
                          type_pos(Y)=jj
follows_nn_string(X)=Z ← type_pos(X)=nn, follows(X,Y)=true,
                          word_to_string(Y)=Z
tfollows_vb_nn(X,Y)=true ← type_pos(X)=vb, tfollows(X,Y)=true,
```

```
                                       type_pos(Y)=nn
tfollows_jj_nn(X,Y)=true ← type_pos(X)=jj, tfollows(X,Y)=true,
                                       type_pos(Y)=nn
```

The first two clauses express the direct successor relations between a generic string and an adjective or a noun, while the last two clauses specify the transitive successor relations for verb-noun and adjective-noun pairs, respectively.

5.4 Rule learning

Logical theories used for the annotation of text are automatically induced from training data by means of the ILP system ATRE (Malerba, 2003). In this application, each concept plays the role of an annotation class (i.e., template slot) and each textual object can be associated with at most one concept, i.e., concepts are considered mutually exclusive. The learning problem solved by ATRE can be formulated as follows:

Given

- A set of *target* predicates $p_1, p_2, \ldots, p_r$ to be learned
- A set of positive (negative) examples E_i^+ (E_i^-) for each predicate p_i, $1 \le i \le r$
- A background theory *BK*
- A language of hypotheses L_H that defines the space of hypotheses S_H

Find

a (possibly recursive) logical theory $T \in S_H$ defining the predicates $p_1, p_2, \ldots, p_r$ (that is, $\delta(T)=\{p_1, p_2, \ldots, p_r\}$) such that the following two conditions hold:

a. for each *i*, $1 \le i \le r$, $BK \cup T \models E_i^+$ (*completeness* property) and

b. $BK \cup T \not\models E_i^-$ (*consistency* property).

The logical theory T is a set of first-order definite clauses (Lloyd, 1987), like those reported above. The set of concepts to be learned is defined by means of a set of literals of the type annotation(X)=*annotation class*. No clause is generated for the concept annotation(X)=*no tag*. Each unit of analysis, which corresponds to a sentence, is represented by means of the set of positive/negative examples related to the sentence as well as the set of ground literals in the BK which describe properties and relations among tokens in the sentence. The set of literals associated to a unit of analysis is called *object* and is formally represented as a ground (i.e., without variables) multiple-head clause. Therefore, ATRE's representation of training data is individual-centered (Blockeel & Sebag, 2003) and this has both theoretical (PAC-learnability) and computational advantages (smaller hypothesis space and more efficient search).

The background knowledge *BK* may also include a set of Horn clauses which define new predicates, not used for the description of training objects but deemed useful for the formulation of the logical theory used in the annotation process. Examples are the *tfollows* predicates defined in the previous section. An example of Horn clause which defines the predicate *char_number_char* is reported in the following:

```
char_number_char(X) ← first_is_char(X), middle_is_numeric(X),
    last_is_char(X)
```

The satisfaction of the completeness and consistency properties guarantees the correctness of the induced theory with respect to the sets of positive and negative examples, but not necessarily with respect to new instances of the target predicates. The selection of the clause

in T is made on the basis of an inductive bias. For example, clauses which cover a high number of positive examples and a low number of negative examples may be preferred to others.
At high-level, the learning strategy implemented in ATRE is *sequential covering* (or *separate-and-conquer*) algorithms (Mitchell, 1997), that is, one clause is learned (conquer stage), covered examples are removed (separate stage) and the process is iterated on the remaining examples. More precisely, a logical theory T is built step by step, starting from an empty theory T_0, and adding a new clause at each step. In this way we get a sequence of theories

$$T_0 = \varnothing, T_1, \ldots, T_i, T_{i+1}, \ldots, T_n = T,$$

such that $T_{i+1} = T_i \cup \{C\}$ for some clause C.
The conquer stage aims at finding the best clause C to add. The search for this clause is made among those that cover specific positive examples, called *seeds*, which have not been covered by T_i yet.
The most important novelty of the learning strategy implemented in ATRE is embedded in the design of the conquer stage. Indeed, the separate-and-conquer strategy is traditionally adopted by single predicate learning systems which generate predicate definitions, that is, sets of clauses with the same predicate in the head. In ATRE, clauses generated at each step may have different predicates in their heads. In addition, *the body of the clause generated at the i-th step may include all target predicates* $p_1, p_2, \ldots, p_r$ *for which at least a clause has been added to the theory* T_i. In this way, dependencies between target predicates can be expressed by learned theories.
The order in which clauses of distinct target predicates have to be generated is not known in advance. This means that the actual dependencies between target concepts which a learned theory can express have to be discovered by the system and is not specified by the user. For this reason, it is necessary to generate clauses with different predicates in the head and then to pick one of them at the end of each step of the separate-and-conquer strategy. Since the generation of a clause depends on the chosen seed, several seeds (at least one, if any, per target predicate) have to be chosen among those still uncovered. Therefore, the search space is actually a forest of as many search-trees (called *specialization hierarchies*) as the number of chosen seeds. In each search tree a directed arc from a node (clause) C to a node C_0 exists if C_0 is obtained from C by a adding a literal (C is specialized into C_0).
The forest can be processed in parallel by as many concurrent tasks as the number of search-trees (hence the name of *separate-and-parallel-conquer* for this search strategy). Each task traverses the specialization hierarchy top-down (or general-to-specific), but synchronizes traversal with the other tasks at each level. Initially, some clauses at depth one in the forest are examined concurrently. Each task is actually free to adopt its own search strategy, and to decide which clauses are worth to be tested. If none of the tested clauses is consistent, clauses at depth two are considered. Search proceeds towards deeper and deeper levels of the specialization hierarchies until at least a user-defined number of consistent clauses is found. Task synchronization is performed after that all "relevant" clauses at the same depth have been examined. A supervisor task decides whether the search should be continued or not, according to the results returned by the concurrent tasks. When the search is stopped, the supervisor selects the "best" consistent clause according to the inductive bias specified by the user (e.g., the clause which covers a high number of positive examples and a low number of negative examples). This search strategy provides us with a solution to the

problem of *interleaving* the induction of distinct target predicate definitions. It also has the advantage that simpler consistent clauses are found first, independently of the predicates to be learned. Finally, the synchronization allows tasks to save much computational effort when the distribution of consistent clauses in the levels of the different search-trees is uneven.

A more detailed description of the search strategy implemented in ATRE and its optimization through caching techniques is reported in (Malerba, 2003; Berardi et al., 2004).

5.5 The architecture of BEE

The BEE[4] (Biomedical Entity Extractor) system was developed to implement the approach described in the previous sections. BEE supports users in:

- defining annotation schema;
- manually annotating texts to provide mining examples for user classes;
- customizing linguistic analysis through dictionary (gazetteers) management;
- automatically generating data for mining;
- using learned theories to perform automatic annotation of new texts;
- visualizing and revising annotation results.

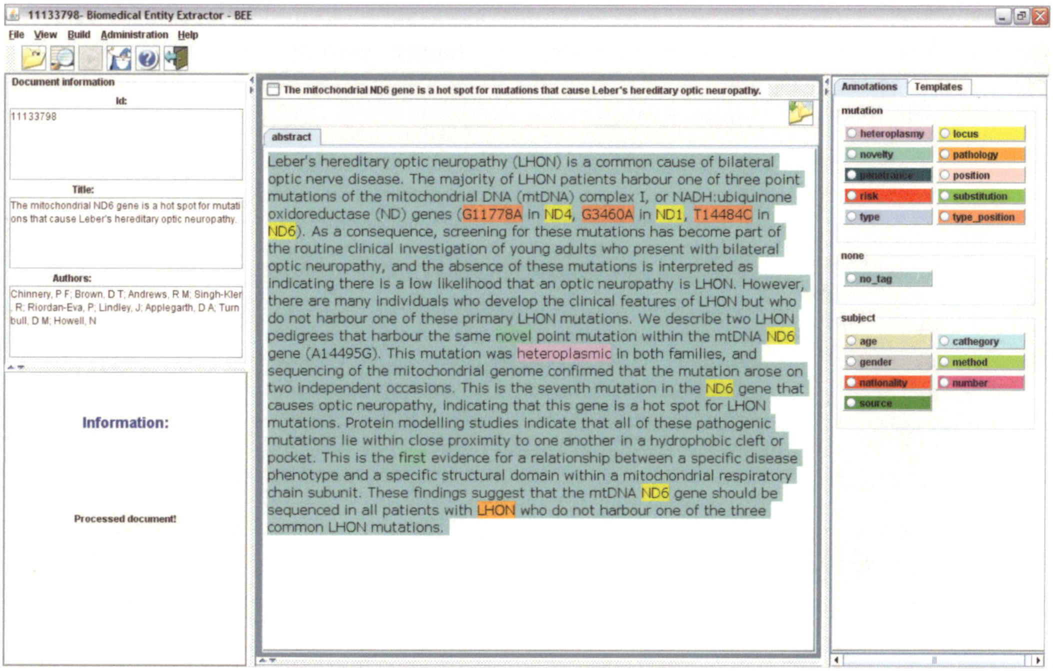

Fig. 1. BEE GUI

The BEE system includes a Graphical User Interface (GUI) which provides the user with facilities to customize the system for the specific information extraction problem. In

[4] http://www.di.uniba.it/~malerba/software/BEE

particular, domain dictionaries are submitted by selecting flat files and assigning a lookup name to each dictionary. Annotation schema are manually defined by grouping user-defined categories of named entities into templates. The GUI includes a wizard which supports the user in managing training sessions, i.e., data selection, choice of concepts to be learned, definition of learning parameters, specification of background knowledge, and running and monitoring learning tasks. Finally, the GUI allows users to manually associate tokens with categories on the basis of text pre-processing results, as shown in Figure 1.
The general architecture of the system is shown in Figure 2. The System Manager works by allowing user interaction and by coordinating the activity of all other components. It interfaces the system with the data persistence layer to store (1) information on texts concerning pre-processing results, feature extraction, associated annotations; (2) linguistic resources (i.e., gazetteers, acronym dictionaries, grammars); (3) annotation schemas of the biomedical problem at hand; (4) learned theories. The User Manager supports operations aiming to customize the system on the specific user-defined biomedical problem. The Text Processor is in charge of data elaboration and mapping into the learning descriptions operations described in Section 5.2 and 5.3. The output of this module allows users to invoke both the Recognition Module and the Learning Module through the GUI. The former is responsible for clause application and automatic association of annotation slots on text, the latter performs all the activities necessary to support learning sessions. Actually, the Recognition Module is able to match body parts of clauses available in the learned knowledge base with descriptions of new texts.

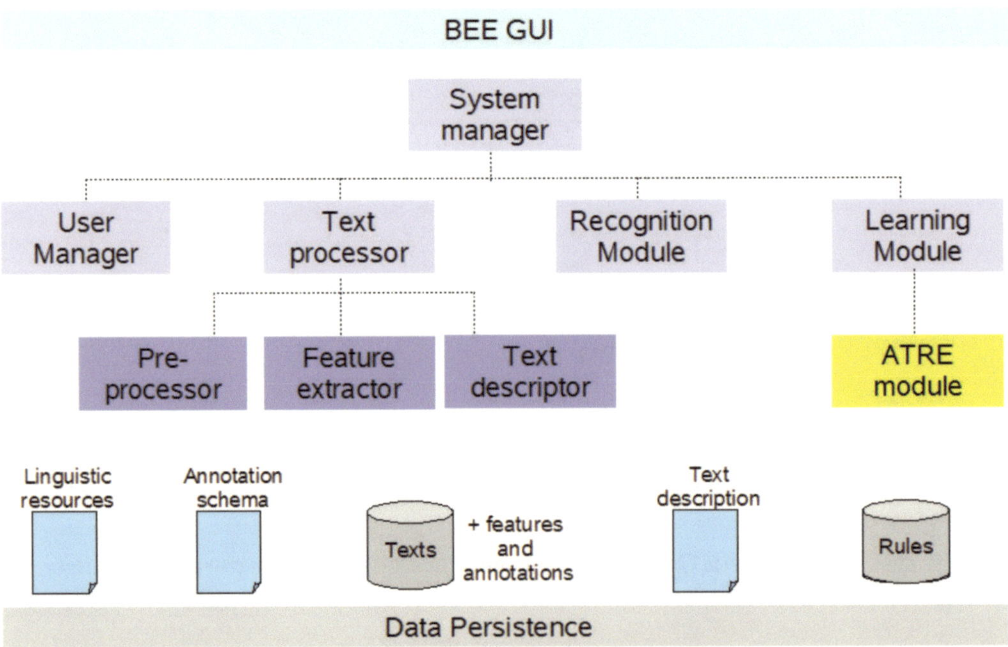

Fig. 2. BEE architecture

BEE is a java standalone application since it is conceived as an integrated environment for information extraction from texts, where curators define the annotation problem, prepare data, revise results, and learning experts manage learning operations. A web service version including the text processor and the recognition module is also available for collaborative environments. This web service is separately trained on application domains and made available together with knowledge bases.

6. Experiments

Fine tuning of the system on the HmtDB case study has been carried out within activities concerning the LIBI[5] (International Laboratory for BioInformatics) project. This projects aims at designing and setting up an advanced IT platform to support a newly-conceived Bioinformatics and Computational Biology laboratory "without walls". This includes tools enabling the deployment and maintenance of genomic, proteomic and transcriptomic databases, as well as the design and execution of new algorithms, and software for the analysis of genomes and their expression products. A collaborative environment has also been developed to boost both knowledge and resource sharing: researchers can share both data analysis tools, in the form of simple or composed (workflow) services and data, which are accessed through data federation mechanisms that allow their dislocation and heterogeneity to be bypassed. Available analysis tools cover not only typical bioinformatics algorithms supporting *in silico* molecular data handling and analyses, but also a suite of general-purpose text and data mining algorithms that enhance analysis capabilities of biological data managed by means of the federated database. Such an environment, where mining tools can benefit from the aggregated view of a plethora of different information sources provided by the federated database, is an ideal candidate where prototyping and testing systems devoted to semi-automated database annotation. To accomplish such a challenging task, data curation is one of the preliminary key steps. To this end, HmtDB has been federated together with other specialized data sources (including PubMed) and interfaced by the BEE miner to support mitochondrial genome curation activities.
We conducted an experiment on 130 full papers concerning mitochondrial mutations carefully selected for the annotation of HmtDB. In this phase, experiments were conducted on the mutation template, where benefits of the proposed learning method can be observed. Conversely, most of the issues of annotating subjects information can be almost fully satisfied by using regular expressions. Entities with a very low distribution of examples (i.e., risk, penetrance, novelty, heteroplasmy) were not considered in the experiment reported in this chapter. From the set of relevant papers, we obtained 368 target sentences out of 1040 sentences. Considering the total number of tokens used to describe sentences, the number of annotated tokens was 890, that is, 2.42 tokens per target sentence and 6.86 per paper, namely about 20.5% of the total number of tokens considered in the experiment. The remaining tokens, i.e., 3461, were considered as non-tagged (i.e., as negative examples for all concepts to be learned). Trainers have tagged a single occurrence of target concepts in the papers by preferring occurrences reported in the neighbourhood of other target concepts to be learned in order to discover intra-sentence dependence.

[5] http://www.libi.it

Performances are evaluated by means of a 5-fold cross-validation, that is, the set of 130 papers is firstly divided into five folds (see Table 3), and then, for every fold, ATRE is trained on the remaining folds and tested on the hold-out fold.

Results were evaluated according to several criteria. For each concept, we computed both the number of omission and commission errors and the value of precision and recall. Omission errors occur when annotations of tokens are missed, while commission errors occur when wrong annotations are "recommended" by some rule. The omission measure is reported as the ratio of the number of omission errors and the number of positive examples, and the commission measure as the ratio of the number of commission errors and the total number of examples. The recall measure is computed as the ratio of positive examples correctly annotated (i.e., true positives) and the sum of true positives and false negatives (i.e., omission errors). The precision measure is computed as the ratio of true positives and the sum of true positives and false positives (i.e., commission errors). The F-measure is the weighted harmonic mean of precision and recall, that is:

$$F - measure = \frac{precision \cdot recall}{precision + recall}$$

Experimental results are reported in Table 4 for each fold, while Table 5 reports accuracy values for each class.

Fold	#sentence	#locus	#position	#substitution	#type	#type_position	#pathology	#no_tag
1	71	37	12	5	8	31	69	650
2	76	39	8	6	5	56	73	735
3	75	49	6	6	7	57	83	712
4	70	35	7	6	10	39	52	633
5	76	42	15	8	13	39	67	731
Total	368	202	48	31	43	222	344	3461

Table 3. Distribution of examples per folds

Fold	#locus		#position		#substitution		#type		#type_position		#pathology	
	om	**com**	**om**	**com**	**om**	**com**	**om**	**com**	**om**	**com**	**om**	**com**
1	10.81	0.26	41.66	0	60	0.25	0	0.25	19.35	0.13	43.48	3.63
2	23.08	0.23	62.5	0.11	66.67	0	0	0	8.93	0.46	43.83	3.06
3	16.33	0.11	66.67	0	50	0	0	0	10.53	1.16	50.6	2.15
4	11.43	0.13	28.57	0	16.57	0	0	0	41.03	0.27	55.77	3.7
5	9.52	0.11	66.67	0.11	50	0	7.69	0	30.77	0.46	44.78	2.12
Avg.	*14.23*	*0.17*	*53.21*	*0.04*	*48.67*	*0.05*	*1.54*	*0.05*	*22.12*	*0.5*	*47.69*	*2.93*
St.D.	*5.58*	*0.07*	*17.24*	*0.06*	*19.24*	*0.11*	*3.44*	*011*	*13.68*	*0.4*	*5.36*	*0.77*

Table 4. Experimental results (percentage values): Average number and standard deviation of omission errors over positive examples and commission errors over negative examples

Category	Precision		Recall		F-measure	
	Avg	St. Dev.	Avg	St. Dev.	Avg	St. Dev.
locus	95.9	1.84	85.43	5.7	90.30	3.72
position	91.67	11.79	46.79	17.24	60.93	16.44
substitution	90	22.36	51.33	19.24	63.74	18.14
type	96	8.94	98.46	3.44	96.98	4.84
type_position	90.13	4.88	77.3	13.73	82.59	8.17
pathology	60.37	9.23	52.06	5.13	55.72	6.09

Table 5. Experimental results (percentage values): Mean and standard deviation of Precision, Recall and F-measure (β=1)

Fold	#locus	#position	#substitution	#type	#type_position	#pathology
1	165/35	36/15	26/11	34/5	191/52	275/116
2	163/30	40/14	25/10	37/5	166/54	271/119
3	153/36	42/13	25/10	36/5	165/33	261/110
4	167/38	41/16	25/11	32/5	183/47	292/120
5	160/37	33/15	23/11	29/4	183/39	277/116
Avg.	*4.62*	*2.65*	*2.35*	*7.01*	*4.07*	*2.37*

Table 6. Complexity of learned theories: number of positive examples over number of covered clauses per concept and average values

Performance variability for some concepts (e.g., *position, substitution, pathology*) among folds is due to different degrees of data sparseness, such as heterogeneity of examples and low percentage of positive observations available. However, the percentage of commission errors is very low with respect to that of omission errors (the system misses annotations rather than suggesting wrong ones) independently of the fold. This means that learned clauses are quite specific. By considering the complexity of learned theories (see Table 6), coverage rate can explain recall values. The best performances are obtained on the *type* class whose examples are the most homogeneous. Conversely, the worst performances are related to the annotation of a *pathology*. Actually, learning tasks for the *pathology* class appear to be intrinsically more complex, since we observe the highest percentage of commission errors despite the highest percentage of positive examples available. As regards the percentage of omission errors, we note that, while this is positively correlated to the number of discovered clauses, it is not correlated to the number of positive examples. This confirms the complexity of this annotation task. Low recall values and overfitted theories reflect difficulties mentioned in Section 4.4 concerning the variety of morpho-syntactic variations on the same pathology name, which leads to heterogeneous representations of examples. By scanning the learned theories, we observe that, for some classes, namely *substitution* and *position*, many clauses do take into account only lexical information specified by the predicate *word_to_string*. Indeed, on these entities the system performs the highest number of omissions and very few commissions. Concerning the *locus* and *type_position* entities, some omission errors were performed, in fact, good values of coverage rate are reported for theories learned for these concepts. By observing learned clauses, we found several clauses depending on lexical information but also some more general clauses as the followings:

```
annotation(X1)=locus ←follows_string_nn(X2)=mutation,
    word_category(X1)=gene, tfollows(X2,X1)=true

annotation(X1)=type_position ← char_number_char(X1)=true

annotation(X1)=type_position ← tfollows_string_nn(X2)=trnaser,
    type_of(X1)=alphanumeric
```

The first clause states that X1 is labelled as *locus* if it belongs to the gene category and it occurs in the sentence after the word "mutation". The second clause states that X1 is labelled as *type_position* if it is an alphanumeric token composed by a char, a number and another char. This is one of the first clauses that ATRE adds to the learned theory and covers many examples. Actually, information on type and position of a mutation is tokens such as A1262G, which means that A is substituted by G at position 1262 of the DNA. The third clause concerns the same concept and states that X1 is labelled as *type_position* if it is an alphanumeric token which is followed by the string "trnaser". This matches patterns where type and position information occurs in the neighbourhood of gene names (e.g., trnaser).
Clauses stating dependencies between these two concepts have been also discovered:

```
annotation(X1)=type_position ← annotation(X2)=locus,
    type_of(X1)=alphanumeric,
    distance_word_category(X2,X1)in[1.0..1.0]
```

It states that X1 is labelled as *type_position* if it is an alphanumeric string at distance one from a token labelled as *locus*.
Results show that annotation of concepts suffering from name mention ambiguity depends on the efficacy of the text pre-processing module in conjunction with the ability to exploit specialized lexical resources. Previous experiments, which are described in (Berardi & Malerba, 2007) where the usefulness of recursive theories is investigated, lead to different results. In particular, for concepts such as *type*, *locus* and *type_position* we got opposite findings since learned theories were very specific and constrained to lexical information. The new gene name dictionaries and the revised method for text tokenization and lexical patterns identification adopted to run experiments described in this chapter are able to keep under control morpho-syntactic variability of terms belonging to these classes.
Other meaningful clauses discovered in this experiment follow:

```
annotation(X1)=position ← annotation(X2)=substitution,
    tfollows_cd_nn(X1,X2)=true
```

This clause states that X1 is annotated as *position* if it is a numeric token that precedes a noun which has been annotated as *substitution.*

```
annotation(X1)=pathology ← follows_string_vb(X2)='trna(asn)',
    tfollows(X2,X1)=true
```

This clause states that X1 is annotated as *pathology* if it follows a verb preceded by the token 'trna(asn)', which is the name of a mitochondrial gene.

```
annotation(X1)=substitution ← first(X1)=a, last(X1)=g
```

This clause states that X1 is annotated as *substitution* if it is a token starting with the 'a' and ending with the 'g' characters, that are two nucleotide symbols. This is a peculiar clause which allows to recognize all the mutations where the *A* base is substituted by the *G* base in a genome.

7. Conclusion

The maintenance of biological databases is currently a problem of great interest because the progress made in many experimental procedures has led to an ever increasing amount of data, mostly buried in textual form. In this chapter, we present a framework for biomedical information extraction from text that integrates a data mining module for extraction rule discovery. Patterns for biomedical entity extraction are induced from a set of manually labelled texts that are relevant for the application at hand. The mining process can exploit domain knowledge and search for dependencies among entities of interest. Application of the approach to the HmtDB annotation case study is described. Results show complexity of some learning tasks and usefulness of automatic text mining strategies. The mining system allows us to discover meaningful patterns among biomedical entities which can subsume some semantic relations, such as the association of a DNA mutation with the responsible gene. We are currently working to extend the framework by integrating a text classification system to automatically perform selection of literature that is relevant for the annotation task, which is an additional time-consuming and tiring task for curators. Since the work confirms that mining annotation rules offers a promising alternative to hand-coding, we plan to investigate approaches which are able to learn accurate models in the case of weakly labelled training data. This can alleviate the cost of producing complete training data which is a main drawback of supervised approaches. Moreover, weakly labelled data can be easily produced by exploiting the huge amount of knowledge already available in biological databases and by coupling it accurately with references that are provided as evidence of stored entries (Craven & Kumlien, 1999).

8. Acknowledgments

This work partially fulfills the research objectives set by the F.I.R.B. 2003 project LIBI (International Labratory of BioInformatics) funded by the MIUR (Italian Ministry for Education, University and Research) under grant RBLA039M7M (http://www.libi.it).

9. References

Accetturo, M., Santamaria, M., Lascaro, D., Rubino, F., Achilli A., Torroni, A., Tommaseo-Ponzetta, M., Attimonelli, M. (2006). Human mtDNA site-specific variability values can act as haplogroup markers. HUMAN MUTATION. vol. 27(9), pp. 965-974 ISSN: 1059-7794. doi:10.1002/humu.20365.

Aitken, J. S. (2002). Learning Information Extraction Rules: An Inductive Logic Programming approach. In F. van Harmelen (Ed.): Proceedings of the 15th European Conference on Artificial Intelligence, pages 355-359, IOS Press, Amsterdam.

Alfarano, C., Andrade, C.E., Anthony, K., Bahroos, N., Bajec, M., Bantoft, K., Betel, D., Bobechko, B., Boutilier, K., Burgess, E., et al. (2005) The Biomolecular Interaction

Network Database and related tools 2005 update. Nucleic Acids Res. 2005 Jan 1;33(Database issue):D418-24.

Andrews, R. M., Kubacka, I., Chinnery, P. F., Lightowlers, R. N., Turnbull, D. M., Howell, N. (1999) Reanalysis and revision of the Cambridge reference sequence for human mitochondrial DNA. Nat Genet 23:147

Attimonelli, M., Accetturo, M., Santamaria, M., Lascaro, D., Scioscia, G., Pappada, G., Russo L., Zanchetta L. & Tommaseo-Ponzetta, M. (2005): Hmtdb, a human mitochondrial genomic resource based on variability studies supporting population genetics and biomedical research. BMC Bioinformatics 1(6) Suppl 4:S4.

Baumgartner, Jr. W. A., Cohen, K. B., Fox, L., Acquaah-Mensah, G., Hunter, L., (2007). Manual annotation is not sufficient for curating genomic databases. Bioinformatics 23:i41-i48.

Berardi, M. , Varlaro, A., Malerba, D. (2004). On the effect of caching in recursive theory learning. In Rui Camacho, Ross D. King, and Ashwin Srinivasan, editors, 14th International Conference on Inductive Logic Programming, ILP 2004, volume 3194 of Lecture Notes in Computer Science, pages 44–62. Springer.

Berardi, M., Malerba, D. (2007): Learning Recursive Patterns for Biomedical Information Extraction. In S. Muggleton, R. Otero, & A. Tamaddoni-Nezhad (Eds.): Inductive Logic Programming: ILP 2006, LNAI 4455, pages 79–93, Springer: Berlin.

Blockeel, H., Sebag, M., (2003). Scalability and efficiency in multi-relational data mining. SIGKDD Explorations, 5(1): 17-30.

Cohen, A.M. & Hersh, W.A. (2005). A survey of current work in biomedical text mining, Brief. Bioinform., 6(1):57-71.

Craven, M., Kumlien, J. (1999): Constructing biological knowledge bases by extracting information from text sources. In: Proceedings of the Seventh International Conference on Intelligent Systems for Molecular Biology, pp. 77–86. AAAI Press, Stanford.

Cunningham, H., Maynard, D., Bontcheva, K., Tablan, V. (2002) Gate: A framework and graphical development environment for robust nlp tools and application. In: Proc. of the 40th Anniversary Meeting of the Association for Computational Linguistics (ACL'02), Philadelphia, USA.

Cussens, J., Nedellec, C. (ed.) (2005): Genic Interaction Extraction Challenge. Proceedings of the 4th ICML Workshop on Learning Language in Logic (LLL05), Bonn, Germany.

Gaizauskas, R. and Wilks, Y. (1998). Information Extraction: Beyond Document Retrieval. Computational Linguistics and Chinese Language Processing 3, 17-60.

Goadrich, M. , Oliphant, L., Shavlik, J. (2004). Learning Ensembles of First-Order Clauses for Recall-Precision Curves: A Case Study in Biomedical Information Extraction. In Rui Camacho, Ross D. King, and Ashwin Srinivasan, editors, 14th International Conference on Inductive Logic Programming, ILP 2004, volume 3194 of Lecture Notes in Computer Science, pages 98-115, Springer.

Hirschman, L., Yeh, A., Blaschke, C., and Valencia, A. (2005) . Overview of biocreative: critical assessment of information extraction for biology. Bioinformatics, 6, 2005.

Horn, F., Lau, A. L., Cohen, F. E. (2004) .Automated extraction of mutation data from the literature: application of MuteXt to G protein-coupled receptors and nuclear hormone receptors. Bioinformatics 2004 20 (4): 557-568.

Horner, DS, Pesole, G. (2003) The estimation of relative site variability among aligned homologous protein sequences. Bioinformatics 2003, 19:600-606.

Jensen, L. J., Saric, J., Bork, P. (2006). Literature mining for the biologist: from information retrieval to biological discovery. Nature Reviews Genetics, Vol. 7, No. 2., pp. 119-129.

Krallinger, M., Erhardt, R.A., Valencia A. (2005) Text-mining approaches in molecular biology and biomedicine. Drug Discovery Today. 2005 Mar 15; 10(6):439-45.

Levi, G., and Sirovich, F. (1976) 'Generalized and-or graphs', Artificial Intelligence, 7, 243-259.

Lloyd, L. (1987). Foundations of Logic Programming, 2nd ed. Springer-Verlag.

Lu, Z., Cohen, K. B., Hunter, L. (2007). GeneRIF quality assurance as summary revision. Pac. Symp. on Biocomput., 12, 269–280.

Malerba D. (2003). Learning recursive theories in the normal ILP setting. Fundamenta Informaticae, 57(1):39–77.

Mitchell, T.M. (1997). Machine Learning. McGraw-Hill.

Muggleton, S. (1992). Inductive Logic Programming. Academic Press, London.

Nédellec, C. (2004). Machine Learning for Information Extraction in Genomics - State of the Art and Perspectives. In: Text Mining and its Applications: Results of the NEMIS Launch Conference Series: Studies in Fuzziness and Soft Computing Sirmakessis, Spiros (Ed.), Springer Verlag.

Nienhuys-Cheng, S.-W., de Wolf, R. (1997). Foundations of inductive logic programming. Springer, Heidelberg.

Pesole, G., Saccone, C. (2001). A novel method for estimating substitution rate variation among sites in a large dataset of homologous DNA sequences. Genetics 2001, 157:859-865.

Porter, M.F. (1997). Readings in information retrieval. An algorithm for suffix stripping, pp. 313–316

Ramakrishnan, G., Joshi, S., Balakrishnan, S., Srinivasan, A. (2007). Using ILP to Construct Features for Information Extraction from Semi-structured Text. In Hendrik Blockeel, Jan Ramon, Jude W. Shavlik, Prasad Tadepalli (Eds.): Inductive Logic Programming, 17th International Conference, ILP 2007, volume 4894 of Lecture Notes in Computer Science, pages 211-224, Springer 2008.

Rebholz-Schuhmann, D., Kirsch, H., Couto, F. (2005). Facts from Text—Is Text Mining Ready to Deliver?, PLoS Biology 3(2): e65

Shah, P.K., Bork, P., (2006). LSAT: learning about alternative transcripts in MEDLINE. Bioinformatics 22(7): 857-865

Shatkay, H., Feldman, R. (2003) Mining the biomedical literature in the genomic era: an overview. Journal of Computational Biology 10, 821–855.

Smeitink, J., van den Heuvel, L. & DiMauro, S. (2001) The genetics and Pathology of Oxidative phosphorylation. Nature Reviews Genetics 2001, 2:342-352.

Srinivasan, P. (2004). Text Mining: Generating Hypotheses from Medline. Journal of the American Society for Information Science, 55 (4), pp. 396-413.

Torroni, A., Rengo, C., Guida, V., Cruciani, F., Sellitto, D., Coppa, A., Calderon, FL., Simionati, B., Valle, G., Richards, M., Macaulay, V., Scozzari, R.: Do the four clades of the mtDNA haplogroup L2 evolve at different rates? Am J Hum Genet 2001, 69:1348-1356.

Wallace, D. C., Brown, M. D. & Lott, M. T. (1999) Mitochondrial DNA variation in human evolution and disease. Gene 1999, 238:211-230.

Yeh, A. S., Hirschman, L., Morgan, A. A. (2003). Evaluation of text data mining for database curation: lessons learned from the KDD Challenge Cup. Bioinformatics, Vol. 19 Suppl. 1

17

Social Data Mining to Improve Bioinspired Intelligent Systems

Alberto Ochoa [1,ض], Arturo Hernández[2], Saúl González[1], Arnulfo Castro[1], Alexander Gelbukh[3], Alberto Hernández[4] and Halina Iztebegovič[5]

[1]Juarez City University,
[ض] CIATEC,
[2]CIMAT,
[3]CIC-IPN,
[4]CIICAp-UAEM,
[5]Montenegro University
[1, 2, 3, 4ض] México
[5]Montenegro

1. Introduction

The proposal of this chapter is to explain the implementation of social data mining to improve results in bioinspired intelligent systems using generation of clusters, associative rules; decision trees, associated models, dioramas and multivariable analysis for obtain knowledge about any issue related with a topic. This kind of intelligent systems using bioinspired computing - specially, group intelligence techniques such as: Ant Colony, Particle Swarm Optimization and Cultural Algorithms- that try to simulate biological processes that occur in the nature. Intelligent agents use this information to make decisions to improve a needed heuristic optimization in different fields such as: negotiation, argumentation or artificial societies simulation.

First in section 2 of this chapter, we approach different concepts related with social data mining and how to use different ways to analyze and model the necessary information to support the correct decision of agents; in next three sections we explain the way to generate a specific behaviour by using group intelligence techniques -ant colony (section 3), particle swarm optimization (section 4) and cultural algorithms (section 5), In section 6, we apply this knowledge in diverse fields and application domains that use a heuristic optimization. In section 7 we compare different cases of studies: Eurovision Voting problem, and the Distribution of Elements. Finally in section 8 we provide our conclusions and outline our future research.

2. Social data mining – basic notions

Social data mining systems enable people to share opinions and obtain a benefit from each other's experience. These systems do this by mining and redistributing information from computational records of social activity such as Usenet messages, system usage history, citations, and hyperlinks among others. Two general questions for evaluating such systems are: (1) is the extracted information valuable? , and (2) do interfaces based on extracted information improve user tasks performance?

We report here on social data mining applications, systems that mine information from the structure and content of web pages and provide an exploratory information workspace interface. We carried out experiments that yielded positive answers to both evaluation questions. First, a number of automatically computable features about web sites do a good job of predicting expert quality judgments about sites. Second, compared to popular web search interfaces, the Topic Shop interface to this information lets users select significantly higher quality sites, in less time and with less effort, and to organize the sites they select into personally meaningful collections quickly and easily. We conclude by discussing how our results may be applied and considering how they touch on general issues concerning quality, expertise, and consensus

The motivation for the social data mining approach goes back at least to Vannevar Bush's *As We May Think* essay. Bush envisioned scholars blazing trails through repositories of information and realized that these trails subsequently could be followed by others. Everyone could walk in the footsteps of the masters. In our work, we have formulated a similar intuition using the metaphor of a path through the woods. However, this metaphor highlights the role of collective effort, rather than the individual. A path results from the decisions of many individuals, united only by where they choose to walk, yet still reflects a rough notion of what the walkers find to be a good path. The path both reflects history of use and serves as a resource for future users.

Social data mining approaches seek analogous situations in the computational world. Researchers look for situations where groups of people are producing computational records (such as documents, Usenet messages, or web sites and links) as part of their normal activity. Potentially useful information implicit in these records is identified, computational techniques to harvest and aggregate the information are invented, and visualization techniques to present the results are designed. Thus, computation discovers and makes explicit the "paths through the woods" created by particular user communities. And, unlike ratings-based *collaborative filtering* systems (Resnick et al., 1994), social data mining systems do not require users to engage in any new activity; rather, they seek to exploit user preference information implicit in records of existing activity. The "history-enriched digital objects" line of work (Hill et al., 1992) was a seminal effort in this approach. It began from the observation that objects in the real world accumulate *wear* over the history of their use, and that this wear – such as the path through the woods or the dog-eared pages in a paperback book or the smudges on certain recipes in a cookbook – informs future usage. *Edit Wear* and *Read Wear* were terms used to describe computational analogues of these phenomena. Statistics such as time spent reading various parts of a document, counts of spreadsheet cell recalculations, and menu selections were captured. These statistics were then used to modify the appearance of documents and other interface objects in accordance with prior use. For example, scrollbars were annotated with horizontal lines of differing length and color to represent amount of editing (or reading) by various users.

Other work has focused on extracting information from online conversations such as Usenet. PHOAKS (Hill & Terveen, 1996) mines messages in Usenet newsgroups looking for mentions of web pages. It categorizes and aggregates mentions to create lists of popular web pages for each group. In (Viegas et al, 1990) have harvested information from Usenet newsgroups and chats and have used them to create visualizations of the conversation.

These visualizations can be used to find conversations with desirable properties, such as equality of participation or many regular participants. (Smith & Fiore, 2001) also extracted information from newsgroups and designed visualizations of the conversational thread structure, contributions by individual posters, and the relationships between posters.
Still other work has focused on extracting information from web usage logs. Footprints (Wexelblat et al., 1999) records user browsing history, analyzes it to find commonly traversed links between web pages, and constructs several different visualizations of this data to aid user navigation through a web site. Pursuing the metaphor of navigation, some researchers have used the term *social navigation* to characterize work of this nature (Munro et al., 1999). Finally, a distinct technical approach was taken by (Chalmers et al., 1998). They used the activity *path* - e.g., a sequence of URLs visited during a browsing session - as the basic unit. They have developed techniques to compute similarities between paths and to make recommendations on this basis - for example, to recommend pages to you that others browsed in close proximity to pages you browsed.

Mining the Web

Most relevant to the concerns of this paper is the work that mines the structure of the World Wide Web itself. The Web, with its rich content, link structure, and usage logs, has been a major domain for social data mining research. A basic intuition is that a link from one web site to another may indicate both similarity of content between the sites and an endorsement of the linked-to site. An intellectual antecedent for this work is the field of bibliometrics, which studies patterns of co-citation in texts (Egghe et al., 1990). Various clustering and rating algorithms have been designed to extract information from link structure.
(Ochoa et al, 2007) was developed a categorization algorithm that used hyperlink structure (as well as text similarity and user's data access) to categorize web pages into various functional roles and using Cultural Algortihms. Before (Pitkow & Pirolli, 1997) experimented with clustering algorithms based on co-citation analysis, in which pairs of documents were clustered based on the number of times they were both cited by a third document Kleinberg formalized the notion of document quality within a hyper-linked collection using the concept of *authority* (Kleinberg, 1998). At first pass, an authoritative document is one that many other documents link to. However, this notion can be strengthened by observing that links from all documents aren't equally valuable - some documents are better *hubs* for a given topic. Hubs and authorities stand in a mutually reinforcing relationship: a good authority is a document that is linked to by many good hubs, and a good hub is a document that links to many authorities. Kleinberg developed an iterative algorithm for computing authorities and hubs. He presented examples that suggested the algorithm could help to filter out irrelevant or poor quality documents (i.e., they would have low authority scores) and identify high-quality documents (they would have high authority scores). He also showed that his algorithm could be used to cluster pages within a collection, in effect disambiguating the query that generated the collection. For example, a query on "Jaguar" returned items concerning the animal, the car, and the NFL team, but Kleinberg's algorithm splits the pages into three sets, corresponding to the three meanings.
Several researchers have extended this basic algorithm. Weight links based on the similarity of the text that surrounded the hyperlink in the source document to the query that defined the topic made several important extensions. First, they weighted documents based on their

similarity to the query topic. Second, they count only links between documents from different *hosts*, and average the contribution of links from any given host to a specific document. That is, if there are k links from documents on one host to a document D on another host, then each of the links is assigned a weight of 1/k when the authority score of D is computed. In experiments, they showed that their extensions led to significant improvements over the basic authority algorithm.

PageRank is another link-based algorithm for ranking documents. Like Kleinberg's algorithm, this is an iterative algorithm that computes a document's score based on the scores of documents that link to it. PageRank puts more emphasis on the quality of the links to a particular document. Documents linked to by other documents with high PageRank scores will themselves receive a higher PageRank score than documents linked to by low scoring documents.

In summary, much recent research has experimented with algorithms for extracting information from web structure. A major motivation for these algorithms is that they can be used to compute measures of document quality. Yet this work has proceeded without much experimental evaluation, leaving two basic questions unanswered: first, what benefits do the more complicated link-based algorithms provide beyond simple link counts? And second, how well do the various link-based metrics (in-links, authority scores, PageRank scores) actually correlate with human quality judgments? We will report on an experiment that investigates these issues.

Information Workspaces

Once information has been extracted, it must be presented in a user interface. Users must be able to evaluate collections of items, select items they find useful, and organize them into personally meaningful collections. (Card et al, 1991) introduced the concept of *information workspaces* to refer to environments in which information items can be stored and manipulated. A departure point for most such systems is the file manager popularized by the Apple Macintosh and then in Microsoft Windows. Such systems typically include a list view, which shows various properties of items, and an icon view, which lets users organize icons representing the items in a 2D space. (Mander et al., 1992) enhanced the basic metaphor with the addition of "piles". Users could create and manipulate piles of items. Interesting interaction techniques for displaying, browsing, and searching piles were designed and tested. Bookmarks are the most popular way to create personal information workspaces of web resources. Bookmarks consist of lists of URLs; typically the title of the web page is used as the label for the URL. Users may organize their bookmarks into a hierarchical category structure. (Abrams et al., 1998) carried out an extensive study of how several hundred web users used bookmarks. They observed a number of strategies for organizing bookmarks, including a flat ordered list, a single level of folders, and hierarchical folders. They also made four design recommendations to help users manage their bookmarks more effectively. First, bookmarks must be easy to organize, e.g., via automatic sorting techniques. Second, visualization techniques are necessary to provide comprehensive overviews of large sets of bookmarks. Third, rich representations of sites are required; many users noted that site titles are not accurate descriptors of site content.

Finally, tools for managing bookmarks must be well integrated with web browsers. Many researchers have created experimental information workspace interfaces, often designed expressly for web documents. (Card et al., 1996) describe the Web Book, which uses a book metaphor to group a collection of related web pages for viewing and interaction, and the Web Forager, an interface that lets users view and manage multiple Web Books. In addition to these novel interfaces, they also presented a set of automatic methods for generating collections (Web Books) of related pages, such as recursively following all relative links from a specified web page, following all (absolute) links from a page one level, extracting "book-like" structures by following "next" and "previous" links, and grouping pages returned from a search query. (Mackinlay et al., 1995) developed a novel user interface for accessing articles from a citation database.

The central UI object is a "Butterfly", which represents an article, its references, and its citers. The interface makes it easy for users to browse among related articles, group articles, and generate queries to retrieve articles that stand in a particular relationship to the current article. The Data Mountain of (Robertson et al., 1998) represents documents as thumbnail images in a 3D virtual space. Users can move and group the images freely, with various interesting visual and audio cues used to help users arrange the documents.

In a study comparing the use of Data Mountain to Internet Explorer Favorites, Data Mountain users retrieved items more quickly, with less incorrect or failed retrieval. Other researchers have created interfaces to support users in constructing, evolving, and managing collections of information resources. SenseMaker (Baldonado et al, 1997) focuses on supporting users in the contextual evolution of their interest in a topic. It attempts to make it easy to evolve a collection, e.g., expanding it by query-by-example operations or limiting it by applying a filter. Scatter/Gather (Pirolli et al, 1996) supports the browsing of large collections of text, allowing users to iteratively reveal topic structure and locate desirable documents.

VIKI system (Marshall et al., 1994) lets user organize collections of items by arranging them in 2D space. Hierarchical collections are supported. Later extensions (Shipman et al., 1999) added automatic visual layouts, specifically non-linear layouts such as fisheye views. (Hightower et al., 1998) addressed the observation that users often return to previously visited pages. They used Pad++ (Bederson et al., 1996) to implement PadPrints, browser companion software that presents a zoomable interface to a user's browsing history there are a number of important issues that deserve further investigation. One direction is to seek new sources for mining information about user preferences. As we have discussed, researchers have investigated hyperlink structure, electronic conversations, navigation histories and other usage logs, and purchasing history. One area with great potential is electronic media usage, in particular, listening to digital music. By observing what music someone is listening to, a system can infer the songs, artists, and genres that person prefers, and use this information to recommend additional songs and artists, and to put the person in touch with other people with similar interests. We took a step in this direction with a system that lets users visualize individual and group listening histories and define new play lists relative to listening history (Terveen et al., 2002). (Crossen et al., 2002) reported on a system that learns user preferences from the music they listen to, then selects songs to play in a shared physical environment, based in part on the preferences of all people present.

As user preferences are extracted from more and more sources, the issue of combining different types of preferences becomes important. For example, PHOAKS extracted preferences about web pages from Usenet messages and presented them to users. As users browsed through this information, PHOAKS tracked which pages users clicked on (another type of implicit preference), and users also could rate web pages (explicit preferences).

Developing general techniques for combining different types of preferences is a challenge. (Billsus et al. 1998) was presented a method for weighting different types of contributions; however, whether this is the best combination method and how to determine appropriate weights are still open issues. It is worth pointing out that the task that TopicShop supports – selecting a subset of items from a large set and then organizing the subset arises – is quite general and occurs in other contexts. For example, of the many people I exchange email with, a small subset are "contacts" whom I wish to keep track of, and organize into groups which I can use to manage my communication. We have applied this intuition in a project with Steve Whittaker, developing a new interface for the ContactMap contact management system (Whittaker et al., 2002). Features about potential contacts including their organization and frequency and regency of communication are extracted from email archives and presented in a table; as in TopicShop, the table can be sorted by any of the columns. And, when users find important contacts, they add them to their "map" (equivalent to the TopicShop Work Area) by dragging and dropping. Contacts on the map are organized by spatial arrangement and color coding. This experience illustrates that the general interaction paradigm of TopicShop can be applied in an altogether different domain. While our experiment compared TopicShop to the state-of-the-art Web directory Yahoo, it may have occurred to the reader that our techniques are suitable for integration with such a system. This is absolutely correct. Both directory systems, which contain categories of web sites typically built by a person, and search engines, which retrieve documents based on their similarity to a query, could benefit. An effective way to apply the results of our research would be to enhance (say) Yahoo by (1) using a WebCrawler/analyzer to augment each manually constructed collection of pages with the sorts of profiles our experiments showed effective, and (2) providing a TopicShop-style information workspace interface. Such a system would combine the advantages of people – applying judgment to select the initial set of collections – and computers – applying analysis techniques to provide enhanced information and to keep the collections up to date. A similar tactic could be taken by a search engine; this would be most efficient for one such as Google that already maintains a database of links between web pages. Finally, note that this argument shows that even a very large, manually constructed set of "seed" pages can be enhanced significantly by providing additional features, grouping pages into sites, and offering a good user interface

3. Behaviour in group intelligence techniques – ant colony

Various biologically inspired approaches to problem solving using a social metaphor have been proposed. For example, both Particle Swarm Optimization (PSO) and Ant Colony Optimization (ACO) have been employed to solve problems in optimization and design. Both approaches employ simple social interactions between agents to produce emergent social structures that are used to solve a given problem. In this paper we investigate the emergence and power of more complex social systems based upon principles of cultural evolution. Cultural Algorithms employ a basic set of knowledge sources, each related to knowledge observed in various social species. These knowledge sources are then combined to direct the decisions of the individual agents in solving optimization problems. Here we develop an algorithm based upon an analogy to the marginal value theorem in foraging theory to guide the integration of these different knowledge sources to direct the agent population. Various phases of problem solving emerge from the combined use of these knowledge sources and these phases result in the emergence of individual roles within the population in terms of leaders and followers. These roles result in organized swarming in the population level and knowledge swarms in the social belief space. Application to real-valued function optimization in engineering design is used to illustrate the principles.

Ant Colony Algorithm

Ant Colony Optimization (ACO) is based on the observation, in the laboratory, of colonies of ants. Investigators found that ants are able to find the shortest path from the source of food to the nest without using visual tracks (Hölldobler et al, 1990). Also it was observed that they were able to adapt to the changes on the environment, for example, using a new path once the previously used stops being feasible due an obstacle.

It is well known that the primary manner how the ants form and maintain a path is by using pheromones. In the ant colony proposed by (Dorigo et al, 1996), an ant is frequently defined as an agent of simple calculations that iteratively constructs a solution to a problem, a problem of trajectory planning. In this model, ants deposit certain amount of pheromones, a chemical substance, whereas they walk, and each ant probabilistically prefers to follow a pheromone-rich direction. Thus, the pheromone and its density through the path are the knowledge that in ACO shares among the individual ants. The partial solutions of the problem correspond to states where each ant is moved from one state to another. ψ corresponds to a more complex partial solution. In each step σ, each ant k calculates a set of feasible expansions to its present state, and then it moves to one of these, according to a distribution of the specified probability as it follows:

$$p^{k}_{\iota\psi} = \begin{cases} \dfrac{\alpha \cdot \tau_{\iota\psi} + (1-\alpha)\cdot \eta_{\iota\psi}}{\sum(\alpha \cdot \tau_{\iota\nu} + (1-\alpha)\cdot \eta_{\iota\nu})}, \text{if } \text{éø} \in tabu_k, \text{éí} \notin tabu_k \\ 0, \text{otherwise} \end{cases}$$

Here the set $tabu_k$ represents a set of feasible movements for ant k and the parameter α defines the relative importance of the path with respect to its attraction.

After each iteration t of the algorithm, trails are updated using the following formula:

$$\tau_{\iota\psi}(t) = \rho\tau_{\iota\psi}(t\text{-}1)+\Delta\tau_{\iota\psi}$$

where ρ is a user-defined coefficient and $\Delta\tau_{\iota\psi}$ represents the sum of the contributions of all ants that use move ($\iota\psi$) to construct their solution. An iterative process increases the level of those cells related to moves that were part of "good" solutions, while decreasing all others.The pseudo-code from (Maniezzo, 2000) describes how the basic Ant Colony Optimization works:

1. (Initialization)
initialize $\tau\iota\psi$, $\forall\iota$, ψ
2. (Construction)
For each ant k do
    repeat
        compute $\eta\iota\psi$, $\forall\iota$, ψ
        choose in probability the state to move into
        append the chosen move to the k-th ant's set $tabu_k$

until ant k has completed its solution
[apply a local optimization procedure]
enddo
3. (Trail update)
For each ant move (ι, ψ) do
Compute $\Delta\tau_{\iota\psi}$ and update the trail values
4. (Terminating condition)
If not (end_condition) go to step 2

ACO is applied extensively to problems of optimization of trajectory planning in many areas like symmetric and asymmetric variants of the travelling agent, as well as problems of partitioning and the associated times of telecommunication networks. What emerges from the social interaction in the colony of ants are the trajectories of high performance according to the defined terms of performance given by certain functions. Some unexpected trajectory characteristics have been demonstrated for certain kinds of problems such as to find the minimum cost path of a general graph. Recently, a number of algorithms inspired in the behaviour of social groups has been used to solve complex problems of optimization. Some of these algorithms include the particle swarm optimization (PSO) (Kennedy & Eberhart, 1995), ant colony (ACO) (Dorigo et al., 1995), and cultural algorithms (Reynolds et al., 2005). These three algorithms use a model based on a population as the base of the algorithm and solve problems by sharing information via the social interaction among agents.

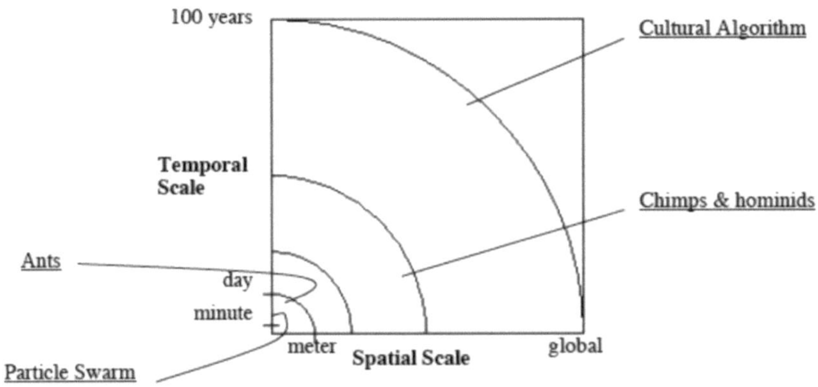

Fig. 1. Scale of Social Interaction.

Figure 1 expresses each of these approaches in terms of space and the continuous time on which the social interactions happen. We must notice that colony of ants and particle swarm are found near the left end of this continuity. For example, in particle swarm, the agents can locally change their speed and direction of movement by the interaction with other agents. In ant colony, the agents locally interchange the information in terms of the density and gradient of pheromone that marks their path. The pheromone is deposited by an ant that moves through the path. The frequency in the use of a path is indicated by the amount of pheromone that has been deposited, considering its degradation in the atmosphere up to a certain level. The cultural algorithms on the other hand allow agents to act reciprocally in diverse ways using several reflective forms of symbolic information present in complex cultural systems. The basic cultural algorithm allows that individuals communicate via a shared space of beliefs. The shared space considers five basic types of information that can be shared mentally or symbolically. It is well known that the scale of interaction within complex systems affects the nature of the structure arising from the interaction of agents within that system (Holland, 1998). Now we examine briefly each one of the three social models for solution of problems in terms of the nature of their social interactions and their own distinctive features.

4. Behaviour in group intelligence techniques – particle swarm optimization

Particle Swarm Optimization (PSO) is a stocastic technique based in the optimization of a population, developed by Kennedy and inspired by the social behavior of the flock of birds or the shoals of fishes. In PSO, the potential solutions, called particles, move through the space of the problem following the trajectories of their optimal neighbors. Each individual particle does not lose either their last better aptitudes or the ones of its neighbors (social vision) within a fixed radius. This information determines its following direction and speed (cognitive vision). PSO is initialized with a particle group at random (solutions) and later looks for optimal degrees putting the day the generations. In each iteration, each particle is bought up to date better following both "values". The first best solution (aptitude) that has reached until now (the value of the aptitude also is stored). This value is called pbest. The other "best" S-value is followed by the optimizer of the particle accumulation, which is the best value obtained until now by any particle in the population. This second better S-value a best global and call gbest. When a particle participates in the population like its topological neighbors, the second best S-value the best premises and lbest is called. After finding better values the particle updates both its speed and position with the following equations (a) and (b):

$$v[]=v[]+c_1*rand()*(pbest[]-present[])+c_2*rand()*(gbest[]-present[]) \quad (a)$$

$$present[] = present[]+v[] \quad (b)$$

v[] is the particle velocity, present[] is the current particle (solution).pbest[] and gbest[] are defined as started before.rand() is a random number between (0,1). c_1,c_2 are learning factors. Usually c_1, = c_2 = 2.

The pseudocode of the initial version of PSO for variables of real value is determined by (Kennedy et al., 2001) of the next way:

```
    For each particle
        initialize particle
    End For
    Do
    For each particle
        calculate fitness value
        if the fitness value is better than the best fitness value (pBest) in history
        set current value as the new pBest
    End for
choose the particle with the best fitness value of all the particles as the gBest
For each particle
   calculate particle velocity according equation      (a)
   update particle position according equation         (b)
End for
   While maximum iterations or minimum error criteria is not attained
```

In order to simulate the individual and interpersonal learning of the cultural transmission (social), PSO manages simplicity and effectiveness (speed of convergence). It has performed well in a variety of test problems. It operates suitably on two dimensions but they can theoretically be extended to multiple dimensions. Due to the simplicity of its social behavior with respect to its results with base in the convergence, ranks of convergence, and other unexpected characteristics have been produced. The unexpected characteristic base is the swarm of particles, or coordinated movement of individuals through the space search towards the optimal solution.

5. Behaviour in group intelligent techniques – cultural algorithms

The Cultural Algorithms (CAs) is a class of computer models derived from the observation of the process of cultural evolution in the nature (Reynolds et al., 2005). ACs has three main components: a population space, a belief space, and a protocol that it describes as the knowledge is interchanged first in both components. The population space can support any population based on a computer model, such as the Genetic Algorithms and the Evolutionary Programming. The basic framework is shown in Figure 2.

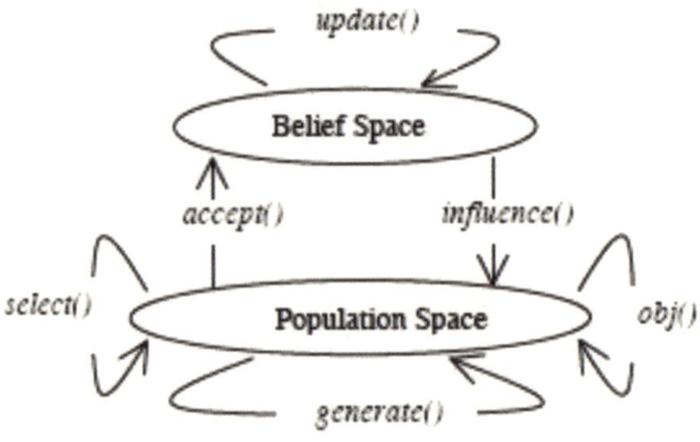

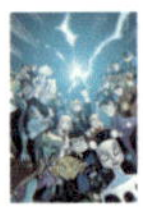

Fig. 2. Conceptual Diagram of Cultural Algorithms.

The cultural algorithms are a dual system of the inheritance that characterizes the evolution in human culture in the macro-evolutionary level, that happen within the space of beliefs, and in the micro-evolutionary level, that happens in the population space. The knowledge produced in the population at micro-evolutionary level is accepted or goes to the space of beliefs, and is used selectively to fit the knowledge structures there. This knowledge can then be used to influence the changes in the population in the following generation.
What differentiates the cultural algorithms from the PSO or the ACO approaches is the fact that cultural algorithms use five basic types of knowledge in the process of resolution of problem instead of only the transmitted value. There is evidence in cognitive sciences that each of these types of knowledge is present in several animal species and it assumes that human social systems support as minimum each of these types of knowledge. The sources of knowledge include the normative knowledge (ranges of acceptable behaviors), the circumstantial knowledge (the units or the memories of right and failed solutions among others), the domain knowledge (knowledge of the objects in the domain, the relations among them, and their interactions), the historical knowledge (temporary landlords of the behavior), and the topographic knowledge (space landlords of the behavior). This set of

categories is seen as complete for a given domain in the sense that all knowledge available can be expressed in terms of a combination of one of these classifications.

6. Evolve computing applying to diverse fields that use a heuristic optimization

The cultural algorithms have been tested with benchmarking problems (Chung et al., 1998) and also have been applied successfully in a diverse number of application areas such as modelling the evolution of agriculture, learning conceptualizing (Morrison et al., 1999), optimization of real-value functions (Jin et al., 1999) , re-engineering of the knowledge bases for the manufacturing assembly processes (Rychlyckyj et al., 2003), modelling systems of price incentives based on agents, distribution of elements in a diorama, in predicting a ranking in Eurovisión, in the simulation of a social model in an intelligent game (Ochoa, Ponce et al., 2007), and combined with Predator/Prey Game for analyzing cultural problems (Ochoa, Quezada et al., 2008) among others. Whereas it is right, the relative complexity of the sources of knowledge and its interaction make difficult to determine because the cultural algorithms work so well. Indicated alternatively, under what conditions some systems indeed can solve a given problem and the belief space can be seen as samples For a right process to solve the problem.

We begin this section examining how cultural algorithms solve problems of resources optimization within an experimental atmosphere. In our research, first we use a simulated atmosphere of the world of cubes, and we adapted it for our experiments. Within this world, the resources are distributed in piles (cones) in the land (Sugarscape style) (Epstein et al, 1996). We can put in the landscape an arbitrary number of cones, each with a size that varies, to produce surfaces of the forage of the complexity that varies. The distribution of cones can be static, dynamic, and deceptive (in which the positioning of some cone hides better areas of agents than they climb the hill). Then the agents build reciprocally social via these several sources of knowledge to find the optimal degree, and in the dynamic atmosphere they don't lose his position, that changes in a certain rate. Then we investigated the appearance of social landlords in both the population space and the belief space when the problem is solved successfully. We use later what we have learned of this experimental atmosphere to solve complex problems in engineering design. Then we observed whether the similar social structures emerge there. We compared the operation of the systems with the optimization of the particles swarm.

Since our problem of the cones world can be described as a search space problem, we used a framework inspired by theoretical results of the biology of populations. Specifically, the agents select diverse sources of knowledge based on which we characterized like "marginal value of información". The inspiration for this comes from the classic work (Charnov, 1976) referring to "marginal theorem of value". In certain situations, the agents who used the marginal value theorem could optimize their product of resource within an atmosphere. Simply stated, the marginal value theorem says that an agent remains within a location in the land until the present resource is minor that the predicted half value. Then one moves to another cell that satisfies each marginal constraint with the value. Here we used an approach to the integration of the knowledge that uses a principle corresponding to "marginal value of knowledge". With this approach, is more probable that an individual uses a strategy that is on the average than it uses other sources of knowledge. Then it was observed that the social organizations emerge in the population space and that the space of

beliefs assures the total success for the system. We use this approach of integration based on marginal value with an evolutionary model of programming for the population and with the five sources of knowledge as the frame of the base to the problems of solution within the simulated atmosphere and of the real world.
We wished to show that the use of the marginal value helps to the integration of the knowledge producing the following emergent structures and behaviors:

1. The appearance of certain phases to solve problems in terms of the relative operation of diverse sources of knowledge in a certain time. We labelled these phases like: heavy, granular, granuloses fine and backward movement. Each phase is characterized by the domination of a set or subgroup of knowledge sources that are the best to generate new solutions in that phase. Indeed, the dominant subgroup of knowledge sources is often applied in a specific sequence within each phase. It appears a type of knowledge that produces new solutions that therefore are operated on the other knowledge source. The transitions between the phases happen when the solutions produced by a phase can be exploded better by the sources of knowledge associated with the following phase.
2. The appearance of groups of individuals that move within the space of the problem as a result of the interaction of the cultural knowledge. From these phases they emerged continuously in static, dynamic, and deceptive atmospheres when the marginal approach and the integration of the s-value used. We call them " cultural groups of populations".
3. Then we observed the group knowledge in a put-level, we called them "clusters of knowledge". Due to this, the sources of the group knowledge in the goal level were produced by the interaction of the sources of knowledge via the marginal value theorem and this one serves to induce a group in the level of population.

7. Cases of studies of data mining to improve evolve computing

Diverse applications inspired in social data mining combined with evolve computing have a great value. In this section, we present two of them in order to compare their contributions; the first is related with a hybrid system that permits to determine the ranking of a debutant country in the Eurovision Song Contest. In the other, it is showed an intelligent tool which accommodate societies in a diorama which performs the accommodations by evaluating cultural and social differences.

7.1 Hybrid system using data mining and particle swarm optimization to determine the ranking of a new participant in Eurovision.

Many problems involve not structured environments which can be solved from the perspective of Particle Swarm Optimization (PSO). In this research we analyze the voting behavior in a popular song contest held every year in Europe. The dataset makes possible to analyze the determinants of success, and gives a rare opportunity to run a direct test of vote trading from logrolling. We show that they are rather driven by linguistic and cultural proximities between singers and voting countries. With this information it is possible to predict the score of a new country, and distribute the votes for a lot of the participants; this paper tries to explain this social behavior.
The Eurovision Song Contest (ESC) held for the first time in Lugano, Switzerland, in 1956, where seven countries competed. Non-European countries can also take part: Israel,

Morocco, Turkey, Armenia and Georgia are now regular participants. In 2008 Azerbaijan and San Marino will participate for the first time. Since 2002, there are 24 slots for finalists, four of which are reserved for the Big Four (France, Germany, Spain and the United Kingdom). Each ESC is broadcasted by television; in 2001 the contest was broadcasted live all around the world. Nowadays, it is watched by several hundred millions of people. The ratings are normalized so that the favorite song gets 12 points, the next one 10, and then 8, 7, 6, 5, 4, 3, 2 and 1. This allows each voting country to give positive ratings to ten other countries. Participating countries cannot vote for their nationals. The order in which candidates perform is randomly drawn before the competition starts. When performance ends, countries are asked to cast their votes. Results are announced country by country, in the same order in which participants performed. Participants are ranked according to their aggregate score. Eurovision have been studied with different perspectives: the compatibility between countries and the political and cultural structures of Europe (Rauhlen, 1997), the persistent structure of hegemony in the Eurovision Song Contest (Suaremi et al., 2006), cultural voting (Yair, 1995) and the analysis about Grand Prix which evaluate many countries participating in different years and with different many of countries competing (Yair et al., 1996), among others. This research is novel because analyze the behavior of all countries when arrived a new country in a new ESC. The objective is to predict the final ranking of Azerbaijan and San Marino, the new contenders in Eurovision Song Contest 2008. The organization of this section is the following. The analysis of the 52 ESC editions to incorporate *a priori* knowledge about the voting patterns and relationships between neighbor countries is explained. Next, the problem statement is defined. The COPSO algorithm is thoroughly explained. Our approach is then tested in the ESC 2007. The experiments and the analysis applied to estimate the final ranking of Azerbaijan and San Marino in ESC 2008 are explained and finally the conclusions are provided.

Eurovision Ranking using Data Mining.

Data mining is the search of global patterns and the existent relationships among the data of immense databases, but that are hidden inside the vast quantity of information (Ochoa A., Meneguzzi, P. Et al, 2006). These relationships represent knowledge of value about the objects that are in the database. This information is not necessarily a faithful copy of the information stored in the databases. Rather, is the information that one can deduce from the database. One of the main problems in data mining is that the number of possible extracted relationships is exponential. Therefore, there are a great variety of machine's learning heuristics that have been proposed for the discovery of knowledge in databases. One of the most popular approaches to represent the results of data mining is to use decision trees. A decision tree provides a procedure to recognize a given case for a concept. It is a "divide and conquer" strategy for the acquisition of the concept (instance). Decision trees have been useful in a great variety of practical cases in science and engineering; in our case we use data mining to characterize the historical voting behavior for each country. Thus, we selected societies that have participated and characterized its behavior based on their previously emitted votes, which allowed to describe in great detail both the society and the individual. The purpose is to explain υij, the vote (that is, the number of points) casted by the people of country $i \in L$ in evaluating the performer of country $j \in L$ ($i \neq j$, since country i can not vote for its own candidate), where L is the total number of participating countries. If countries i and j ($i \neq j$) exchanged their votes, without taking into account any other feature, the voting equation could simply be written

$$v_{ji} = \alpha_{ij} v_{ij} + u_{ij} \tag{1}$$

Where α_{ij} is a commitment parameter, and v_{ij} a random disturbance. If exchanges of votes were "perfect", and both countries kept their commitment, α_{ij} would be equal to 1. More generally, such an equation should contain variables k={1,…,K representing the characteristics (language of songs –English, French, Italian-, lyrics, music, genre and others) of a performer (singer or band) from country *i*, and variables representing the performances of the country *i* along its T*i* participations in the ESC.

$$v_{ji} = \alpha_{ij} v_{ij} + \beta \sum_{k=1}^{K} x_{ik} + \gamma \sum_{t=1}^{T_i} z_{it} + u_{ij} \tag{2}$$

where β and γ are parameters to be estimated. The part associated with beta parameter is related with the attributes of performance of a song (music, lyrics, language among others) and her/his/their interpreter(s). The part associated with gamma parameter is the related with the performance of a country during the ESC's participations (example: Armenia has participated in 2006 and 2007). A problem arises with the fact that it will appear on the other side of the equation for the observation concerning the vote of country i for the singer representing country j. This can be dealt with in several ways. First, and this is the easiest way, instead of using v_{ij} in the right-hand side, one can use the vote cast in previous competition, say v_{ij}^{-1}, though one could think that countries would not necessarily keep their commitment over time. An alternative is to use only half of the observations along all ESC editions; thus, every v_{ij} that appears in the right-hand side of the equation is not used in the left-hand side.

The voting equation is estimated by linear methods. The influence of the order in which musicians appear in competition has often been outlined. The exogenous order in which candidates perform is thus included as determinant. Other variables include (a) a dummy for host country, determined by the citizenship of the previous year's winner-the variable takes the value 1 for the performer whose citizenship is the same as that of the host country-, (b) the language (Gelbukh et al, 2007), in which the artist sings (English, French, Spanish, Italian, in other), (c) gender of the artist, and (d) whether the artist sings alone, in a duo or in a group. The last group of variables will include linguistic and cultural distances between voters and performers, and may dispense us from using variables that characterize voters. National culture differences are represented by the four dimensions studied in (Ginsburgh et al., 2005). These studies identified and scored the four following dimensions that make for "cultural distances":

Power Distance: It measures the extent to which the less powerful members of a society accept that power is distributed unequally; it focuses in the degree of equality between individuals;

Individualism: It measures the degree to which individuals in a society are integrated into a group; it focuses on the degree a society reinforces individual or collective achievements and interpersonal relationships;

Masculinity: It refers to the distribution of roles between genders in a society; it focuses on the degree a society reinforces the traditional masculine work role of male achievement, control, and power;

Uncertainty avoidance: It deals with the society's tolerance for uncertainty or ambiguity, and refers to man's search for truth.

Table 1: Correlations between Cultural Distances and Linguistic

	Language	Power	Indiv.	Masc.	U. A.
Language	1				
Power	0.205	1			
Indiv.	0.254	0.111	1		
Masc.	-0.092	0.031	-0.128	1	
U. A.	0.319	0.567	0.404	0.083	1

Table 2: Cultural Distances vs Contender Characteristics

	(a)	(b)	(c)	(d)
Quality	0.911	0.914	0.901	0.905
	(0.03)	(0.03)	(0.03)	(0.03)
Logrolling	0.028	0.022	0.018	0.016
	(0.01)	(0.01)	(0.01)	(0.01)
Order	0.003	0.002	0.004	0.003
of perf.	(0.01)	(0.01)	(0.01)	(0.01)
Host	0.177	0.191	0.155	0.171
country	(0.24)	(0.24)	(0.24)	(0.24)
Sung in	0.14	0.193	0.101	0.135
english	(0.14)	(0.14)	(0.14)	(0.14)
Sung in	0.353	0.354	0.343	0.347
french	(0.17)	(0.17)	(0.18)	(0.18)
Male	0.139	0.148	0.147	0.154
singer	(0.13)	(0.13)	(0.13)	(0.13)
Duet	0.223	0.147	0.203	0.174
	(0.20)	(0.20)	(0.20)	(0.20)
Group	0.1	0.08	0.087	0.079
	(0.13)	(0.13)	(0.13)	(0.13)
Language	-	-1.142	-	-0.634
		(0.22)		(0.24)

Table 1 illustrates the correlations between the cultural distance and native languages for the countries (Gelbukh & Sidorov, 2006) that are present in our sample. Uncertainty avoidance is correlated with three other variables, but otherwise, distances seem to pick up very different dimensions of people's behavior. One of the most interesting characteristics observed in this experiment were the diversity of the cultural patterns established by each community. The structured scenes associated with the agents cannot be reproduced in general, so time and space belong to a give moment. They represent a unique form, needs and innovator of adaptive behavior which solves a followed computational problem of a complex change of relations. The generated configurations can metaphorically be related to the knowledge of the behavior of the community with respect to an optimization problem (to make alliances to obtain a better ranking). Columns (a) to (d) of Table 2 contain the results of an OLS estimation of equation 2. We first observe that quality always plays a very significant role, which should of course not be surprising. Logrolling is significant only in (a), in which no account is taken of linguistic and cultural distances. It ceases to be in all the other equations once linguistic and/or cultural distances are also accounted for. Note that even when the coefficient is significantly different from zero, its value is very small. Order of appearance plays no role, while among the other variables, the only one which has some influence is "sung in French". Though not all distance coefficients are significantly different from 0 at the level of 5 percent of probability, they all pick negative signs (the larger the

Table 3: Performance Rates

Country	2008	2007
Armenia	0.87	0.64
Ukraine	0.81	0.77
Georgia	0.79	0.61
Serbia	0.78	0.55
Azerbaijan	0.77	-
Ireland	0.68	0.69
Belarus	0.66	0.61
Sweden	0.65	0.64
Turkey	0.63	0.6
Finland	0.62	0.51
Malta	0.61	0.58
Russia	0.60	0.59
Albania	0.59	0.58
Greece	0.58	0.55
Israel	0.57	0.53
Slovenia	0.56	0.54
Bosnia & Herzegovina	0.55	0.51
Hungary	0.54	0.51
Poland	0.53	0.52
Croatia	0.52	0.51
Latvia	0.51	0.49
Belgium	0.49	0.47
France	0.48	0.46
Romania	0.46	0.43
Germany	0.45	0.42
Spain	0.44	0.37
FYR Macedonia	0.43	0.42
United Kingdom	0.42	0.43
Bulgaria	0.40	0.41
Norway	0.39	0.38
The Netherlands	0.37	0.39
Iceland	0.36	0.35
Estonia	0.35	0.34
Portugal	0.34	0.37
Lithuania	0.33	0.34
Moldova	0.32	0.36
Denmark	0.31	0.33
Cyprus	0.30	0.28
Montenegro	0.29	0.21
Switzerland	0.25	0.26
Czech Republic	0.22	0.21
San Marino	0.14	-
Andorra	0.11	0.08

distance, the lower the rating). The Table 3 presents the expected performance rates for 2008. The performance rate tries to predict the country rank through environment variables observed along 52 previous ESC editions. The Table 3 shows the performance rate of the last ESC where Ukraine had the highest rate. In the ESC 2007 the winner was Serbia which had a performance rate of 0.55, below the top-10. The performance rates were estimated based on the characteristics listed in Table 4 and the country performance along previously participations in every ESC edition. For example, in ESC 2007 participated 42 countries hence it was more complex to obtain a second place than in 1981 for example, when only 20 countries participated. Obviously, for the new contenders, Azerbaiyan and San Marino, there is not historical information available. The information obtained through data mining, denotes a similar behavior of countries into the same neighborhood and with similar characteristics (language, territorial extension, religion, in others). Thus, the historical performance for Azerbaijan was calculated from Armenia, Georgia, Bosnia & Herzegovina and Turkey; and for San Marino was calculated from Italy, Switzerland, Andorra, Monaco, Malta and Luxembourg. The parameters used by the model to calculate the performance rate are: β=0.4 and γ=0.6. The model used to calculate the values of Table 3 is the following:

$$r_i = 0.4\sum_{k=1}^{7} x_{ik} + 0.6\sum_{t=1}^{T_i} z_{it} \tag{3}$$

Where T_i is the number of ESC editions that country i has participated. Equation 3 is a synthesis of the voting model presented in Equation 2. The missed term $\alpha_{ij}v_{ij}$ represents the voting behavior expected between countries i and j. A robust model was developed adding probability terms that reflect the voting history between a judge country I and a contender country $j(v_{ij})$. The complete model and its implicit problem are explained in the next section.

Problem Statement.

The objective of this study is to estimate the position rank of the new contenders, Azerbaijan and San Marino. This implies to estimate the final voting matrix, where every cell j, i represents the score given to contender i by country j; that is v_{ji}. For attaining a well prediction, the model should controls the voting behavior between judges and contenders taking into account the historical performance that reflects the cultural empathy, the commonality of regions, the returning voting patterns, in others. The estimated performance rate could guide the model towards an optimal voting configuration according to the current expectations of the experts.
The next objective function posses these two important features of the ESC, the voting behavior and the performance rate explained in the previous Section. Notice that Equation 3 is part of Equation 4.

$$\text{Maximize } f = \sum_{i=1}^{C}\sum_{j=1}^{N} c_{ij} + 4\sum_{i=1}^{C}\sum_{k=1}^{S} p_{ik} + \frac{2}{max_S}\sum_{i=1}^{C} s_i * r_i \tag{4}$$

Subject to:

- Country j can not vote for itself.
- Country j just can vote one time for contender i.
- Country j just can give a score k to only one contender i.

Where N is the number of voting countries, C is the number of contenders, S is the number of available scores S={12,10,8,7,6,5,4,3,2,1} and max_s=12 is the maximum score. The first two terms represent the performance of the final ranking. In the first term of equation 4, c_{ij} is the probability that a score k was given by country j for a contender country i. Table 5 shows an example of the probabilities c_{ij} of Finland for score s=12. Along 52 ESC editions, Finland has received 19 times a score of 12 points from 11 different countries. Sweden and Iceland are the countries which have voted more times for Finland, both with 3 editions. Therefore, they are the countries with highest probabilities C_{ij}. In the second term of Equation 4, P_{ik} is the probability that a country i receives a score k from country j. Table 6 shows an example of the probabilities p_{ik} of Finland with Germany. Finland has received 16 votes from Germany. In 4 times, Germany has given a score of 1 point to Finland; thus, it is the score with highest probability p_{ik}. For the last term of Equation 4, s_i represents the scores sum got by a contender country i from every country $j \neq i$; and r_i represents the expected performance rate of the country i in the competition (see Table 3). The probabilities c_{ij} and q_{ij} were calculated based on the previous ESC editions. The probabilities for Azerbaiyan and San Marino were calculated observing the behavior of the voting along 52 ESC editions between a mature country and a new contender.

Table 4: Contender Characteristics

Characteristic	Quality Factor
Language	0.30
Lyric and Topic	0.25
Musical Arrangement	0.20
Musical Genre	0.15
International Fame	0.10
Sex of Singer	-0.10
Number of Singers	-0.15

Table 5: Example of Country Voting Probability

Contender (i)	Country (j)	Score (k)	Frequence (f_j)	c_{ij} f_j/TF_k
Finland	Denmark	12	1	0.0526
Finland	Estonia	12	2	0.1053
Finland	Germany	12	2	0.1053
Finland	Greece	12	1	0.0526
Finland	Iceland	12	3	0.1579
Finland	Ireland	12	1	0.0526
Finland	Norway	12	1	0.0526
Finland	Poland	12	2	0.1053
Finland	Sweden	12	3	0.1579
Finland	Switzerland	12	1	0.0526
Finland	U. Kingdom	12	2	0.1053
			$TF_k = 19$	1.0000

Table 6: Example of Score Voting Probability

Contender (i)	Country (j)	Score (k)	Frequence (f_k)	p_{ij} f_k/TF_j
Finland	Germany	12	2	0.1250
Finland	Germany	10	1	0.0625
Finland	Germany	7	1	0.0625
Finland	Germany	6	1	0.0625
Finland	Germany	5	3	0.1875
Finland	Germany	4	1	0.0625
Finland	Germany	3	1	0.0625
Finland	Germany	2	2	0.1250
Finland	Germany	1	4	0.2500
			$TF_j = 16$	1.0000

The model explained in this section, implies to solve a combinatorial problem which attempts to estimate the final voting table of ESC 2008 (for predicting the position rank of Azerbaijan and San Marino). The constrained optimization problem has two parts. In the first part, the problem is to find the optimal combination that maximizes the sum of probabilities (first two terms of Equation 4). This implies 43 voting countries (subject to the mentioned constraints) which must assign 10 different scores (*S*) to 25 contender countries, resulting 2.99E+14 possible combinations. In the second part, the total sum of the votes obtained by every contender country is calculated. The vote sums (s_i) are used to calculate the weighted sum presented in Equation 4 (third term). This implies again to find the optimal combination out of 2.99E+14 possible solutions. The maximization of both parts of the problem generates a tradeoff between the voting behavior and the performance rate. For solving the current optimization problem, we use a simple and innovative PSO used on constrained optimization problems which is thoroughly explained in the next section.

Constrained optimization via PSO.

Particle Swarm Optimization (PSO) (Kennedy & Eberhart, 1999) is an algorithm inspired by the motion of a bird flock. Each member of the flock is called "particle". In PSO, the source of diversity, called variation, comes from two sources. One is the difference between the particle`s current position xt and the global best GBest (best solution found by the flock), and the other is the difference between the particle's current position xt and its best historical value PBest (best solution found by the particle). Although variation provides diversity, it can only be sustained for a limited number of generations because convergence of the flock to the best is necessary to refine the solution. The velocity equation combines the local information of the particle with global information of the flock, in the following way.

$$\begin{aligned} v_{t+1} &= w * v_t + \phi_1 * (P_{Best} - x_t) + \phi_2 * (G_{Best} - x_t) \\ x_{t+1} &= x_t + v_{t+1} \end{aligned} \quad (5)$$

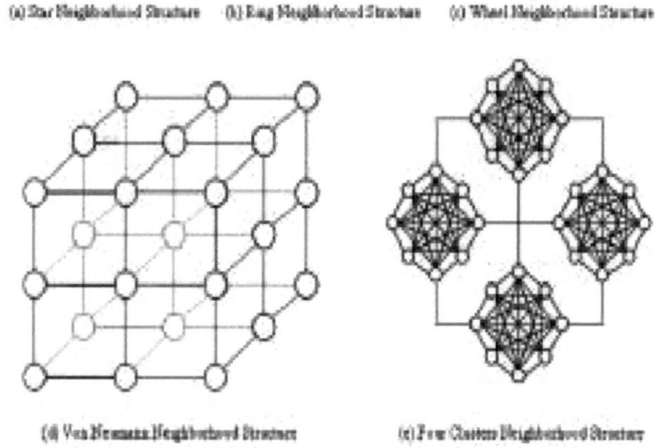

Fig. 3. Neighborhood strctures for PSO

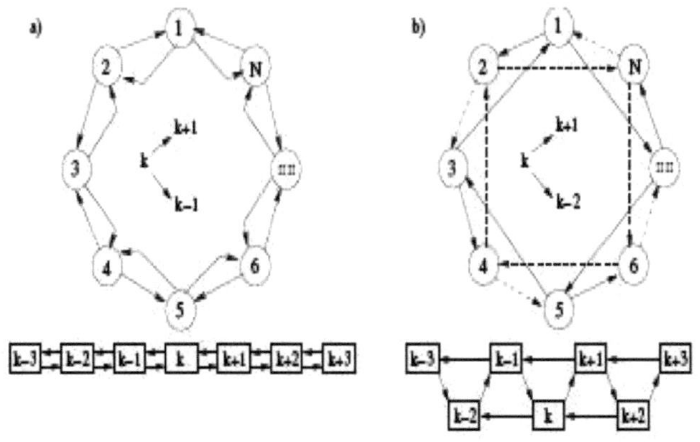

Fig. 4. Ring neighborhood structures. a)Doubly-linked ring (original PSO). b) Sigly-linked ring

A leader can be global to all the flock, or local to a flock's neighborhood. Flock neighborhoods have a structure that defines the way information is concentrated and then distributed among its members. The most common flock organizations are shown in Figure 1. The organization of the flock affects search capacity and convergence. The original ring structure is implemented by a doubly-linked list, as shown in Figure 4-a. COPSO uses an alternative ring implementation, the singly-linked list, shown in Figure 4-b. This structure improved the success of experimental results by a very important factor.

Experiments ESC 2007: Model Validation.

In order to know the performance of the proposed model, it was tested in estimating the final ranking of the countries which competed for the first time on the ESC 2007: Czech Republic, Georgia, Montenegro and Serbia. In the ESC 2007, these 4 countries competed in the unique Semi-Final stage against other 24 countries for obtaining just 10 places to the Final stage. In the Final stage, 14 countries were waiting for competing against the first 10 places of the Semi-Final. The 14 finalists were composed by the "Big Four" (Germany, Spain, France and United Kingdom) and the first 10 places of the ESC 2006. The list of contenders for every stage is available in the web host of the ESC 2008. For estimating the voting matrix, 30 runs of each experiment, Semi-Final and Final, were performed to obtain a better estimation of the final ranking. In every run, 350,000 function evaluations were performed. For the Semi-Final stage, the result of every run is a voting matrix and a rating list from 1 to 28. The average along the 30 runs was calculated for every contender. Next, the average ranking was obtained to determine the 10 countries which were going to contend in the Final stage. Three measures were calculated from the 30 runs: average, median, and interquartile range. The interquartile range has a comprehensiveness of 50% around the median value (second quartile Q2), which is calculated through the lower quartile Q1 (first quartile) and upper quartile Q3 (third quartile). In descriptive statistics a quartile is any of the three values which divide the sorted data set into four equal parts, so that each part represents 1/4 of the sampled population. The difference between the upper and lower quartiles is called the interquartile range. The results of the Final stage for Georgia and Serbia. In ESC 2007, Georgia obtained the 12th position in the Final stage, which is a value into the estimated interquartile range and very close to the average value predicted along 30 runs. Nevertheless, the predictions for Serbia are far away to the reality. Serbia was the winner of the ESC 2007. Maybe, no ESC experts had guessed that a new contender would win the contest. The ESC 2007 results showed how hard is to estimate the ESC's behavior. In the next section, the estimation of our approach for ESC 2008 is presented.

Experiments ESC 2008.

This year, the ESC consists of three stages: 2 Semi-Finals and Final. 43 countries will be represented in the Eurovision Song Contest -Belgrade 2008. Five of them are automatically qualified for the Final: The "Big Four" (France, Germany, Spain and United Kingdom) and the winner of the ESC 2007, Serbia (host country). On January 28th was determined which 19 countries are represented in the First Semi-Final, and which 19 in the Second Semi-Final. France, Germany, Spain, United Kingdom and Serbia will be voting in one of the two Semi-Finals. Germany and Spain will vote in the First Semi-Final, and France, United Kingdom and Serbia in the Second Semi-Final. The objective of this experiment is to predict the final ranking for Azerbaijan and San Marino. Azerbaijan and San Marino will compete in the First Semi-Final for winning a place in the Final stage. For this experiment 30 runs were performed with 350,000 function evaluations. The results of the First Semi-Final indicate that Azerbaijan could attain a place in the Final stage. The results for both Azerbaijan and San Marino are contrasting because Azerbaijan obtained the first place and San Marino the last place at the First Semifinal.

Televoting Results

Contestants	Total Score	France	Ireland	Iceland	Spain	United Kingdom	Denmark	Germany	Switzerland	Belgium	Cyprus	Netherlands	Sweden	Turkey	Israel	Greece	Portugal	Norway	Finland	Slovenia	Bosnia-Herzegovina	Croatia	Estonia	FYR Macedonia	Hungary	Latvia	Lithuania	Malta	Poland	Romania	Russia	Azerbaijan	Ukraine	Albania	Andorra	Belarus	Bulgaria	Moldova	Czech Republic	Armenia	Georgia	Serbia	Montenegro	San Marino
Romania	45	4	3	0	12	0	0	0	0	0	3	0	0	0	6	0	4	0	0	0	0	0	0	0	0	0	0	0	0		0	0	0	0	0	0	0	12	0	0	0	0	0	1
United Kingdom	14	0	8	0	0		0	0	0	0	0	0	0	0	0	0	0	0	0	0	0	0	0	0	0	0	0	0	0	0	0	0	0	0	0	0	0	0	0	0	0	0	0	6
Albania	55	0	0	0	0	0	0	0	8	0	0	0	0	1	0	10	0	0	0	4	1	8	0	12	0	0	0	0	0	0	0	1	0		0	0	0	0	0	0	0	0	7	3
Germany	14	0	0	0	0	0	0		2	0	0	0	0	0	0	0	0	0	0	0	0	0	0	0	0	0	0	0	0	0	0	0	0	0	0	0	12	0	0	0	0	0	0	0
Armenia	199	12	0	1	10	0	0	6	0	12	10	12	2	10	8	12	0	0	0	5	6	0	0	1	0	0	0	0	12	4	12	0	7	2	0	7	8	2	12		12	5	1	8
Bosnia and Herzegovina	110	2	2	0	0	0	2	5	7	0	0	7	10	6	0	0	0	10	6	10		12	0	5	0	0	0	0	0	0	0	3	0	0	0	0	0	0	1	0	0	12	10	0
Israel	124	6	0	0	0	0	0	3	1	5	2	3	0	0		1	0	3	8	3	5	2	0	0	3	0	3	0	5	6	6	7	5	4	0	4	2	6	0	6	3	7	5	10
Finland	35	0	0	7	0	0	0	0	0	0	0	0	7	0	0	0	0	4		0	0	0	10	0	0	1	0	0	2	0	0	0	0	0	4	0	0	0	0	0	0	0	0	0
Croatia	44	0	0	0	0	0	0	2	3	0	0	0	0	0	0	0	3	0	0	8	10		0	2	0	5	0	0	0	1	1	0	1	0	0	0	0	0	0	2	1	3	2	0
Poland	14	0	10	0	0	4	0	0	0	0	0	0	0	0	0	0	0	0	0	0	0	0	0	0	0	0	0	0		0	0	0	0	0	0	0	0	0	0	0	0	0	0	0
Iceland	64	0	0		4	6	12	0	0	0	0	0	8	0	4	0	7	8	7	0	0	0	0	0	0	2	0	6	0	0	0	0	0	0	0	0	0	0	0	0	0	0	0	0
Turkey	138	10	0	0	0	8	4	10	6	10	0	10	0		0	0	0	2	4	0	8	0	0	7	5	0	0	0	0	8	2	12	4	10	0	3	5	0	0	0	6	0	0	4
Portugal	69	8	0	6	8	0	0	4	10	6	0	5	0	0	0	0		0	0	0	0	3	0	0	0	0	0	0	0	0	0	0	3	0	10	0	0	0	0	0	0	1	0	5
Latvia	83	0	12	4	2	10	6	0	0	0	0	0	3	0	0	0	8	0	0	0	0	4	7	0	0		10	7	0	0	0	0	0	0	2	0	0	0	3	0	2	0	3	0
Sweden	47	0	0	3	1	0	8	0	0	0	1	0		0	1	0	0	7	5	0	0	0	2	0	1	0	1	12	0	0	0	0	0	3	0	0	0	0	0	0	0	2	0	0
Denmark	60	0	1	12	0	3		0	0	0	0	0	5	0	0	0	5	12	0	0	0	0	3	0	2	7	2	4	0	0	0	0	0	0	0	0	0	0	2	0	0	0	0	2
Georgia	83	0	0	0	0	0	0	0	0	0	7	0	0	4	2	4	1	0	0	0	0	0	5	0	0	8	5	5	0	0	7	10	8	0	0	6	0	3	4			0	0	0
Ukraine	230	0	6	5	7	5	7	0	0	1	6	0	0	8	10	6	12	0	3	2	3	7	4	4	6	10	6	10	10	3	8	10		8	6	10	7	7	8	5	10	6	4	0
France	47		0	8	0	2	5	0	0	0	0	0	4	0	0	0	0	1	2	0	0	0	6	0	0	3	8	0	1	0	0	0	0	0	3	0	0	0	0	4	0	0	0	0
Azerbaijan	132	0	0	0	0	0	0	1	0	7	0	2	0	12	3	3	0	0	0	1	0	0	0	8	12	4	7	0	7	2	10		10	0	7	8	3	8	10	0	7	0	0	0
Greece	218	3	4	0	3	12	3	12	5	8	12	6	1	7	5		0	0	0	6	7	5	1	3	8	0	0	2	3	12	3	6	2	12	8	2	10	4	5	8	4	8	6	12
Spain	55	5	0	0		1	1	0	4	4	4	0	0	3	0	8	10	0	1	0	0	0	0	0	0	0	0	0	0	0	0	0	0	1	12	0	0	0	0	1	0	0	0	0
Serbia	160	7	0	2	0	0	0	8	12	0	5	8	6	0	0	5	0	6	0	12	12	10	0	10	7	0	0	1	4	7	4	2	0	5	0	1	4	1	6	3	0		12	0
Russia	**272**	1	5	0	5	0	0	7	0	3	8	1	0	5	12	7	6	5	10	7	4	6	12	6	10	12	12	8	6	10		8	12	6	5	12	6	10	7	12	8	10	8	0
Norway	182	0	7	10	6	7	10	0	0	2	0	4	12	2	7	2	2		12	0	2	1	8	0	4	6	4	3	8	5	5	5	6	7	1	5	1	5	0	7	5	4	0	7

Fig. 5. The final Scoreboard of ESC 2008.

The average median and interquartile range for the 30 runs were calculated by determine the results of the Final stage. The experiments predict a 7th place for Azerbaijan in the ESC 2008. Also, the results estimate an interquartile range equal to 4, that is a final ranking from 3rd to 11th. The final position of Azerbaijan was 8th place, and the final Scoreboard of ESC 2008 is showed in Figure 5, Azerbaijan is the 20 th row, and is emphasized using a blue box.

Conclusions.

The prediction of future events is a hard task, also impossible in several topics. There are several methods that have been used as an auxiliary tool, for building estimation models (Data Mining, Regression models, Support Vector Machines, Neural Networks). In this work, data mining and evolutionary computation are combined for predicting the behavior of the European society in a music contest. A huge set of models to predict the final ranking of the Eurovision Song Contest can be found in its web host. These works do not have focussed their attention in model the behavior of the European society when a new country competes for the first time in the ESC. Our approach propose a model that includes two main features: voting behavior and cultural characteristics. The model incorporates historical information about the vote assignation, that European society has performed along previously ESC editions. Besides the model includes information about intrinsic characteristics of the contender that represents a country (language, lyrics, genre, in others). The prediction performance was judged the last 24th May, 2008 when Eurovision Song Contest - Belgrade 2008 was developed. Next year this research is oriented to obtain the ranking of a returned country: Slovakia which doesn't compete since 1998. We will utilize our proposed model and the information of another returned country Monaco who returned to ESC after 25 years in 2004 and its linguistic neighboor Czech Republic.

7.2 A hybrid methodology for classifying elements in a Social Diorama

Evolutionary computation is a generic term used to make reference to the solution of planned and implemented computational problems based in models involving an evolutionary process. Most of the evolutionary algorithms propose biological paradigms, and the concepts of natural selection, mutation and reproduction. Nevertheless, other paradigms exist that can be adopted in the creation of evolutionary algorithms. Many environment problems are not structured, that can be considered from the perspective of cultural paradigms; the cultural paradigms offer a wide range of categorized models that don't know the possible solutions to the problem - a common situation in the real world.

The intention of the present subsection is to apply the computational properties of the cultural technology; in this case of corroborating them by means of mining data to propose the solution to a specific problem, adapted from the modeled literature about societies. Combined to this, we analyzed the location of a representing individual in a society with respect to the social similarity of his neighbors, in a form of a popular representation denominated diorama. The set of study conformed by 87 societies allowed us to analyze the individual characteristics without affecting the total sense of the diorama, and gave us the opportunity to emulate the distances that separate each one and also group them into the cluster that they belong to. Demonstrating that characteristic linguistics exists and culture that approximates them as well as they move apart. By means of this information it is

possible to predict the best diorama, redistributing the individuals that are part of it. This article tries to explain this representation of social behavior.
The Cultural Algorithms are an approach of Evolutionary Computing, which use the culture like a vehicle to store excellent and accessible information to all the members of the population during many generations. Like in a human society, the cultural changes act as time advances; this provides a line base for the interpretation and documentation of individual behaviour within a society (Desmond et al., 1995). The Cultural Algorithms were developed to model the evolution of the cultural component through the time and to demonstrate how it learns and acquires knowledge. In agreement with this conception, the cultural algorithms can be used to lead the process of the self-adaptation within evolutionary systems in a variety of application areas (Callogerodóttir & Ochoa, 2007). The basic cultural algorithm can be described by means of the following pseudo code (Figure 6).

```
Begin
    t=0;
    Initialize POP(t); /* Initialization of population */
    Initialize BLF(t); /* Initialization of believing space */
    Repeat
            Evaluate POP(t);
            Vote (BLF (t), Accept (POP(t))));
            Adjust (BLF (t));
            Evolve(POP(t), Influence(BLF(t)));
            t = t +1;
            Select POP(t) from POP(t-1);
    Until (Term condition is reached)
End
```

Fig. 6. Pseudo code base of Cultural Algorithms.

Initially a population of individuals that define the solution space, which is represented like a set of solutions within the space search, is generated randomly to create the first generation. In our example, the solution space contains a list of the attributes that can be used in the classification procedure. The space of beliefs is emptiness. For each generation, the Cultural Algorithm will be able to evolve a population of individuals using "frame" Vote-Inherit-Promote (VIP). During the phase of vote, the members of the population are evaluated to identify their contribution to the space of beliefs by using the acceptance function. These beliefs contribute in most of the solution of the problem and are selected or put to voting as they contribute to the present space of beliefs. The belief space is modified when the inherited beliefs are combined with the beliefs that have been added by the present generation, this is made using a reasoning process that allows updating the space of beliefs. Next, the updated space of beliefs is used to influence the evolution of the population. The belief space is used to influence the rest of the population and the acceptance of its beliefs is modified. During the last phase a new population is reproduced using a basic set of evolutionary operators. This new population might be evaluated and the cycle continues successively, until all the population has the same space of beliefs (Tang et al., 2006). Cycle VIP finishes when a condition of completion is introduced. This condition is usually reached when only a small or no change is detected in the population through several generations or when certain knowledge in the space has emerged from beliefs, as it is appreciated above in Figure 6.

Diorama: the social net representation.

A social network is a social structure that can be represented making use of different types of diagrams. The two most common types are the graph and the diorama. The graph is a collection of objects called vertices or nodes that are connected by lines edges or arcs. The nodes represent individuals which sometimes are denominated actors and the edges represent the relations that exist between these actors. The relations can be of different type, like financial interchanges, sexual friendship, relations, or places of tourism, for example. The social networks can be classified in: Dyadic: They only indicate absence or existence of relation between two actors. Valued: The extent of relation can be moderate in terms of order or weight, for example: number of sexual encounters between two persons. Transitive: The relation between actor A and B is always reciprocal. (Example: both read the same Blog habitually.) Directed: In this case an actor A has a relation with actor B, but, that does not imply that B has the same relation with A. (Example: to lend money) The representation of a social network can consist of one or more graphs where these graphs conceptualize the network, that is, the representation is made mainly on the basis of the relations that exist among the actors who conform the network. On the other hand dioramas are representations elaborated with materials or elements in three dimensions, which sometimes represent a scene of the real life. They are located in front of a curved bottom that can be painted in such a way that it simulates real surroundings and also they can be enhanced with illumination effects. In this subsection, we focus our attention in a practical problem of the literature related to Social Modeling, the accomplishment of a diorama, which allows us to understand the position that keeps a society with respect to others. The capacity to establish the locations in the diorama, allows us to establish "the negotiation of the best position" for the given set of societies. The solution to this problem could be given by a sequence of generations of agents, denoted "community". The agents can only reassign a position with respect to the other societies, according to previous behaviors (Ochoa, Ponce, et al., 2007) as seen in figure 7. A diorama can accommodate plant, animals, people, and battles among other things. In the case of the social networks, a diorama, unlike the graphs, characterizes the social network, that is, in a dyoram one of the actors who conform the network according to their roll and to the position imagines each that they have within the same one. The development of the social networks requires on one hand, the conceptual development, and on another, the development of discreet mathematical measures that allow ontological to explore the human systems from a sustained concept and in the data. But it is necessary to prioritize the conceptual development and the categories of the social network system, and at the same time thinking about the mathematical model.

Distributing elements within a diorama.

From the point of view of the agents, the problem of optimization is very complex, taking into account that the best location of a representing individual for a society, with respect to other representatives, is not known. In the proposed algorithm for the cultural change, the individuals in the space of beliefs (beliefspace) through their best paradigm (BestParadigm) are put to zero to represent the fact that culture increases the amount of expectations associated with the location of a society with respect to others, giving an incentive to the behavior associated with the best paradigm (BestParadigm). We selected 87 societies described in (Memory Alpha, 2008) and characterized their social behavior with base in seven attributes: emotional control, ability to fight, intelligence, agility, force, resistance, and speed. These characteristics allow us to describe as much the society as the individual. The development of this tool was based on our desire to share the intuitive understanding about the treatment of a new class of systems, where individuals are able to have empathy, a reserved characteristic to live beings.

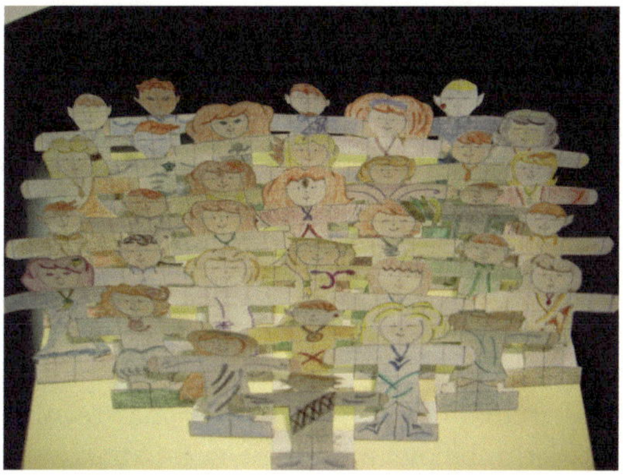

Fig. 7. Representation of 33 Societies (Memory Alpha, 2008) using a Rols Dyoram.

Complementary Methodology

Data mining is the search of global patterns and the existent relationships among data in immense databases, but that are hidden inside the vast quantity of information. These relationships represent valuable knowledge about the objects that are in the database. This information is not necessarily a faithful copy of the information stored in the databases. Rather, is the information that one can deduce from the database. One of the main problems in data mining is that the number of the possible extracted relationships is exponential. Therefore, there are a great variety of machine's learning heuristics that have been proposed for the knowledge discovery in databases. We included in our research the so called decision tree.

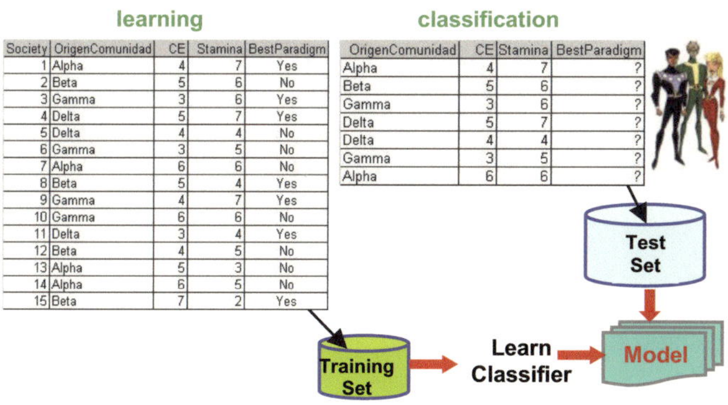

Society	OrigenComunidad	CE	Stamina	BestParadigm
1	Alpha	4	7	Yes
2	Beta	5	6	No
3	Gamma	3	6	Yes
4	Delta	5	7	Yes
5	Delta	4	4	No
6	Gamma	3	5	No
7	Alpha	6	6	No
8	Beta	5	4	Yes
9	Gamma	4	7	Yes
10	Gamma	6	6	No
11	Delta	3	4	Yes
12	Beta	4	5	No
13	Alpha	5	3	No
14	Alpha	6	5	No
15	Beta	7	2	Yes

OrigenComunidad	CE	Stamina	BestParadigm
Alpha	4	7	?
Beta	5	6	?
Gamma	3	6	?
Delta	5	7	?
Delta	4	4	?
Gamma	3	5	?
Alpha	6	6	?

Fig. 8. Proposed decision tree, used to characterize the cultural and social similarity inside each society.

One of the most popular approaches to represent the results of data mining is to use decision trees (Ochoa, Ponce, et al., 2007). A decision tree provides a procedure to recognize a given case for a concept. It is a "divide and conquer" strategy for the acquisition of the concept (instance). Decision trees have been useful in a great variety of practical cases in science and engineering (Zolezzi, Aandraison & Ochoa-Zezzatti); in this case we used data mining to characterize the individuals of each society (agents' community) and to understand how they obtain the best paradigm, as shown in figure 8.

Experiments

In order to achieve the most efficient arrangement of individuals in a social network, we developed an atmosphere to store the data of each one of the representing individuals of each society. This was made with the purpose of distributing in an optimal manner each of the evaluated societies. One of the most interesting characteristics observed in this experiment was the diversity of the cultural patterns established by each community. The structured scenes associated with agents cannot be reproduced in general, since they only represent a little moment in the space and time of the different societies. This represents a unique form and innovation of adaptive behavior which solves a computational problem. It does not cluster societies based only on their external appearance (genotype), but try to solve a computational problem that involves a complex change among the existing relations. The generated configurations can be metaphoric related to the knowledge of the behavior of the community with respect to an optimization problem (to belong culturally to a cluster with other similar societies that are not in the same quadrant (Memory Alpha, 2008)). The main experiment consisted of detailing each of the 87 communities, with 500 agents, and one condition of unemployment of 50 generations. This allowed us to generate different scenes for the best possible diorama, which was obtained after comparing the different cultural and social similarities from each community to determine the existing relations among them. The developed tool classified each of the societies belonging to each quadrant, with two tonalities, the strong tone for societies that included linguistic identity, and a smooth tone for societies only with a cultural identity. This permitted to identify changes in the time with respect to the other societies (see Figure 9).

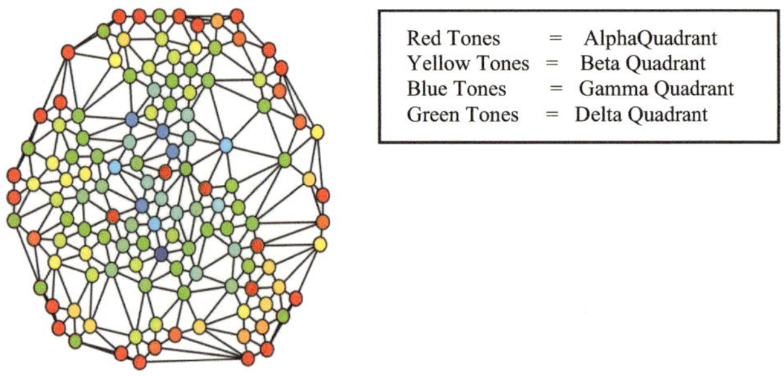

Fig. 9. Graph constructed by means of the use of Cultural Algorithms and Clusterization (Social Data Mining).

Using Cultural Algorithms we improved substantially the understanding of how to obtain the "best paradigm", because we classified properly the agent communities based on an approach that keeps their relation attributes. This allowed us to understand that the concept of "negotiation" exists with base in the determination of the function of acceptance on the part of the rest from the communities to the proposed locations for the rest of the same ones.

The Cultural Algorithms offer a powerful alternative for optimization problems and redistribution of clusterization. For that reason, this technique provides a quite comprehensible panorama of the cultural phenomenon represented (Ochoa, Ponce, et al., 2007). This technique allowed us to visualize the possibility of generating experimental knowledge created by the community of agents for a given application domain. The analysis of the level and degree of cognitive knowledge of each community is a desired aspect to evaluate for the future work. The answer can reside between the similarity that exists in the communication between two different cultures and how these are perceived. On the other hand, to understand the true similarities of different societies, based on the characteristics that group them in a cluster as well as those that make them unique, demonstrates that the small variations go beyond phenotypes characteristics and are mainly associate to tastes and similar characteristics developed through the time (Vukčević & Ochoa et al., 2007).
A new Artificial intelligence can take care to analyze individually these complexities that each society has, without forgetting that still they need methods to understand original and particular characteristics of each society.

8. Conclusion and the future research.

Social Data Mining try to improve the proposed solution by many evolving compute techniques (Ant Colony, PSO, and Cultural Algorithms) and provides knowledge by obtain the best solution in the search space. There are an important number of questions that deserve additional research. One will be to find new information sources to mine users preferences. An area with great potential is the electronic usage of media, specifically, digital music. By analyzing what kind of music is someone listening, a system can deduce the songs, the singers and the genders the person prefers, and by using this information recommending additional songs and artists, to get the person in touch with people of similar interests. We made an approach on this direction with a system that allows users to view individual and historical group listening lists and define with this information new listening lists (Ochoa, 2007). These systems learn of the user preferences based on the listened music, after songs are selected to be played on a shared physical environment, based on the preferences of the whole participants.

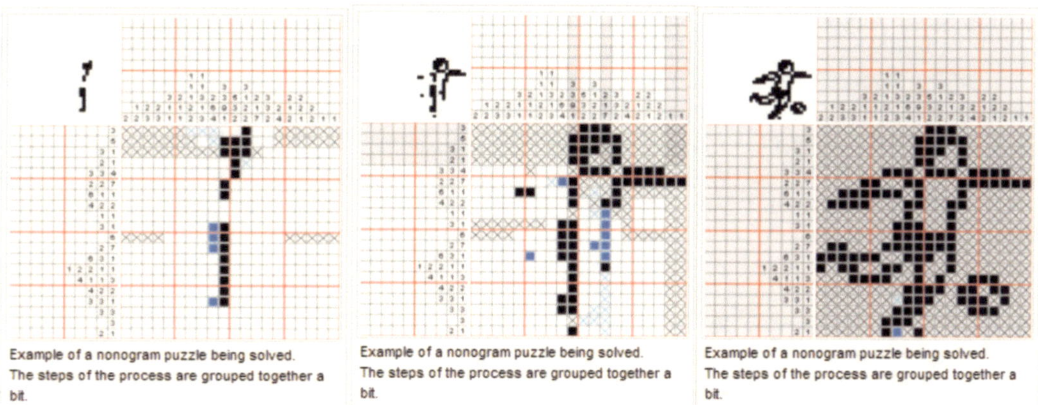

(a) (b) (c)

Fig. 10. Phases of solution of Japanese Puzzle using Data Mining and Cultural Algorithms.

Future research are Japanese Puzzles, which are a complex and combinatorial problem (see Figure 10). By using social data mining and cultural algorithms we believe it is possible to resolve them with less epoches; current benchmark has a restriction of 100*100 cells but using these two techniques we believe it is possible to overcome this restriction and obtain better results than those obtained by applying only genetic algorithms. In (González & Ochoa, 2008) is presented an approach to this novel research.

8. References

Abrams, D., Baecker, R., and Chignell, M. Information Archiving with Bookmarks: Personal Web Space Construction and Organization, in *Proceedingsof CHI'98* (Los Angeles CA, April 1998), ACM Press, 41-48.

Baldonado, M.Q.W., and Winograd, T. An Information-Exploration Interface Supporting the Contextual Evolution of a User's Interests, in *Proceedings ofCHI'97* (Atlanta GA, March 1997), ACM Press, 11-18.

Bederson, B.B., Hollan, J.D., Perlin, K., Meyer, J., Bacon, D., and Furnas, G. 1996. Pad++: A zoomable graphical sketchpad for exploring alternate interface physics. *J. Visual Lang. Comput.* 7, 3–31.

Billsus, D. & Pazzani, M. Learning Collaborative Information Filters, in *Proceedings of the International Conference on Machine Learning* (Madison WI, July 1998), Morgan Kaufmann Publishers.

Callogerodóttir Z. & Ochoa A. Optimization Problem Solving using Predator/Prey Games and Cultural Algorithms In Proceedings of NDAM'2003, Reykiavik; Iceland.

Card, S.K., Robertson, G.C., and Mackinlay, J.D. The Information Visualizer, an Information Workspace, in *Proceedings of CHI'91* (New Orleans LA, April 1991), ACM Press, 181-188.

Card, S.K., Robertson, G.C., and York, W. The WebBook and the Web Forager: An Information Workspace for the World-Wide Web, in *Proceedings of CHI'96*(Vancouver BC, April 1996), ACM Press, 111-117

Chalmers, M., Rodden, K., and Brodbeck, D. The Order of Things: Activity- Centred Information Access, In Proceedings of 7th International Conference on the WWW, 1998. (Brisbane Australia, April 1998), 359-367.

Charnov, E. L. Optimal Foraging: the Marginal Value Theorem". *Theoretical Population Biology*, 9, 129-136, 1976.

Chung, C. & Reynolds, G. R. CAEP: An Evolution-based Tool for Real-Valued Function Optimization using Cultural Algorithms. *International Journal on Artificial Intelligence Tools,* 7(3), 239-291, 1998.

Crossen, A., Budzik, J., and Hammond, K.J. Flytrap: Intelligent Group Music Recommendation, in Proceedings of IUI'2002 (San Francisco CA, January 2002), ACM Press.

Desmond, A. & Moore J. Darwin–la vida de un evolucionista atormentado. Generación Editorial; Brazil, 1995.

Dorigo, M., Maniezzo, V. & Colorni, A., 1996, "Ant System: Optimization by a Colony of Cooperating Agents". IEEE Transactions on Systems, Man and Cybernetics-Part B, 26(1), 29-41.

Egghe, L and Rousseau, R. *Introduction to Informetrics: Quantitative methods in library, documentation, and information science*. Elsevier, New York, NY, 1990.

Epstein, J. & Axtell R. *Growing Artificial Societies*. MIT Press/Brookings Institue, Cambridge, MA, 1996.

Gelbukh, A. & Sidorov G. Alignment of Paragraphs in Bilingual Texts Using Bilingual Dictionaries and Dynamic Programming. In Proceedings of CIARP 2005: 824-833

Gelbukh, A.; Sidorov, G. & Chanona-Hernández, L. Lexical-Based Alignment for Reconstruction of Structure in Parallel Texts. In Proceedings of NLDB 2007: 401-406
Ginsburgh, V. and Noury A.. Cultural voting: The Eurovision Song Contest. http://ssrn.com/abstract=884379, 2005.
Gónzalez S. & Ochoa A. Resolution of Japanese puzzles using Data Mining and Cultural Algorithms. (Accepted paper) In Proceedings of COMCEV'2008, México; 2008.
Hightower, R.R., Ring, L.T., Helfman, ,J.I., Bederson, B.B., and Hollan, J.D., Graphical multiscale Web histories: A study of PadPrints. in *Proceedings of Hypertext '98* (Pittsburgh PA, June 1998). ACM Press, New York, NY.
Hill, W.C., Hollan, J.D., Wroblewski, D., and McCandless, T., Edit Wear and Read Wear, In: *Proceedings of CHI'92*. (Monterey CA, May 1992), ACM Press, 3-9.
Hill, W. C. and Terveen, L. G. Using Frequency-of-Mention in Public Conversations for Social Filtering. in *Proceedings of CSCW'96* (Boston MA, November 1996), ACM Press, 106-112.
Holland, J. H. Emergence in Evolve Compute. Addison-Wesley Press, Reading, MA, 1-10, 1998.
Hölldobler, B. & Wilson, E. O. *The Ants*. Springer-Verlag, Berlin, 1990.
Jin, X.. & Reynolds, G.R. Using Knowledge-Based Evolutionary Computation to Solve Nonlinear Constraint Optimization Problems: a Cultural Algorithm Approach. In *Proceeding of the 1999 CEC*, 1672-1678, 1999.
Kennedy, J. & Eberhart, R. C. Particle Swarm Optimization. In *Proceeding of the IEEE International Conference on Neural Networks*, Perth, Australia, IEEE Service Center, 12-13, 1995.
Kennedy, J. and Eberhart, R. The Particle Swarm: Social Adaptation in Information-Processing Systems. McGraw-Hill, London, 1999.
Kennedy, J.; Eberhat, R.C.; & Shi, Y. Swarm Intelligence. Morgan Kaufmann Publishers, San Francisco, CA, 2001.
Kleinberg, J.M. Authoritative Sources in a Hyperlinked Environment, in *Proceedings of 1998 ACM-SIAM Symposium on Discrete Algorithms* (San Francisco CA, January 1998), ACM Press.
Mackinlay, J.D., Rao, R., and Card, S.K. An Organic User Interface for Searching Citation Links, in *Proceedings of CHI'95* (Denver CO, May 1995), ACM Press, 67-73.
Mander, R., Salomon, G., and Wong, Y.Y. A 'Pile' Metaphor for Supporting Casual Organization of Information, in *Proceedings of CHI'92* (Monterey CA, May 1992), ACM Press, 627-634.
Maniezzo, V. Ant Colony Optimization: An Overview, 2000.
Marshall, C., Shipman, F., and Coombs, J. VIKI: Spatial Hypertext Supporting Emergent Structure, in Proceedings of ACM ECHT '94, (Edinburgh, Scotland, September 1994). ACM Press,13-23.
Memory Alpha. memory-alpha.org (Star Trek World), 2008.
Morrison, R. & De Jong, K. A Test Problem Generator for Non-Stationary Environments. In *Proceedings of Congress on Evolutionary Computation*, IEEE Press, 2047-2053, 1999.
Munro, A.J, Höök, K., and Benyon, D (Eds.) *Social Navigation of Information Space*. Springer, 1999.
Ochoa, A. et al. Explain a Weblog Community, in *Proceedings of HAIS'2007* (Salamanca, Spain), 2007.
Ochoa A., Meneguzzi P. et al. Italianitá: Discovering a Pygmalion effect on Italian communities using data mining. In Proceedings of CORE'2006.
Ochoa A., Ponce J. et al. Baharastar – Simulador de Algoritmos Culturales para la Minería de Datos Social. In Proceedings of COMCEV'2007, México, 2007.

Ochoa A., Quezada S. et al. From Russia with disdain: Simulating a civil War by means of Predator/Prey Game & Cultural Algorithms. (Accepted paper) MICAI'2008; México, 2008.

Pirolli, P., Schank, P., Hearst, M., and Diehl, Scatter/Gather Browsing Communicates the Topic Structure of a Very Large Text Collection, in *Proceedings of CHI'96* (Vancouver BC, April 1996), ACM Press, 213-220.

Pitkow, J., and Pirolli, P. Life, Death, and Lawfulness on the Electronic Frontier, in *Proceedings of CHI'97* (Atlanta GA, March 1997), ACM Press, 383-390.

Rauhlen, M.. Culture's Consequences. Beverly Hils, California: Sage, 1997.

Resnick, P., Iacovou, N., Suchak, M., Bergstrom, P., Riedl, J. GroupLens. An Open Architecture for Collaborative Filtering of Netnews. In: Proceedings of CSCW'94 (Chapel Hill NC, October 1994), ACM Press, 175-186.

Reynolds, R. G. & Saleem, S. M. "The Impact of Environmental Dynamics on Cultural Emergence". *Perspectives on Adaptions in Natural and Artificial Systems*. Oxford University Press, 253-280, 2005.

Robertson, G., Czerwinski, M., Larson, K., Robbins, D.C. Data Mountain: Using Spatial Memory for Document Management, in Proceedings of UIST'98 (San Francisco CA, November 1998), ACM Press, 153-162.

Rychlyckyj, N.; Ostrowski, D.; Schleis, G. & Reynolds, R. G. Using Cultural Algorithms in industry. In *Proceedings of the 2003 IEEE Swarm Intelligence Symposium*, 187-192, 2003.

Shipman, F., Marshall, C., and LeMere, M. Beyond Location: Hypertext Workspaces and Non-Linear Views, in Proceedings of ACM Hypertext '99, ACM Press, 121-130.

Smith, M.A., and Fiore, A.T. Visualization Components for Persistent Conversations, in Proceedings of CHI'2001 (Seattle WA, April 1998), ACM Press, 136-143.

Suaremi, T., Shikari, K., & Hal Shayera. Understand social groups using artificial intelligence techniques. In Proceedings of NDAM'2006, Reykiavik, Iceland, 2006.

Tang, H. et al. The Emergence of Social Network Hierarchy Using Cultural Algorithms, VLDB'06, Seoul, Korea, 2006.

Terveen, L.G., McMackin, J., Amento, B., and Hill, W. Specifying Preferences Based On User History, in Proceedings of CHI'2002 (Minneapolis MN, April 2002), ACM Press.

Viegas, F.B. and Donath, J.S. Chat Circles, in Proceedings of CHI'99 (Pittsburgh, PA, May 1990), ACM Press, 9-16.

Vukčević I., Ochoa A. & Đraguljovič, H. Similar cultural relationships in Montenegro. WKDD'2007, England, 2007.

Wexelblat, A. and Maes, P. Footprints: History-Rich Tools for Information Foraging, in Proceedings of CHI'99 (Pittsburgh PA, May 1999), ACM Press, 270-277.

Whittaker, S., Jones, Q., and Terveen, L. Persistence and Conversation Stream Management: Conversation and Contact Management, in Proceedings of HICSS'02.

Yair, G.. Unite unite Europe: The political and cultural structures of Europe as relected in the eurovision song contest. Social Netwroks, 17(2): 147-161, 1995.

Yair, G. & Maman, D. The persistent structure of hegemony in the ESC. Acta Sociologica, 39:309-325, 1996.

Zolezzi, D.; Aandraison, D. & Ochoa-Zezzatti, A. A model to explain the extinction of San Benedicto Rock Wren using Cultural Algorithms. In Proceedings of OCAAI'2007. Bakú, Azerbaijan, 2007.